A Handbook on African Traditional Healing Approaches & Research Practices

Second Edition

Edited by
Njoki Wane & Erica Neeganagwedgin

Nsemia

First Edition: November 2013
Second Edition: July 2014
Edited by: Njoki Wane & Erica Neeganagwedgin
Cover Design Concept: Isaac Darko
Cover Design: Danielle Pitt
Layout Design: Kemunto Matunda

Published by Nsemia Inc. Publishers (www.nsemia.com); Oakville, Ontario, Canada

Note for Librarians: A cataloguing record for this book is available from Library and Archives Canada

ISBN: 978-1-926906-33-1 paperback

DEDICATION

To all those who seek to heal and restore balance in the world.

To all past, present and future indigenous healers for their contribution to wellness of society.

Notes on the Second Edition

The chapter titled *The State of Traditional Medicine in Zimbabwe* that was in the First Editon has been removed. As well, author biographies have been updated accordingly

Acknowledgements

We would like to take this opportunity to thank all the contributors to this anthology. Thank you for your patience and your commitment to Indigenous Ways of knowing. Thank you to all the various reviewers who made different comments on different drafts of this work. In addition thank you to all those who participated in editing the work: Michelle, Natasha, Brendan. Thank you to all the students who have taken Dr. Wane's course: *Sociology of Indigenous Approaches to Health and Healing Practices: Implications for Education.* Thank you to our families for your ending support of our academic work.

Last, but not least, *asante sana Mungu* (Thank you so much our Creator) for being with us every step of the way as we worked on this anthology.

TABLE OF CONTENTS

Part B: Practical Examples of Indigenous Healing

Preface

Kai ner Maa Pitanta, Toronto

The need to reclaim the ancestral wisdom of Africa is paramount to the survival and well-being of not only the African people, but also the world. The interpretation and understanding of Indigenous wisdom must come from those who carry the voices of this misunderstood science within their ancestral memories. It must be made clear and irrefutable that the contributions of Indigenous people are based on sound theoretical principles that have formed the foundation of Western scientific progress. Studying the interaction and movement of different kinds of energy has always been critical to Indigenous people's understanding of healing. The Western interruption of our healing systems precluded a deliberate distortion of the Indigenous people's sublime understanding of energy and matter in its homicide of Indigenous culture. How can a healer seek to restore order without knowing the fundamental structural energy and material underpinnings of natural phenomena?

Western science cleverly co-opted Indigenous practices and replaced them with terms such as psychology, whose core meaning, "psychologia," was the study of the science of the soul and of spirits. It is the Indigenous person's reverence for the scientific expression of natural law and its communication to us in the form of mathematics, chemistry, biology, music, and more that leads her/him to deify the manifestation of its inherent ordering of matter and energy from its original eternal matrix to the physical experience of life. We have always understood the coexistence of the material and immaterial as necessary dualities that feed and need each other.

This book represents a global movement. Western notions of representing modernity are suffering the inevitable karmic consequences of failing to see the connections between physical, emotional, and spiritual healing, and of failing to see how traditional healing systems created and sustained balance and order in families and communities. We have always known that divine law and scientific law are connected, and more important than just knowing this, we live it. How else could we collaborate with our ancestors? This book reaffirms our need to view life cosmologically. From this cultural viewpoint, we can begin to remove the colonial veil covering the truth of Indigenous practices and understand millennia-old techniques such as divination as sound predictive mathematical processes rooted in binary principles.

In this handbook, Wane and Neeganagwedgin provide writings that challenge us to examine the outworn cultural paradigms that hold us back from continuing on a spiritual/cultural transformation and from recognizing ourselves as Divine Beings. This movement requires traditional healing to embrace the principles of best practice if we are truly to resume our responsibility as the spiritual caregivers of the Earth.

Foreword

Natasha Burford
University of Toronto
Septembcr, 2013

The book you hold in your hand is a gift that I wish I'd had during the time of a health crisis in my early life. It is a book that cannot only heal your body; it can also heal your soul. The information on the pages reveals time-tested treatments and may just be the very thing you need to read for your specific situation.

At 19, my life changed radically when I was diagnosed with SLE, Systematic Lupus. I was physically active, healthy, and very spiritual. Suddenly bedridden for months, I felt like my whole world had crashed. My doctor prescribed antibiotics, steroids, antidepressants, and even sleeping pills to give me some type of normality. With all the various side effects from the conventional medicine given to me, I decided to try visiting a naturopathic doctor. That is when things started getting better. I was reintroduced to many ancient foods, some of which my parents had used in their countries of Jamaica and Trinidad and Tobago. I soon became a vegan and only ate organic fruits, vegetables, and grains. I saw a profound difference in my health, as well as my mood. However, it was difficult keeping up with such a regimented diet, so I slowly retreated back to my poor food choices; and yes, my health was once again impacted. Now at 37, with three children, I try to eat better. However, I really did not embrace the need to eat healthy until another major crisis hit in my life. My father was diagnosed with cancer and I saw first-hand how alternative medicine and my family's strong spiritual beliefs were able to heal him. After the "required" chemotherapy damaged his kidneys and advanced his disease, the doctors gave my dad two weeks to live. They sent him home from the hospital simply to die. My family and I desperately, but courageously, decided to take my dad off of all the medicines the doctors had prescribed—which were merely painkillers—and only give him vitamins, Indigenous foods, love, and continuous prayers. It has been over two months now and my dad is doing better than ever. Whether you are young or old, understanding the importance of how to heal yourself is crucial to gaining peace of mind.

When I first started my community organization to mentor young women, I saw the growing need to encourage healthy lifestyles. I was then invited to lead an education organization as executive director before returning to my teaching position. Now I aim to teach about healing, both physically and spiritually, in a plethora of ways. It was this awareness that inspired me to pursue my Master's Degree, at which time I met professor Wane during her class in Cultural Knowledges at OISE and was automatically inspired to work with her. She shared her knowledge with the class in a way that was different from other professors because she was open to truly learning from her diverse students. Further, she was patient, graceful, and embodied love. She opened my desire to know my Indigeneity, my culture. This was a gap within me that I did not know existed. It began my journey of my own healing. Her teaching has enriched my life. For this, I am forever grateful.

When I read the pages of this book, I was astonished that the information contained on these pages isn't more easily and readily accessible. It is no secret that the introduction of the European influence in Africa and all over the world has had a detrimental impact on Indigenous knowledge. This book enables us to return to the teachings of Ancient Indigenous practitioners who taught their patients basic knowledge about herbs, healing, and ceremonial practices *before* this knowledge was disrupted. It reintroduces us to nature as the foundation of healing.

In chapter five we learn that *food is medicine* and we explore healthy eating within the sphere of Indigenous knowledge.

This book describes Indigenous foods before the impact of colonialism and globalization hit our local food stores. It beautifully interweaves environmental and spiritual health through captivating experiences as well as musical arts as a type of healing practice.

As shown throughout the experiences of the various authors, many different countries cover a wide array of healing practices, rarely found together in one book.

It is refreshing to be given a global perspective of African traditional healing and community wellness. This book is a must read for anyone who believes they can blindly trust the foods we eat and the medicines that are "supposed to" heal us. It is enlightening to know that there are natural cures for everything and that we have had the answers to many of our illnesses from the beginning of time. This book has completely changed the way I think about health and healing practices. It has given me an overview of various healing practices throughout the African continent and has allowed me to gain invaluable knowledge that I am able to implement regarding my health and the health of my family simply by the foods that we eat. I am blessed that my dad and I both still have time to do something about it.

Recognizing that the health industry is a multi-billion dollar industry, it is vitally important that every person be fully knowledgeable about health practices and the various options for health care. With the rate of illnesses and premature death in North America, there is

Introduction

Njoki Wane & Erica Neeganagwedgin

> There is a reawakening of traditional healing...The modern-day phenomena of the Lifestyle of Health and Sustainability (LOHAS) and embodied Complementary and Alternative Medicine (CAM) consumer markets speak powerfully to this reawakening based on the need for traditional healing philosophies and environmental correctness. (Pesek, Helton, & Nair, 2006, p. 115)

Indigenous healing practices are unique because all physical, mental, and spiritual phenomena are studied, practiced, and taught to a whole community (Battiste, 2000; Dei, Hall, & Rosenburg, 2000; Wane, 2005; Waterfall, 2002b). Ancient Indigenous practitioners taught their patients basic knowledge about herbs, healing, and ceremonial practices. However, due to colonizing forces and the growing impetus of migration to urban centers, this knowledge was disrupted. To support or refute Pesek's above quote, we must consider the role that healing plays in larger issues of tradition. For instance, there is no single way to describe African tradition, let alone the complex, multidimensional, and multilayered healing practices and approaches within that tradition. How do we describe this complex system? Should we be looking for common themes found among different ethnic groups in Africa? This book aims to make sense of African traditional healing practices and knowledge in all their dynamic complexity. We also acknowledge that African traditional healing practices and forms of belief have been in existence for over three million years (Rassmussen, 2006).

Traditional healing practices correct the internal imbalances through which disease manifests within an individual, and emphasize the re-establishment of an individual's harmony with his/her environment and the natural cycles to which all life is subject. Given the impact of globalization and ongoing colonial imposition, Indigenous societies are faced with a myriad of physical, psychological, and spiritual distresses (Antone, Miller, & Myers, 1986; McMichael, 2000). Globalization poses new threats to health in areas such as microbiology, physiology, and chemistry; these threats include the introduction of new viruses and pollutants, as well as global climate change (McMichael, 2000).

Globalization, immigration, and demographic changes have increased the interconnectedness of people with regard to social, political, economic, technological, and cultural exchanges. However, globalization has generally led to the dominance of Western views of health and mental health, as well as the policies and interventions associated with them. In other words, the integration of 'foreign' values and ideas has been more apparent in non-Western countries. But as globalization continues to characterize the world we live in, it is imperative for researchers, practitioners, clinicians, educators, and those in training to abandon their sense of self-sufficiency and actively increase their understanding of traditional healing practices. This book brings together chapters that illuminate the development of health and well-being from an Indigenous perspective, while also interrogating the Eurocentric and Western cultural hegemonic practices of knowledge production in the field of health care and in the ways of engaging with the wellness programme.

There is a paucity of research publications on African Indigenous healing practices in this area of study. While existing books have mainly examined theories and interventions pertaining to international or global health care and psychology, or general cross-cultural strategies for ethnic minorities living in Western countries, many have not attempted to bring into focus the vast array of research on African traditional healers and healing. We believe there are very few texts available to the growing numbers of health care practitioners, social workers, medical doctors, psychiatrists, counsellors, and psychotherapists who take an interest in the development of people's physical and mental health concerns, particularly those of people of African descent.

The Handbook of African Traditional Healing Approaches & Research Practices is a collection of essays demonstrating the continuing interest in, and importance of, Indigenous ways of knowing. The authors examine African Indigenous healing practices from different viewpoints in various African countries, including Kenya, Ghana, South Africa, Uganda, Zimbabwe, Rwanda, and Tanzania. While the collection does not cover the multiplicity of African experiences, it shows that there are core common themes among African peoples and societies when it comes to traditional ways of providing healing and wellness to communities.

The essays are arranged into two main sections. Those in Part A examine Indigenous healing practices from theoretical and practical perspectives, while those in

Part B examines two prevalent themes: respect for ancestors and the significance of community wellness. In "African Indigenous Healing Practices," Njoki Wane asserts the importance of Indigenous knowledges and their connection to African healing practices. The author argues that the continued importance of traditional healing practices in the lives of many African people is proof of resistance to colonialism and its efforts to wipe out those practices.

Akwasi Asabere-Ameyaw, George Dei, and Kolawole Raheem, in their essay, "A Sociological Study of Traditional Medicine and Herbal Pharmacology in Africa: Research Issues, Challenges, and Possibilities," provide an extensive review and analysis of the ways in which traditional medicine and plant pharmacology are incorporated into African schools. The authors argue for the importance of examining traditional medicine from a sociological perspective. The authors' work shows the need to examine sociological perspectives legitimately and call for Indigenous ways of knowing to be taken seriously, to be seen as relevant and valid in academia.

"Conceptualizing Illness from an Islamic Perspective," by Sumaya Laher, notes that Islam is a major religion on the African continent and explores the differences and commonalities between Islamic worldviews on illness.

In "Capture the Spirit to Become a True African Medical Practitioner," Meki Nzewi discusses the intricacies involved in practising traditional African healing and medical practices. Nzewi asserts that African worldviews are embedded in Indigenous healing practices, and that such worldviews look at healing and wellness using various understandings of physical, community, and physiological health. To reinforce this notion, the author points out that African Indigenous healing is twofold in that there are public health and individual health practices.

Mary Ashiedu's "Food as Medicine: Indigenous Dietary Practices in Africa" examines the impact of Westernized diets on the health of Indigenous people. The author asserts that when Western forms of diet replace Indigenous foods systems, people develop non-communicable diseases. She calls for the reclamation and revival of Indigenous food systems as medicines for the body.

Tom Ndege and Joash Abere Migosi, in their essay, "The Tragedy of Modernity: Traditional Healers of Kakamega Forest in a Brand New Order," look at the connection between modernism and Indigenous worldviews, using the Kakamega Forest as a case study. The authors provide an examination of the impact of colonially imposed worldviews on traditional healing practitioners, their patients, and practices.

In "Bringing Traditional Healers Back into the Conversation," Immaculate Wamimbi Tumwine cites Uganda as a model country where collaboration exists between traditional healers and conventional medical practitioners. The author argues that there is a change in the perception of traditional medicine due to the failures and gaps in conventional means of healing, as well as the issue of inaccessibility highlighted by other authors in this book. Tumwine calls for the need for the government to be a more active participant in recognizing the importance of traditional healing practices.

Emilio Ovuga's work, "The Concepts of Traditional Healing Practices Amongst the Acholi and Madi in Northern Uganda," points to the difficulties and significance of providing health care to people in rural Africa. Ovuga shows that one of the reasons people continue to turn to traditional medicines and healers is that they are often more accessible than doctors practising modern medicine. Ovuga provides case studies of practitioners who claim to be able to cure or heal many illnesses, as well as the various methods and ways in which curing and healing occur. He concludes by urging traditional healers and conventional health practitioners to work collaboratively.

Regine King and Izumi Sakamoto, in "Healing Psychosocial Trauma in Societies Recovering from Massive Violence: The Case of Rwanda," argue that the Western approaches for dealing with postwar conflict are limited and do not fit African postwar contexts. The authors highlight the colonial impact and influence on Indigenous ways of healing and African thought systems, and call for a more integrative psychosocial model, blended with current local models, in an attempt to promote healing and wellness.

Edna Ayree and Roy Moodley's essay, "Chewing Kola Nuts in Canada: An Analogue of African Traditional Healing Practices and Modern Psychotherapeutic Methods," focuses on the role traditional African healing has played both on the African continent and with the African diaspora living in Canada. The authors call for an integration of traditional healing practices into psychotherapy.

Edmund J. Kayombo's essay, "An Act Governing Traditional Medicine Practices: An Experience in Tanzania," examines the longstanding use of traditional medicine in Tanzania, looking at the necessity of bringing together traditional African healing practices and conventional medicine, despite the fact that they are informed by different legal systems.

Erica Neeganagwedgin and Simon Murangiri's essay, "Healing Practices of Kenyan Traditional Healers: A Dialogue/Interview," is an examination of the parallels between healing practices on the African continent and those of the diaspora in the Caribbean.

Eleanor Ross' "Spirituality and Ethics in South African Traditional Healing: Implications for the Helping Professions" looks at the links between African traditional healing systems and spirituality. The integration of both African and Western approaches are discussed as well as the implications for current healthcare approaches in South African contexts.

Finally, in "Ethno-medicinal Practices among the Indigenous Acholi Community of Uganda," Francis Akena speaks about how the Acholi people of Northern Uganda heavily respect and rely on the traditional medicine practices of their culture. Akena explains some of the rituals in this unique community and how the conventional, modern health system can benefit from the rich, ancient knowledge of the Ugandan traditional practices.

This anthology reflects the value of Indigenous healing practices. It shows that traditional medicinal practices are important aspects in the lives of African people, both historically and today. Traditional healing practices are intricately tied to African people's ancestral knowledge, history, traditions, and overall understanding of wellness. While African thought systems on healing are varied, they are nonetheless rooted in a much more multidimensional understanding of humanity. Throughout the book, we are reminded of the importance of looking beyond conventional ways of healing and that although we now live in modern times, traditional healing and medicines continue to play a vital role in our lives as well as in the pursuit of physical, mental, spiritual, and emotional well-being.

References

Antone, B., Miller, D., & Myers, B. (1986). *The power within people.* Tribal Sovereignty Associates.

Battiste, M. & Youngblood Henderson, J. (2000). *Protecting Indigenous knowledge and heritage: A global challenge.* Saskatoon, Saskatchewan: Purich Publishing.

Dei, G. J. S., Hall, B., & Goldin Rosenberg, D. (2000). *Indigenous knowledges in global contexts: Multiple readings of our world.* Toronto: University of Toronto Press.

McMichael, P. (2000). *Development and social change.* London, UK: Pine Forge Press

Pesek, T., Helton, L., & Nair, M. (2006). Healing across cultures: Learning from traditions. *EcoHealth, 3*(2), 114-118.

Rassmussen, S. (2006). *Those who touch: Tuareg medicine women in anthropological perspective.* DeKalb, IL: Northern Illinois University Press.

Rassmussen, S. (2001). *Healing in Community.* N.p.: Bergin & Garvey Press.

Wane, N. (2005). Claiming, writing, storing, sharing African Indigenous knowledge. *Journal of Thought, 40*(2), 27-46.

Waterfall, B. (2002a). Native people and the social work profession: A critical exploration of colonizing problematics and the development of decolonized thought. *Journal of Educational Thought, 36*(3), 1-23.

Waterfall, B. (2002b). Reclaiming identity: Native wombmyn's reflections on womb based knowledges and spirituality. In N. Wane, E. Lawson, & K. Deliovsky (Eds.), *Back to the Drawing Board: African Canadian Women and Feminism* (pp. 292-308). Toronto: Sumach Press.

Part A
Theory and Practice

Chapter One

AFRICAN INDIGENOUS HEALING PRACTICES

Njoki Wane, University of Toronto

Introduction

> To be attracted to an ancient way of life is to initiate one's personal spiritual emancipation...the road to correcting ills goes through the challenging path of ritual....To ritualize life, we need to learn how to invoke the spirits or things spiritual into our ceremonies... Invocation suggests that we accept the fact that we ourselves don't know how to make things happen...we seek strength from spirits or Spirit by recognizing and embracing our weakness. (Somé, 1993, pp. 67, 97)

Somé's quotation provides pointed suggestions in terms of emancipation of the spirit and how to sustain it through the ritualization of life. The mention of an ancient way of life automatically provokes the notion of duality between contemporary existence and something of the past, such as witchcraft or witchdoctors. In this paper, ancient refers to the timelessness of spiritual ways of knowing that had no name, yet people adhered to as central to their lives. In contemporary times, that thing is referred to as spirituality, or as many African people refer to it, the connecting force between the living, the dead, and those to come. The purpose of this paper is threefold. I will first examine the differences between various traditional healing practices, including herbal healing (using plant leaves, tree barks, roots, and flowers), emotional or spiritual healing, ritualistic healing, energy healing, and community healing. I will then explore the healing practices of African peoples in relation to their physical, mental, emotional, and spiritual illnesses. Lastly, I will analyze any contributions that African Indigenous healing practices have made to the knowledge and understanding of contemporary healing practices. This paper does not deal with issues of witchcraft as examined by different anthropologists, such as Geschiere (1997). I base my discussion on the following questions: What is Indigenous healing and African Indigenous healing in particular? What causes sickness in our bodies, minds, and spirits? How is this knowledge acquired? I situate this discussion in the theoretical framework of Indigenous knowledge.

Indigenous Knowledge as a Theoretical Framework

Indigenous knowledge is a lived experience that is informed by ancestral voices, cultures, local languages, songs and proverbs. It is an outcome of interactions that occur among families and communities, and it is constantly changing (Castellano, 2000; Wangoola, 2000). All of the learning and teachings are intertwined within the context of everyday interactions. Members of the community generate this form of knowledge, and then pass it on to the next generation through storytelling, observation, songs, ceremonies, and traditional rituals. There are many definitions of what constitutes Indigeneity, but most scholars agree that Indigenous knowledge is defined in relation to a particular group's common history, traditions, culture, and language. According to Dei (1993), Indigenous knowledge is a "holistic and inclusive form of knowledge in that it encompasses mental, intellectual, spiritual, and physical and contributes to the development of the individual self and the interconnections between the self and society within the Earth" (p. 28). Furthermore, Indigenous knowledge encompasses both individual and collective stories. As Solomon (1990) writes, people in Indigenous groups use their stories to understand their relationships with the cosmos. Indigenous knowledges are embodied in that they are embedded as a memory in Indigenous people's bodies, water, and land (Jousse, 2000; Solomon & Wane, 2005). The Indigenous knowledge theoretical framework speaks to traditional healing practices that were interrupted—but not destroyed—by colonization and are regaining momentum as a celebration and re-recognition of the richness of African culture, and as a resistance to colonialism. Tsey (1997) sees ethno-medicine as both a decolonizing and anti-colonial tool. He says, "For Indigenous people in developed countries such as Aboriginal Australians and the Maori in New Zealand, resurgence of traditional medicine is part of anti-colonial struggle and pride in cultural identity" (as cited in Bradym, 1995, p. 1065). This chapter celebrates ancient traditional healing practices as a way to reclaim what was, and what should have been, if there were no interruptions in people's lifestyles. It is an acknowledgement that traditional healing is both an ancient medicine and the medicine of the future; it is timeless (Wane, 2002).

General Overview

Since the advent of colonialism, African communities bore marks of Western knowledge. This is because, despite the presence of 'formal' political independence, colonial knowledge has found a place to grow and spread in the consciousness of the colonized, creating a dissonance in the spirit and disconnection from one's roots (Wane, 2002). These processes began during the colonial era and were fostered by an educational system that sought to replace Indigenous ways of knowing with colonial ways. This is captured eloquently by Somé (1993):

> At the colonial school I had been told that the rituals my people performed to heal were devilish and inspired by Satan....What I learned from my white teachers was...poisonous and even dangerous to me and others...It was as if literacy destroyed the ability to learn the Indigenous knowledge that I was trying to reclaim. (p. 8)

These 'evil' practices were often the African Indigenous healing practices and those who bore the brunt of the attack were the traditional healers who were, and still are, misrepresented as being evil, misguided, and workers of the devil. Often, these practices were considered evil because there was no word to explain in English how the healing was taking place, no way to verbalize the process that led to healing. This is a pattern in the colonizing missions. Whenever the colonizers could not make sense of a particular way of life or dogma that they encountered, they referred to it as evil, witchcraft, barbaric, primitive, and sub-standard. What the colonizers missed was the ritualistic and methodical response of Indigenous healers whenever they were confronted with the illness of an individual or a community. In addition, the colonizers failed to take note of how members of the community took charge of their own well-being. Every member of the family performed continuous purification, meditation, and wellness practices to maintain the harmony of his/her soul, body, and mind. Everything they did was sacred and Creator–directed, from their work to their clothing, from their relationships to their homes, and from their sacred groups to their governments. Like the Hunzas of the Himalayas today, Africans for centuries were non-policed, peaceful people who, through the maintenance of balance among all relationships, sustained a harmonious environment (Afua, 2000; Arewa, 1998).

African traditional healers, in particular, were the first to experience the repressive new system of the colonial government, not only through the fear created by the introduction of new religions and modern medicines, but also through the destruction of people's spirits as well as their physical environment. The colonial government felt that these traditional practitioners were a reminder of past ways of life and thus a threat to their new autonomy and power. The settlers created laws that forbade any mode of practicing traditional healing, whether through herbs or spiritual. The worst destruction came via the introduction of commercial farming, which necessitated clearing thousands of acres of Indigenous vegetation and forests. In the process, most of the medicinal plants that healers used for their curative practices were destroyed. The destruction of the habitats for both human and animal populations amounted to taking the very lifeline of Indigenous people. Without access to the curative Indigenous plants, a whole community was condemned to a sure death penalty. As Megan Vanghan (1991) has pointed out, any form of report or account of African people by colonial administrators, anthropologists, natural historians, missionaries, and medical or health officials, painted Africans as 'pathological others' in need of being rescued from themselves. This was a complex and well planned political agenda that had to be implemented to pave the way for the establishment of the Western medical system. As Marsland (2007) states, "the early missionaries believed that medical services were an important tool in their efforts to convert Africans to Christianity" (p. 758).

A classic stereotype constructed by the colonialists was that of the 'witchdoctor.' This pejorative label erroneously described diviners as doctors/witches, whose mysterious practices were often seen to be analogous with 'black magic.' This was probably due to the "colonial construction of African 'otherness' and essential 'primitiveness' which persists to this day" (Wane, 2002, p. 276). Amutabi (2008) describes how 'othering' processes homogenize and universalize experience, causing the "wrong conclusions [to be] were drawn about Africa" (p. 151). Amutabi (2008) emphasizes the need for Africans to write their stories in order to correct the misconceptions of their Indigenous healing practices. However, there is still a scarcity of scholarly work being done by Africans about traditional healers, despite the urgent need, as eloquently stated by Amutabi (2008):

> In Kenya...little has been written about Indigenous medicine and the health practices of alternative healers, but this did not stop the government from incorporating the Indigenous medical system

> into Kenya's health system. Because of budgetary implications, the government has been unsuccessful in its mission of availing medical services to the majority of the people, and this has provided an opening for the flourishing of the alternative health care system. (p. 153)

In most African countries, however, the fear of governmental reprisals has caused the decline in traditional healing practices and has forced most traditional healers to do their work very quietly, within a circle of trusted supporters. However, with the new resurgence of ethnic practices and medicine all over the world, traditional healing practices are gradually gaining ground and are making a slow, but sure, resurgence.

African Healing Practices

African Indigenous healing has been variously defined as a process of restoration, a journey of recovery, or a process of bringing order. Being healed, according to Carlson and Shield (1990), means living in peace. Indigenous healing is about being aligned with natural spiritual law and is grounded on spiritual guidance embodied in the Creator—the giver of life, harmony, balance, cosmic order, peace, and healing. For many Indigenous knowledge practices around the world, healing operates in the context of a relationship to four constructs: spirituality (Creator, Mother Earth, and Great Father); community (family, clan, and tribe/nation); environment (daily life, nature, and balance); and self (inner passions, peace, thoughts, and values) (Portman, Tarrel, Garret, & Michael, 2006). As taught and practiced by our ancestors, if any of our actions result in disequilibrium, we have to find ways of healing and purifying the environment, our relationships, and ourselves. The holistic healing approach used by Indigenous African healers to diagnose and offer or recommend treatment requires a wide range of physical, emotional, psychological, social, and spiritual engagements.

Indigenous healing is one of the oldest forms of structured medicine, that is, a system that has an underlying philosophy and set of principles by which it is practiced. It is the medicine from which all later forms of medicine developed, including Chinese medicine, Graeco-Arabic medicine, and modern Western medicine. Traditional healing was originally an integral part of all Indigenous cultures and societies, and although archaeological evidence for its existence dates back to only around 6000 B.C., its origins probably date back from well before the end of the last Ice Age. There were, and still are, some regional differences between the principles and philosophies of different African traditional healing methods, but there are also many fundamental similarities that arise from the profound knowledge of the natural laws that all life is subject to and the understanding of how these laws influence living things. Ill health is usually due to an abnormal imbalance, either of the organism within its environment or within the organism itself. Therefore, traditional healing practices work to not only correct internal imbalances, through which disease can manifest in an individual, but also to emphasize re-establishing an individual's harmony with his/her environment and relationship with the natural cycles of life. In theory, African Indigenous healing practices' main purpose is the removal of dissonance and distortions and to restore equilibrium or bring back balance into one's life or environment. As noted by Kakar (2003):

> [I]mpurities of the mind not only lead to mental distress and illness but also physically translated manifest themselves in the body as disease. The removal of the cause—the impurities—also means the cessation of the effect: distress and disease. A purified mind makes for a pure body, however, is not simultaneous with that of the mind but delayed till the impure precipitates of the mind, including karmic traces from the past lives, have worked themselves out (p. 661)

In some cases, the symptom of the sickness is a manifestation of healing itself. For example, when one has diarrhoea, that symptom is itself a process of healing. The body has rejected foods that do not agree with the system, hence the need for removal. While Western medicine usually tries to stop this symptom, African Indigenous healing focuses on assisting the body with removing the harmful matter, rather than stopping its symptomatic expression. In relation to restoring balance, there are things that can be done beyond the physical. For example, in the case of the so-called 'spirit causes' of diseases, Tsey (1997) states that "despite the ability of malevolent spirits to cause the individual misfortune, including illness, this can only happen if the individual or the community create the necessary conditions which allow the spirits to act" (p. 1073). Thus, Indigenous healing may also mean having a clear mind, a spiritual way of thinking including freedom from rage, anger, and hurt, and belief in the Creator, yourself, and other people. Through these connections and accumulations, community becomes important in the health processes. Katz (1982) states that, "Healing is a fundamental integrating and enhancing force, far greater than curing or the application of medicine" (p. 347). As noted by Rasmussen (2008), African Indigenous healing is about more than just health:

> In Africa, as elsewhere, there are new universal concerns on how humans can influence their social, natural, and spiritual environments. Thus understanding health knowledge, belief and management, requires moving beyond medicine and including philosophical questions about the nature of knowledge, moral issues such as concepts of person and causation: who is to blame for what has gone wrong, and reflections about destiny, often manifested in not solely organized religion, but also cosmology, myth, and philosophy. (p. 5)

For complete healing to take place, any society has to pay attention to their community and search for various methods of healing at all levels. Van der Merwe (2008) states that African Indigenous practices focus on the relationships between one another. Therefore, individuals are aware of the fact that "I am, because you are," where "I am" is regarded as the product of his or her fellow community members' ancestral spirits and supernatural forces, represented by "you are." The relationship is not only with human beings but also with other animated and unanimated beings. In other words, healing is a developmental process aimed at achieving balance within oneself, with others, with other creatures, nature, the universe, and spiritual worlds. Recognition of interconnectedness is important in the process of restoring harmony at all levels on the Earth and the universe. Mphande and James-Myers (1993) state that recognition of the principle that all things have an inherent intelligence ('know-how') as an expression of the Creator allows us to understand through observations of nature and the world around us that we are one with the course of good, that it exists within us and we are within it. Healing could also be defined as a form of intervention in the form of bodywork, massage, trance, or rituals. According to Somé (1999), healing is central among African peoples. This is because African ancestors learned very early that human beings are vulnerable to physiological and biological breakdown and, when this happens, it affects all aspects of people's existence (p. 21). Everyone is born with a purpose or mission to be achieved and the healers' power to heal is a gift from the Creator. Among Embu people, for example, the mission can be explained as an endowment from Ngai (meaning "Creator" in Kiembu/Kikuyu) (Wane, 2002).

The environmental surroundings play a vital role as part of the relationship between community and health. Regarding current environmental crises and illness, Hill and Kandemwa (2006) point out:

> African people believe that the natural world is inspirited, and they know there are consequences to the violence we do to the natural domain.... Look at what we are doing to the earth today. It is a dumping place for our poisons. Some nuclear weapons are hidden in the earth. The water and the air are polluted. No wonder we have so many diseases today. They were not sent by God or our ancestors. We are making those diseases ourselves. We do not own the land; the land owns us. We do not own the universe; the universe owns us. (pp. 154, 158)

Many African traditional healers are not surprised at how different and sometimes mysterious diseases rampage through the African continent. People's relationship to the natural world and its laws determine their well-being the well-being of the community. Despite its rich resources, many African states see themselves as poor, dependent, and in need of rescue. This view, in itself, has created bad karma as well as a void in people's lives. The outcome has been fear and anxiety, which has resulted in all kinds of sickness. The dependency syndrome has forced many African nations to depend on handouts that are foreign to people's way of life as well as their bodies. This syndrome has thus resulted in the depletion of people's immune systems and mutation of their generative genes that can no longer be sustained from foreign foods and medicines. Many African nations have forgotten that nature is the foundation of Indigenous life and that without it concepts of community, purpose, and healing would be meaningless (Hill & Kandemwa, 2006, p. 155).

Nature, according to Malidoma Somé (1999, p. 57), is the foundation of healing, and hence the importance of the natural world around us. He is making reference to the trees, hills, mountains, rocks—that is, everything that was here before humankind. This means we can find within nature all the materials needed for healing. Nature is a source of life's circle and a site for education in a broader sense. Furthermore, our ancestors passed down Indigenous healing practices to the following generations, knowledge that they learned from other living creatures such as domestic animals, birds, wild animals, plants, etc. For example, our ancestors observed what animals did and ate, and then applied what they saw to their own healing practices. Other examples can be found in practices such as bathing in salts and the use of herbs, food, roots, etc. Some herbalists had an ability to literally talk or communicate with herbs. In addition, they also learned from other herbalists who were able to identify poisonous plants by observing which plants gorillas or domestic animals avoided while grazing (Kareru, Kenji, Gachanja, Keriko,

& Mungai, 2007). Herbalists also observed the nectar of the flowers that birds and bees avoided. This avoidance meant that the plants and their products were toxic. In addition, plants with thorny leaves were regarded as 'male,' and were considered to be naturally poisonous (p. 85).

Traditional healers see the universe as operating under natural laws that manifest according to specific rules. Among African Indigenous peoples, there is a strong belief that the purpose of life and the nature of disease cannot be understood without knowledge of these laws and their correspondences. Many Indigenous communities know that the natural world is an integral part of their world. It is therefore important to begin healing by reconnecting with the natural world because nature is "our first home, the foundation of our community, the dwelling place of the spirits who watch over us and long to be reconnected with us" (Somé, 1999, p. 57). The term "traditional healer" refers to a person involved in one of a broad range of practices, including herbalism and spiritualism. Traditional healers may include diviners (shamans, priests or priestesses, oracles, spirit mediums, and ceremonial specialists), herbalists, or religious-based healers. Healers do not attend formal institutions of learning but rather tend to learn their art through apprenticeship. However, this is now changing, as some institutions of higher learning are offering courses in alternative medicine or holistic healing approaches. Knowledge is based on practices, explicable or not, used in diagnosing, preventing or eliminating physical, mental, or social disequilibrium and relies on experience and observation handed down from generation to generation.

The African healing practices are unique because all physical, mental, and spiritual phenomena are studied, understood, practiced, and taught to its whole community (Afrika, 2004). There is a need for us to understand that there is a deep structure underlying the current streams of our physical existence and the events in our lives are not random or meaningless but are actually a result of "unseen intelligence supported by a loving universe of helping spirits" (Noble, 2001, p. 197). Somé (1999, p. 57) notes that the spirit world constantly intrudes on our daily lives. He provides us with an example of how a spiritual person in Africa in search of a job will not seek for credentials first, but for spiritual guidance, and then the credentials. The spiritual guidance is usually sought through a medicine person.

In addition, although causation of illness was historically often categorized either as natural or supernatural, Konadu (2007) points out

> In the minds of many healers, so called supernatural was natural and the dichotomy often established by theoreticians and other

> academics is an artificial one that has no real meaning in the life and practice of the people but more so in the minds of those who organized reality in adversarial or antithetical terms. (p. 64)

This point is taken up by Rasmussen (2008), who cites Karp and Masolo (2000): "in Africa, the spiritual realm is never far from the material world in social life and philosophical consciousness, and there is a complex, dynamic interaction between diverse forces: human, superhuman, and nature" (p. 4). Some African traditional healers are characterized by their ability to communicate with ancestral spirits. It is believed that the ancestral spirits, who are said to be responsible for sending visions and giving information to the healer, are an intangible force or power that the healer is connected to. Whatever the ancestors are, the impact they have in people's lives is paramount. Traditional healers can accommodate different belief systems into their healing art and thus have a syncretic approach to healing. They are flexible in their methods of healing. They may take esoteric approaches, or even a psychotherapeutic approach if necessary, and may make referrals to any number of different health care alternatives.

Different Modes of Healing

Malidoma Somé summarizes traditional healing practices as those that:

> take into account the energetic or spiritual condition that is in turmoil, thereby affecting the physical condition. If you focus only on the physical translation of the underlying energetic disorder, then you are ignoring the source of the physical illness. If you address only the physical problem, then you end up perhaps with a cure, which fixes the physical condition, providing a momentary sense of victory over debilitation. This act denies the needs of the energy, the adjustment of the spirit needed to make the cure last. Sooner or later, this disordered energy will figure out a new way to affect the physical body often in a new and more virulent manner than it did originally. If you instead address the energy of the mind and spirit, whose status is affecting the physical body, then you are likely to heal truly. Hence, in the wisdom of Indigenous concepts of healing, all healing must begin by first addressing the energetic problems. (Somé, 1999, p. 30)

Traditional healing practices are holistic in nature because of the basic understanding that there is no separation between mind, body, and spirit. Every human being is an integrated entity and cannot survive in pieces; healing practices are thus to be implemented in an integrated way. Sickness, whether physical, mental or emotional, cannot be treated efficiently by concentrating on the part of the body that is not functioning. There is an emphasis on restoration of the natural harmony of the body through an integrated and holistic manner. Traditional healing focuses on the total individual—the person—not the illness.

All traditional healers work differently with each person who seeks their assistance; the healers may use their herbs, ceremonies, and powers differently for each individual. However, what is interesting is the fact that healers are guided by the wisdom that all organs are related to each other and the functions of the environment (Afrika, 2004). The healer's role is not to 'cure' the illness, but to enhance the inner power or coping mechanisms that one has to react to the illness, and to help one realize his/her own ability to heal.

In the following sections we will categorize and discuss various modes of healing practices. However, it is important to mention that these categories are not clearly distinguished. These modes of healing are interconnected, and healers often practice across these categories. Moreover, because these healing practices are grounded in the dynamic everyday lives of people that may require treatment from various modes, it is necessary to look at these modes intersectionally. While categorization of these modes is necessary for examining them in the academy and may be of heuristic value, it is also often problematic from the local people's point of view in that it limits or ignores the dynamic of Indigenous healing practices. These dynamics need to be kept in mind.

a) Herbal Healing

Ancient African Indigenous practitioners taught their patients about herbs and healing (Afrika, 2004). Notably, given that healing is a part of life, elders include it in their everyday teaching of their children. As a result, almost all African families living in rural settings, where herbalists are often still active, acquire basic knowledge of health and healing. Omonzejele (2008) mentions that "good health for the African is not a subjective affair" (p. 120) but a "community" affair. This community is not exclusive but rather inclusive, consisting of wider communities. Prince and Geissler (2001), reporting on their findings among the Luo of Kenya, show that there is no discrimination when it comes to passing on healing knowledge. They state that:

> There is no clear differentiation between the practices of healers and those of lay people, and there is no clear boundary between a novice's participation in a healer's practice, and the way many children participate in the normal medical activities of Luo homestead. (p. 448)

In addition, they also found that all the children (86 children, aged 10-15 years) in a Luo community where they conducted their research, have "a wide range of plants used for medicine and that many could treat themselves for common ailments (stomach ache, fever, headaches, colds, coughs, and injuries)" (p. 448). In this community, children who are not willing to learn herbal knowledge from their grandmothers have a choice; adults do not force them to learn.

My research (Wane, 2002) among the Embus of Kenya emphasized the same point. I still remember that while growing up in rural Kenya, whenever any of my siblings got sick, my parents did not take them to the hospital. My mother used certain leaves, barks of trees, and roots from the bushes for treatment of different types of sicknesses. I can still recall my mother being called to deliver our neighbours' babies. In every home, there was a healer. However, with the mass migration to urban centers and environmental changes such as the destruction of nature, most people have lost touch with any Indigenous healing practices. While deforestation limits the herbs that herbalists can use, foreign plants brought by European colonizers have also had a negative impact on the Indigenous plants used by herbal healers. In a study of herbalists in Keiyo district in Kenya, Jungerius (1998) states "deforestation and the establishment of small-holder agriculture are less serious for their trade than the replacement of Indigenous trees by plantations with exotic species" (pp. 51, 55). Not only does this create a distance from healing practices, but these healers might lose the ability that we mentioned above, to talk with herbs, forfeiting this intimate part of the healing process.

An important aspect of traditional healing that until recently has been overlooked or superseded by the conspicuous ritual and spiritual component of the healing practice is the efficacy of the active ingredients in the medicinal plants the healers use. There is renewed pharmacological interest in African medicinal plants. Although some scholars, such as Amutabi (2008), mention it, this renewal has emerged due to the increased availability and accessibility of traditional healers in a globalized world. Also, the inability of Western medicine to cure some common diseases, such as malaria, HIV/AIDS, etc., has made people seek traditional healers and alternative methods.

b) Spiritual Healing

African traditional healers are characterized by their ability to communicate with and learn from ancestral spirits. It is believed that the ancestral spirits, who are said to be responsible for the initiation, for illness, and for sending visions and giving information to the healer, coalesce into an intangible power that the healer is connected to (Somé, 1999). Diviners are mostly holistic healers who have the special ability to see deep into the human condition, and a mystical connection with 'greater knowing.' Diviners use this revelatory connection to guide people to live healthier and happier lives.

Divination, one technique the healers use, usually functions as a treatment for social problems. Divination is a practice that is used to deliberately initiate a process of accessing and collecting information. Using randomly arranged symbols and the brain's capacity for analogical thinking, associations can be made that are ordinarily inaccessible. Divination appears to be used to gain healing knowledge through access to what is described as the greater transpersonal field of information. In most African societies, it is the diviner's work to discover the hidden causes behind misfortune and prescribe appropriate action. This action is usually in the form of healing, using plant remedies or other forms of rituals (Hammond-Tooke, 1998). The diviner attends to all of the facets that make up the human condition and uses psychotherapeutic, spiritual, and medical methods to affect a cure. Many factors influence the diviner's choice of healing, including the patient's belief system, the amount of money available, and the seriousness of the illness. For diseases and other medical complaints, patients often resort to both Western doctors and traditional healers.

c) Energy Healing

African Indigenous practices entail natural methods of treatment because natural resources have nurtured human beings since the beginning of time. In order for healing to be effective, it must be connected to the world of nature. Traditional healing practices are always integrated and involve a combination of herbal medicine, rituals, nutritional therapy, physical therapeutics, or the laying of hands as explained by Camara Laye (1990) about his mother:

> I know when I describe [my mother's] powers, you will smile unbelievingly...But I can tell you what I saw with my own eyes. Are there not things everywhere around us that we cannot explain? Late afternoon some men came and asked my mother to use her powers to get a horse on its feet. It was lying in the field and

> refused to move...She went up to the horse, lifted her hand, and said slowly and loudly: 'From the day of my birth I had knowledge of no man until the day of my marriage. And from the day of my marriage I have had knowledge of no man other than my husband. If these things are true, then I command you, horse, rise up!' And we all saw the horse get up at once and follow its master quietly... Where did these powers comes from? (pp. 30-31)

Touch, or energy healing, as described by Rasmussen (2006), conveys messages, either consciously or unconsciously, "with unintended but powerful consequences read differently by the receiver" (p. 59). Kizinger (1997), writing about therapeutic touch in child birth, says that "the practitioner centers his/her own thought and is sensitive to receiving and sending nonverbal messages or energy through the hands" (pp. 209-229). Among the African people, there is a strong belief that energy is present in all matter that embodies the natural laws and universal creative force. This energy manifests itself in the physical world in the form of concrete entities called elements and may be found in different parts of the world. This energy has different names in different cultures; for example, in China it is called *Qi*, in Japan *Ki*, in India *Prana*, while in the Pacific cultures it is known as *Mana* and in the Embu language, it is referred to as *Mwaki* (Wane, 2002). However, despite the fact that this energy may have different names, the underlying attributes of this energy are very much perceived in an identical way in all cultures. Living beings are considered to manifest a higher level of this energy while inanimate objects manifest it in a much more limited and basic way. African Indigenous healers believe that this energy can be disturbed in living beings through thoughts and emotions, harmony with natural cycles, and the quality of one's lifestyle, diet, air, water, and environment. Living the philosophy of harmony and respect for nature and people, African ancestors honoured the Creator and the accompanying divine manifestations in women, men, and all of nature. These ancestors saw nature and their environment both as an expression of the Creator and as an inspiration for self-healing. They actively incorporated the use of the four natural elements (water, earth, air, and fire) into their daily and ritual practices (Sawandi, 2002). Among Embu people, for instance, fire (or *mwaki)* is energetic and consuming, air is active and enlivening, water is formless and controlling, and earth is solid and nurturing. These attributes represent different levels of energy and determine not only the appearance of material objects, but also the inherent nature of living things. Through the blessing and consumption of the four elements, our ancient ancestors protected and strengthened their bodies, minds, and spirits from disease (Afua, 2000; Arewa, 1998, as cited by Wane, 2002). In most Indigenous communities, this translates into a system of individual constitutions and temperaments which represent inherent and acquired characteristics and which must be taken into account to ensure that the correct treatment is used for a given person.

In addition, in some African communities, there are different ways to enhancc the energy, such as dancing at ceremonies. According to Katz (1982), when n/um boils it scatters throughout the dance like the sparks that shower from a roughly stirred fire. Not only is n/um accessible to all, but its very activation includes, rather than excludes, all people present (p. 365). Moreover, the dance promotes social cohesion through the manageable release of hostility (p. 350), and "establishes community, and it is the community, in its activation of n/um, that heals and is healed" (p. 351).

Another example of energy enhancement among many African people is in the rhythm created from drums. For thousands of years, people of African ancestry have known the powerful healing energy of the drum. When certain drums are played, not only do you hear the sound of the rhythm, you also feel the energy and vibrations coming from them. Playing the drum is a great way to relieve the stress of everyday life and will help to improve overall health—mentally, physically, and spiritually. Interestingly, Mphande and James-Myers (1993) mention that European psychiatrists have recently discovered the effects of imagery and rhythm in the healing process, a combination of strong dance with rhythms and use of roots that has been recognized by the traditional doctors for a long time.

Along with rhythm, languages or words (both spoken and unspoken) in the form of chants, for instance, contain the power of healing with their vibrating energy. Abdou (2007) states that "it is precisely in the semantic analysis of the gesture and the effects of the sacrifice and the speeches uttered during the healing process, that one understands that the speech contains a peculiar power" (p. 34).

d) Ritual Healing

There is a strong belief that each time there is need for healing, it is because something in the physical world is a manifestation of some deterioration at an invisible level. Many African Indigenous healers believe that what goes wrong in the visible world is only the tip of the iceberg. Somé (1993) argues that in order to correct a dysfunctional state of the visible world, "one must locate its hidden area, its symbolic dimension, work with it first, and then assist in the restoration of the physical world....

Ritual is the mechanism that uproots these dysfunctions" (p. 25). These rituals fix things already gone wrong. It is also strongly believed that the inherent healing practices found among people of African ancestry were gifts given to them by the Creator. These gifts were used during the times of good health and prosperity as well as during the times of adversity. Each community was provided with sacred traditions of how to look after itself and how to extract medicines from plants or other aspects of the earth. This is because a true community begins in the hearts of the people (Somé, 1993). These sacred traditions were executed through ceremonies or rituals. The rituals were avenues that would clear the minds of the elders from the everyday engagements. These rituals were meant to direct the thoughts or the mind and call attention to the moment.

In contemporary societies, there is an emphasis on research and its outcome. Many times, the research cannot explain certain phenomena or sicknesses and the effort to bring back the order exacerbates the situation. The existence of order and its importance in a material sense is easy to understand. In some African Indigenous communities, the rituals to bring back order are holistic and require preparation and a calmer approach. The elders involved require very specific preparation. This could entail the need to be centered, to still one's thought and listen to the inner spiritual aspects that are capable of being sensitive to the unseen forces of the universe. The stillness of the inner self may be achieved through different methods, which vary from society to society. Among some African societies, this is achieved through fasting, vigils, meditation, offerings, prayer, or visits to sacred sites. A trip to sacred grounds may culminate in the offering of foods, drinks, or the touching of the soil, the trees, or anything that is considered sacred. Among the Embu people, fig (Mugomo) trees are very sacred and most of the Indigenous rituals and offerings were/are carried out under the shade of the trees.

e) Community Healing

As for community healing, each society has its own techniques for bringing balance to the community and its environment. These practices are based on the traditional beliefs of a particular group of people or community and the importance of maintaining harmony. When there is no harmony, disequilibrium occurs, and there is disconnection with universal powers. There are many questions to be answered by the community in regard to healing: who is considered a healer, how did they acquire their skills and healing knowledge, and how should a patient 'pay' for a treatment he/she receives? In some communities, both women and men play an important role, as Omonzejele (2008) describes:

> A medicine woman is just as powerful as her male counterpart, because there is no significant difference between a medicine man and woman. In the communities where they practice, they are accorded equal respect. (p. 121)

However, in some African communities, gender plays an important role in healing. For example, Rasmussen (2006) describes women's role in knowledge production regarding healing in Tuareg society. Women healers are considered to be the only people who know trees, which, according to Ag Solimane (1999) represent humidity and moisture, a symbol of life (p. 67). This knowledge is passed down from mother to daughter (Rasmussen, 2006, p. 119). Thus, as Rasmussen (2006) explains, Tuareg medicine women "offer a local cultural variation on wider spread human themes: the vitality and power of self-regeneration of trees, central in rituals, medicines, folk tales, myths, and poems (p. 118).

Among African Indigenous peoples, healing practices do not entail written instructions, but knowledge acquired through intuition, practice, or spiritual guidance. In most instances, healing traditions are passed from one generation to the next through visions, stories, and dreams. According to the Abdou (2007):

> Dreams (doosii) are altogether a real activity. It is through dreams that different Kaawo spirits (Kaawo-bunùunveil)...reveal causes of their disease, tell them the names of roots of certain plants (dâa-gbinâ) that may form part of the remedies (tìr bukatà) and also teach them magic formulae (nôo-muinr); so dreamlike activity has undoubted implications in the healing process. (p. 28)

Konadu (2007, p. 161) mentions healers who also acquire their knowledge through travel and through the national and international exchange of ideas—There is clear evidence of wide dissemination of information, extensive traveling by healers to gain new knowledge (as cited in Warren, 1982, p. 95), and in particular during lengthy trading periods.

Until the monetary mode of exchange was introduced by colonialism, traditional healers did not ask for pecuniary compensation. Many healers do indicate that they do not use their healing knowledge for monetary benefit, but for creating a "better community." Mandaza (2006) explains it as "guidance from spirits." He says:

> When it comes to healing, I was surprised because my spirits told me never to charge anybody a fee. I received people who could have paid me for my services. I also received poor people with nothing at all but who were very sick. In a dream I was told to heal all of them. The ancestors said, 'There are my people. They are suffering.' (p. 98)

This is seen in many African communities. For example, Tsey (1997) states, "There are different charges for different people depending on circumstances" (p. 1070). Then, Rasmussen (2006) says, "They pay me anything according to capacity" (p. 80). Finally, Omonzejele (2008) states that it is at the "discretion of his patients to pay him (healer) whatever they wish after they have been healed" (p. 124). Some patients do not give him anything but he is pleased to see them healed. According to him, traditional medicine is a vocation for service and not just another job.

Conclusion

The African Indigenous healing knowledges that our ancestors passed down throughout history are complex and dynamic in their forms and the ways in which they have accumulated. These knowledges emphasize the importance of harmony and balance while the contemporary world is distracted and losing touch with these qualities, resulting in wars, natural disasters, illness, economic bankruptcy, and so on. With the imposition of Western colonial knowledge on Africans' lives, these ndigenous healing knowledges, which entailed rich ancient wisdom, have been ignored and suppressed. However, this chapter describes and celebrates the richness of our Indigenous knowledges, discussing the need to start re-thinking our relationships with other human beings, creatures, nature, and the universe, and re-learning how to heal ourselves. This process also asks us to go beyond the Western individualized and trichotomized notions of body, mind, and soul, a process necessarily for decolonizing the contemporary world.

References

Afrika, L. O. (2004). *African holistic health: Disease remedies, holistic sex laws, AIDS & herpes treatments, cocaine detox, foods to avoid, recipes, relationships, self diagnosis, complete remedy.* Brooklyn, NY: A & B Distributors & Publishers Group.

Afua, Q. (2000). *The sacred woman: A guide to healing the feminine body, mind, and spirit.* New York: One World Ballantine Books.

Amutabi, M. N. (2008). Chapter 7: Recuperating traditional pharmacology and healing among the Abaluyia of Western Kenya. In T. Falola & M. M. Heaaton (Eds.), *Health knowledge and belief system in Africa* (Revised ed., pp. 149-170). Durham, NC: Carolina Academic Press.

Arewa, C. S. (1998). *Opening to spirit: Contacting the healing power of the chakras and honouring African spirituality.* London: Thorsons Publishers.

Carlson, R., & Shield, B. (1990). *Healers on healing.* New York, NY: Penguin Putnam, Inc.

Castellano, M. B. (2000). Updating Aboriginal Traditions of Knowledge. In Dei, Hall, & Rosenberg (2000 pp.21-36) Indigenous Knowledges in Global Context. Multiple Readings of Our World. University of Toronto Press Incorporated, Toronto.

Dei, G. (1993). Indigenous African knowledge system: Local traditions of sustainable forestry. *Singapore Journal of Tropical Geography, 14*(1), 28-41.

Geschiere, P. (1997). *The modernity of witchcraft: Politics and the occult in postcolonial Africa.* Charlottesville, VA: University of Virginia Press.

Hammond-Tooke, D. (1998). *Rituals and medicines: Indigenous healing in South Africa.* Johannesburg, South Africa.

Hill, M. O., & Kandemwa, M. A. (2006). *Twin from another tribe: The story of two shamanic healers from Africa and North America.* Wheaton, IL: Quest Books.

Jousse, M. (1925/2000)."Oral-style," "memory" and "the counting necklace." In P.

Denis (Ed.), *Orality, memory, and the past: Listening to the voices of black clergy under colonialism and apartheid* (pp. 65-84). Pietermaritzburg, South Africa: Cluster Publications.

Jungerius P.D (1997). Indigenous knowledge of landscape–ecological zones among traditional herbalists: a case study in Keiyo District, Kenya. *GeoJournal* Volume 44, Issue 1, pp 51-60.

Kareru, P. G., Kenji, G. M., Gachanja, A. N., Keriko, J. M., & Mungai, G. (2007). Traditional medicines among the Embu and Mbeere peoples of Kenya. *African Journal of Traditional, Complementary and Alternative Medicines, 4*(1), 75-86.

Kakar, S. (2003). Psychoanalysis and Eastern spiritual healing traditions. *Journal of Analytical Psychology, 48*(59), 659-678.

Katz, R. (1982). Accepting "boiling energy": The experience of !Kai-healing among the !Kung. *Ethos, 10*(4), 344-368.

Kizinger, S. (1997). Authoritative touch in childbirth: Cross-cultural approach. In R. E.

Davis-Floyd & C. F. Sergent (Eds.), *Childbirth and authoritative knowledge: Cross cultural perspectives* (pp. 209-232). Los Angeles: University of California Press.

Konadu, K. (2007). *Indigenous medicine and knowledge in African society.* New York: Routledge.

Laye, C. (1990). *Dark child* (Reissue edition). New York: Farrar, Strauss & Giroux Adult.

Marsland, R. (2007). The modern traditional healer: Locating 'hybridity' in modern traditional medicine, Southern Tanzania. *Journal of Southern African Studies, 33*(4), 751-765.

Mphande, L., & James-Myers, L. (1993). Traditional African medicine and the optimal theory: Universal insights for health and healing. *Journal of Black Psychology, 19*(1), 25-47.

Noble, V. (2001). Letting nature take its course. *Women and Therapy, 224*, 193-208.

Omonzejele, P. (2008). African concepts of health, disease, and treatment: An ethical inquiry. *Explore: The Journal of Science and Healing, 4*(2), 120-126.

Prince, R., & Geissler, P. W. (2001). Becoming "one who treats": A case study of a Luo healer and her grandson in Western Kenya. *Anthropology & Education Quarterly, 32*(4), 447-471.

Rasmussen, S. J. (2006). *Those who touch: Tuareg medicine women in anthropological perspective.* DeKalb, IL: Northern Illinois University Press.

Rasmussen, S. J. (2008). Introduction: Health knowledge and belief systems in Africa. In T. Falola & M. M. Heaton (Eds.), *Health knowledge and belief systems in Africa* (pp. 3-29). Durham, NC: Carolina Academic Press.

Sawandi, T. (2002). *African medicine: A guide to Yoruba divination and herbal medicine.* Scarborough, ON: RGL Enterprises Int'l. Inc.

Somé, M. P. (1993). *Ritual: Power, healing and community.* Portland, OR: Swan and Raven.

_____. (1999). *The healing wisdom of Africa: Finding life purpose through nature, titual, and community.* New York: Tarcher/Putnam.

Solomon, A., & Wane, N. (2005). Indigenous healers & healing in a modern world. In R. Moodley & W. West (Eds.), *Integrating traditional healing practices into counseling and psychotherapy* (pp. 52-60). London: Sage Publications.

Solomon, A. J. (1990). *Songs for the people—Teachings on the natural way.* Toronto: New Canada Press.

Tsey, K. (1997). Traditional medicine in contemporary Ghana: A public policy analysis. *Social Science and Medicine, 45*(7), 1065-1074.

Van der Merwe, J. C. (2008). Chapter 2: The relevance of worldview interpretation to health care in South Africa. In T. Falola & M. M. Heaton (Eds.), *Health knowledge and belief systems in Africa* (pp. 55-66). Durham, NC: Carolina Academic Press.

Vaughan, M. (1991). *Curing their ills: Colonial power and African illness.* Palo Alto: Stanford University Press.

Wane, N. N. (2002). African women & spirituality: Harmonizing the balance of life. 2002. In N. Wane, K. Deliovsky, & E. Lawson (Eds.), *Back to the drawing board: African Canadian feminism* (pp. 275-278). Toronto: Sumach Press.

Wangoola P. (2000). Mpambo, t*he African Multiversity: A Philosophy to Rekindle the African Spirit.* In George Dei, Budd Hall, and Dorothy Goldin Rosenberg (Eds). *Indigenous Knowledges in Global Contexts: Multiple Readings of Our World.* University of Toronto Press.

Chapter Two

A SOCIOLOGICAL STUDY OF TRADITIONAL MEDICINE AND HERBAL PHARMACOLOGY IN AFRICA: RESEARCH ISSUES, CHALLENGES AND POSSIBILITIES

Akwasi Asabere-Ameyaw, University of Education, Winneba, Ghana
George J. Sefa Dei, OISE, University of Toronto
Kolawole Raheem, University of Education, Winneba, Ghana

Abstract:

This chapter will address some of the key issues and challenges in the study of traditional medicine and plant pharmacology as Indigenous forms of knowing. It reviews the existing literature to set the context for identifying the challenges and possibilities of using such knowledge forms to promote science education in African schools. The authors argue that the contribution of traditional medicine and Indigenous herbalists to community health care needs more attention and that national development, as a whole, cannot simply be assumed. The linkages need to be theorized and operationalized and the sociological dimensions fleshed out for an understanding of the society-nature-culture nexus. By identifying some key questions, the chapter hopes to broach the challenges and possibilities of field research in providing relevant knowledge for the theorization of Indigeneity as valid ways of knowing in the academy. This chapter is informed by the findings of longitudinal research in Ghana undertaken by the Centre for School and Community Science and Technology Studies (SACOST) at the University of Education, Winneba, Ghana, beginning in 2007-2008, examining traditional plant medicine in local contexts. Among the key questions for discussion are: What are the philosophical and epistemological bases of traditional medicine and local plant pharmacology as Indigenous knowledge systems? How can such knowledge be studied? How do we deal with issues of custodianship of these knowledges? How can these knowledges be communicated across communities, including schools? What are the ethnic, gender, age, class, and intergenerational dimensions of these knowledge forms? And how do we introduce these knowledges into the school science curriculum? In the discussion, of particular interest is how to reach a synthesis of traditional science (e.g.,

Indigenous medicine) and Western science (e.g., Western medical practice) in the teaching of school science. The chapter finds that there is a need for the integration of traditional medicinal knowledge into the school science and social studies curriculum. The chapter concludes that research knowledge could be helpful in developing appropriate instructional and pedagogical approaches to the teaching of traditional plant medicine. Teasing out traditional ways of science from a variety of sources, including intergenerational communication, gendered dimensions of traditional knowledge, traditional cultural custodians, and traditional herbalists, should inform research intent on promoting knowledge transfer from traditional and modern practices of science. This would also enhance the socio-cultural and political contexts of traditional medicine and plant pharmacology as potential sources of content for science in African schools.

Introduction

This chapter addresses some of the key issues and challenges in the study of traditional medicine and plant pharmacology as Indigenous forms of knowing. It reviews the existing literature to set the context for identifying the challenges and possibilities of using such knowledge forms to promote science education in African schools. By identifying some key questions regarding the study of local pharmacology, the chapter hopes to broach the challenges and possibilities of field research in providing relevant knowledge for theorization of Indigeneity as valid ways of knowing in the academy.

In theorizing local plant pharmacology as Indigenous ways of knowing, certain key questions need to be broached: What is the philosophical and epistemological basis of traditional medicine/local plant pharmacology? How can such knowledges be studied? How do we deal with issues of custodianship of these knowledges? How can these knowledges be communicated across communities, including schools? What are the ethnic, gender, age, class, and intergenerational dimensions of these knowledge forms? And how do we introduce these knowledges into the school science curriculum?

It is widely recognized in Africa that there is a need for the integration of traditional medicinal knowledge into the school science and social studies curriculum (see Asabere-Ameyaw, Dei, & Raheeem, 2009), and it is also argued that knowledge about local plant pharmacology can be helpful in developing instructional and pedagogical approaches appropriate to the teaching of traditional plant medicine. We need to tease out the traditional ways of knowledge transfer including intergenerational communication and gendered dimensions of traditional knowledge, and work with traditional cultural custodians, traditional herbalists, and medical practitioners to understand the socio-cultural and political contexts of their work.

Indigenous knowledge is primarily about the epistemology of everyday life as evidenced in the interactions of the social, biological, physical, material, political, and symbolic realms of everyday existence. Like every body of knowledge, Indigenous knowledge has its own ontological, conceptual/philosophical, methodological, and axiological groundings. The study of Indigenous knowledge highlights local understandings of the society, nature, and culture interface. The environment is interpreted in the broad sense of its physical and metaphysical connections. The nature of social reality as materially consequential for the body also highlights the interconnections of body, mind, and soul. Indigenous knowledge therefore speaks of the inseparability and inter-dependence of selves and the collective on culture, nature, and material attributes of society. We come to know about ourselves and our worlds by heralding the mind, body, and spirit connections with the larger connectedness of society, culture, and nature. In doing so, we create a holistic existence.

Indigenous knowledge is also based on a cosmological understanding that the elements of the universe are interrelated and intertwined (e.g., the mental, physical and spiritual, material, political, economic, etc.). We cannot simplistically atomize and particularize the everyday living experience. The everyday experience and the social world are not always subject to the certainty of knowing. Indigenous people's use of their cultural knowledge system is derived from living in close relations as well as an appreciation of nature and society. Hence, the Indigenous knowledge system is typically comprised of an understanding of the successful ways by which a people deal with their environments and surroundings.

Nakata (2007) notes the expansive territory covered by the global discourse on Indigenous knowledge as spanning ...across a range of interests such as sustainable development, bio-diversity and conservation interests, commercial and corporate interests, and Indigenous interests. It circulates at international, national, state, regional and local levels in government, non-government, and Indigenous community sectors and across a range of intellectual, public, private, and Indigenous agendas. It is dispersed across various clusters of Western intellectual activity such as scientific research, documentation and knowledge management, intellectual property protection, education, and health. It is, according to (Nakata, 2007, p.2), "politically, economically and socially implicated in the lives of millions of people around the globe."

In Indigenous communities, such knowledges can be found in their story forms—myths, fables, tales, and folklore. They can be found in other forms of material culture, such as symbolic ornaments and body ware and the meanings encoded in cultural artifacts. They can also be found in local cultural resource knowledge and practices associated with traditional pharmacology/plant medicine, farming technologies and agricultural methods, environmental management, soils and vegetation classification, arts and crafts, cultural norms, belief systems, social organization of families and kin groups, cultural festivals, and cultural products (e.g., weaving, pottery, poetry, folklore, music, as well as ornaments creatively fashioned from Indigenous materials, etc.).

The dominance of so-called 'modern science knowledge' has largely led to an untenable situation in which Indigenous knowledge is ignored, neglected, or misapplied. Yet from time immemorial, many Indigenous communities have used their own locally-generated knowledge to change and improve their circumstances (e.g., health needs, local governance, and natural resource management). Traditional/Indigenous knowledge of medicinal plants (including information on the different kinds and functions of plants) has been developed on the basis of careful observations and experimentation in local habitats. This knowledge goes back into ancestral times and they are continually subjected to daily improvements and adaptations. Such a body of knowledge about traditional pharmacology is often contextualized in the community's historical experience with local health and illness situations and has been confirmed by their common usage and societal norms.

Indigenous knowledge also recognizes the important role of local peoples in preserving ecological balance and biodiversity. There are customary laws (e.g., cultural taboos, rites, rituals, etc.) governing individual and community use and relationships to social and natural environments. These customary practices and belief systems are a form of a built-in protection mechanism for over-exploitation of natural resources (Asabere-Ameyaw & Anamuah-Mensah, 2006). Local ecological sustainability works when Indigenous peoples maintain ownership status of their resources, where they can freely adopt local strategies of conservation, regeneration, and distribution and control of resources.

Literature and Context

Over the years, plant and herbal medicine has become an important part of medical treatment in communities, especially in the developing countries. In fact, it can be argued that in any given rural community, an individual who falls sick or is ill is faced with some options seeking treatment. One of these is the use of herbal medicine, or what has been referred to as 'phytomedicine.' As an important source of health diagnosis, prevention, and treatment, this knowledge base deserves careful study in order to understand the Indigenous philosophies that sustain the practice. According to the World Health Organization (WHO), phytomedicine can be defined as herbal or plant "preparations produced by subjecting plant materials to extraction, fractionation, purification, concentration, or other physical or biological processes" (as cited in Okigbo & Mmeka, 2006, p. 83). Plant medicines may be prepared for direct consumption or serve as the source for other herbal products. Such plant or herbal products may contain inert ingredients in addition to the active ingredients (Okigbo & Mmeka, 2006; WHO, 2001).

A number of published works define herbal medicine as part of the general group of remedies termed alternative or complementary medicines. Alternative or complementary medicine is understood as health care systems, practices, and products outside of conventional medicine or the orthodox health care system (see Arcury, Grywacz, Bell, Neiberg, Lang, & Quandt, 2007; Barimah & Teijlingen, 2008; Chao & Wade, 2008). A broader definition given by the World Health Organization described it as "the sum total of all the knowledge and practices, whether explicable or not, used in diagnosis, prevention and elimination of physical, mental and social imbalance and relying exclusively on practical experience and observation handed down from generation to generation, whether verbally or written" (WHO, 2003, p. 1). As Darko (2009) notes, interrogating these definitions reveals a conflicting outlook on the term by a number of writers. Ernst and Fugh-Berman (2002) enthuse that alternative medicine may refer to holistic, natural, non-toxic, integrative, gentle medicine. Others employ the words unproven, unscientific, fringe, and non-traditional. This gives alternative medicine both positive and negative images. The term "alternative medicine" is more widely used in the United States (Arcury et al., 2007), "complementary medicine" is commonly applied in the UK (Arcury et al., 2007), and "herbal medicine" is the preferred term in much of Africa (Barnes et al., 2004). Herbs are the most commonly and popularly used category of complementary and alternative medicine (see Arcury et al., 2007; Barnes et al., 2004; Bruno & Ellis, 2005). Herbs are readily available; they can be grown at home, gathered, purchased at supermarkets, pharmacies, and health food stores. They are available in natural forms as extracts and pills (Arcury et al., 2007).

There are a number of reasons for the use of herbal medicines, especially in so-called developing countries. Okigbo and Mmeka (2006) point to consumers' preference for natural therapies; sustained and historic interest in alternative medicine; the belief that phytomedicine is devoid of side effects (since millions of people all over the world have been using phytomedicine for thousands of years); the belief that phytomedicine is used for the treatment of certain diseases where conventional medicine fails; improvement in the quality; proof of the efficacy and safety of phytomedicine; and the high cost of orthodox medicine. Therapeutically, phytomedicine is believed to have more benefits than orthodox medicine. Phytomedicine is also believed to have fewer side effects than orthodox drugs. It is argued that, while phytomedicine acts by regulating and balancing vital parts of the body, orthodox pharmacological products with sedative and axiolytic actions are likely to be accompanied by undesirable side effects like uncoordinated motor skills and drowsiness (Okigbo & Mmeka, 2006).

It is generally acknowledged that using phytomedicine has economic benefits. Today, most pharmacological companies are scrambling to benefit from both the therapeutic and economic benefits of herbal medicine. According to Gunasena and Hughes (2000), employment opportunities are created through the production, processing, and sale of phytomedicine products in many countries. Calixto (2000) and Blumenthal (1999) also note that

> the European market alone reached $7 billion in 1997; the German market corresponds to about 50% of the European market, about $3.5 billion which represents about $42.90 per capita; the market in France corresponds to about $1.8 billion, Italy follows with $700 million, UK has $400 million, Spain and [the] Netherlands have market sales of $300 million and $100 million respectively. The US phytomedicine trade reached about $3.2 billion in 1996 and 5 billion in 1999. (as cited in Okigbo & Mmeka, 2006, p. 88)

It has further been reported that the Asian market reached $2.3 billion and the Japanese made $2.1 billion (Grunwald, 1995). China exported $400 million worth of traditional Chinese medicines out of China in 1993.

A recurring challenge for many communities is the integration of herbal medicine and orthodox/modern health practices. Patients' usage of either phytomedicine or orthodox medicine is based on the nature of health problems often encountered and the perceived success of each of the systems to adequately care for the health needs of its users. The experience with the two forms of healing systems has also determined local preferences. Most people developed an interest in herbal medicine because it succeeded in areas where conventional health care failed. It is believed that taking prescription and herbal medicines together is more effective than taking either alone (Ernst & Fugh-Berman, 2002; Kuo, Hawley, Weiss, Balkrishnan, & Volk, 2004; Krause, 2008; Ryder, Wolpert, Orwig, Carter-Pokras, & Black, 2008). For this reason, most countries have put in measures to utilize resources from both systems.

It's clear in many Southern countries that just a few have access to modern medical services. The majority use traditional remedies. Consequently, the formalization of the traditional health sector has implications for equity in health care, coverage of primary health care, and financing (Bodeker, 2001). According to Bodeker (2001), Asia, especially China and South Korea, has seen the most progress in integrating its traditional health systems into the national policy. These changes occur in diverse ways. While China integrated the system in response to the need for mobilizing all health care resources, India and South Korea pursued these changes through the politicization of the health sector and ensuing change in national policy. These changes are carried out in two basic policy models. These are the integrated and parallel approaches. In the integrated approach, the modern and traditional medicines are integrated through medical education and practice; China and Vietnam practice this system. The parallel approach has modern and traditional medicine separated within the national health system; India and South Korea practice this system.

The World Health Organization has outlined some general principles believed to accelerate the integration of the two systems, especially in Africa. These include: a) 'political recognition' for the development of traditional medicine; b) the 'development of policy, legal and regulatory framework to promote herbal medicine'; c) promoting 'scientific research on traditional medicine and collaboration work'; d) ensuring that 'intellectual property rights are protected'; e) disseminating 'appropriate information to the general public on the use of traditional medicine'; and, f) providing a 'good economic environment for the thriving of traditional herbal medicines' (see Okigbo & Mmeka, 2006, p. 89). In the West African sub-region, traditional plant medicine is becoming more and more popular among both the elite and non-elite in the society. There are, for example, high-class research centres for herbal medicine in Ghana. In

Nigeria, plant medicine has also been scientifically improved to the extent that orthodox medical practitioners recommend some of them to their patients. The importance of traditional medicine has been highlighted by scholars (see Odugbemi, 2008) who categorically stated that there is an urgent need for conservation of medicinal plants by educating citizens on the importance of planting and replanting for traditional medicine.

There are mounting challenges to the use of herbal medicine. For many years, the argument has raged over whether or not traditional medicine has the efficacy and potency often claimed by its practitioners. Another challenge centers on claims by practitioners that it is able to cure disorders that have been classified terminal by orthodox medicine. These include ailments that are very difficult to manage using orthodox medications such as diabetes, epilepsy, asthma, and HIV/AIDS (Erah, 2008). Other writers have alluded to additional challenges to phytomedicine. According to Elujoba, Odeleye, and Ogunyemi (2005), development of drugs from their natural source is a much more difficult task in phytomedicine than orthodox or synthetic medicine development. Formulation of phytomedicine, particularly in raw or crude-drug form, requires specialized experts who are trained and experienced in its processes. It is further argued that the lack of standardization and quality control of the herbal drugs used in clinical trials are major challenges facing herbal practitioners (Calixto, 2000; Makhubu, 2006). Calixto (2000) and Ernst (1999) also note the risk of side effects due to toxicity, over-dosage, interaction with conventional drugs, manufacturing problems such as misidentification of plants, failure of good manufacturing practice, and contamination as a result of field microbial contamination. Calixto (2000) and Makhubu (2006), among many others, also point out the imprecise diagnosis and dosage of phytomedicine as a major challenge. Other manufacturing problems include poor packaging, chemicals used, existing environmental conditions (temperature, light, etc.), adulteration of plants, and inaccurate preparation and dosage (Elujoba et al., 2005). It is also noted that for the most part, little or no collaboration exists among traditional and orthodox medical practitioners. This has resulted in the loss of valuable ethno-medical knowledge that the traditional medicine practitioner may have. Makhubu (2006) has rightly asserted that, in fact, one of the greatest challenges to the development of herbal medicine is building domestic trust in the products. In other words, it sometimes becomes difficult to convince the local community to accept the efficacy and safety of medications from herbal practitioners. McGee (1998), Elujoba (2003), and Makhubu (2006) have stated that the absence or inadequate record of plant species available, as well as the indiscriminate depletion of forests and plants that hold the core to phytomedicine, account for the loss of many plant medicine species. Coupled with the fact that most traditional healers are advancing in age and dying with untapped knowledge, this represents tremendous challenges for the survival of such Indigenous knowings.

While the existing literature is informative about the challenges and tensions of community health care systems as they search for ways to address health concerns, there is a need for more research to understand the local resource knowledge base, particularly herbal medicines, from the vantage point of local practitioners and users. It is our argument that understanding local cultural resource knowledge bases through more in-depth qualitative studies of communities is needed. It's our argument that more in-depth qualitative studies of communities are needed to better understand local cultural resource knowledge bases. We broach science education that focuses on Indigenous knowledge as a valid way of knowing.

A Ghanaian Case Study

There is a tremendous amount of research on plant medicine in the Ghanaian context (Anamuah-Mensah & Asabere-Ameyaw, 2002; Asabere-Ameyaw, Dei, & Raheem, 2009). Anfom (1989) long ago outlined the challenges of herbal medicine practice in Ghana. The author first identified the several types of traditional healers and moved further to examine the differences in the training procedures and practices for both traditional and orthodox medical practitioners (see Darko, 2009). Acheampong (1989) and Addae-Mensah (1989), while tracing the history of phytomedicine, also identified three major practitioners in Ghana: a) the "properly trained and very competent herbalists" who give less recognition to the spiritual causes of diseases, b) herbalists who give much emphasis to spiritual causes of disease, and c) the itinerant herbalists who usually peddle their herbs from house to house or at bus stations (see Darko, 2009). In using herbal medicine, it is noted that the beliefs and practices of Indigenous people are intrinsically considered to be part of people's everyday life. Darko (2009) has traced the link between individual illness and its relation to the supernatural as well as to Ghanaian traditional religion.

Even though traditional health systems play a significant role in attending to the health needs of Ghanaians, Anfom's (1989) work has identified a host of setbacks when analyzing a number of case studies of patients treated by traditional healers. These obstructions include attaching superstition to every health occurrence that may have been caused by environmental factors (e.g., poor sanitary surroundings). It is also noted that most practitioners overemphasize the efficacy and potency of herbal medicine. Furthermore, extreme individualism and elements of secrecy on the part of practitioners also serve as drawbacks. Anfom (1989) further mentions the effects of colonialism on the role and authority of the traditional healer. Some traditional practitioners are described as having lackadaisical attitudes toward their practice and, therefore, have other jobs as farmers, artisans, fishermen, and civil servants. The high "illiteracy rate" among practitioners is seen as another setback (see Darko, 2009). Though the government has embarked on many projects seeking to integrate orthodox and herbal medicine, these efforts have not reached the intended objectives.

This chapter builds on the existing Ghanaian and African literature and works to tease out the Indigenous philosophies that ground plant medicine as Indigenous knowing. While the primary focus of this chapter is on plant/herbal medicine and its uses, we were also interested in the broader area of traditional medicine. We make a distinction between traditional medicine and plant/herbal medicine. The former is seen as a more comprehensive care, involving the preparation of medicines from plant and animals sources, as well as a traditional health practitioner's recourse to social and spiritual/supernatural forces to effect prevention, diagnosis, and cure of diseases. On the other hand, plant/herbal medicine is the preparation of medications solely derived from plant sources (see Asabere-Ameyaw, Dei, & Raheem, 2009). A Centre for School and Community Science and Technology Studies research study conducted at the University of Education in Winneba, Ghana (see SACOST, 2007) notes that "in herbal medicine diagnosis is limited to physical symptoms and, in a few cases, results of laboratory tests...[while]....diagnosis in traditional medicine looks beyond physical symptoms for causes of diseases" (p. 1). When a diagnosis based on physical symptoms fails to lead to a cure, traditional medical practitioners will fall on spiritual and social resources to determine the remote cause of illness and accordingly effect treatment and prevention. Generally, these knowledge systems [traditional medicine and plant herbal medicine] are not so distinct from each other. Looking at our communities today, the differences are increasingly becoming blurred.

The Study and the Method

As discussed by Asabere-Ameyaw, Dei, and Raheem (2009), in the 2007-2008 school year we began a longitudinal study of local plant pharmacology in Ghana. The project was designed with three main research phases, each consisting of a number of specific research activities—pilot study, extensive field research and data analysis, and dissemination of findings. We began phase one by training student researchers to help the principal investigators to conduct a pilot study. The pilot study was intended to field test the survey with in-depth interview research questions in two metropolitan cities/centres where we hoped to secure a full representation of the diverse Ghanaian ethnic groups. We administered field questionnaires to a total of twenty-nine (29) practitioners. Then we selected six (6) key practitioners to conduct in-depth interviews. A list of survey questions was prepared to ascertain the nature, extent and use of traditional plant medicines in Ghanaian communities. The questionnaire sought responses to simple, open-ended questions. The in-depth qualitative studies focused on five (5) major questions to guide the conduct of interviews on the use and application of traditional plant medicine in local communities. These were:

- Local subjects' understandings of the content, practice, use, relevance, and educational implications of traditional plant medicine as local cultural resource knowledge.
- An examination of the intricate ways local subjects reflect on and articulate the practice, uses, and effectiveness of traditional medicinal plants.
- The extent to which social difference (ethnicity, gender, class, language, as well as intergenerational differences in age) can be read from the study of local cultural resource knowledge.
- The understanding of the epistemological and philosophical groundings of local plant pharmacology and the implications for educational practices, pertaining to classroom and household pedagogy, instruction, and school curriculum.
- Uncovering hitherto other [unknown] uses of traditional plant medicine in the study communities.

To meet these learning objectives, the study sought to address the following four (4) research questions:

a) What does a general survey (through the administration of a questionnaire) on the extent and uses of traditional plant medicine in selected Ghanaian communities tell us about the practice and use of traditional medicine and for which particular ailments?

b) What can we learn regarding the effectiveness of traditional plant medicine and how do we learn it from in-depth qualitative interviews with a select sample of local community users and practitioners of herbs?

c) What are the particular teachings that inform the understanding of traditional medicine as an Indigenous form of knowing?

d) How can the current research information be used to collaborate with Indigenous herbalists, local educators, and other stakeholders to undertake a wider comparative study of the sociological, pedagogical, and instructional aspects of traditional medicine and herbal pharmacology in the larger African contexts?

In 2009, we undertook further research focusing on the northern and upper west regions of Ghana, visiting several local communities for a careful documentation of plants and herbs used for treating common ailments and photographing these for the purpose of teaching and learning. We conducted individual and group interviews with close to a dozen herbalists, highlighting some key social, cultural, and environmental aspects of their work in plant medicine.

The Study Findings: The Qualitative Data Analysis

We have chosen to highlight the narratives quotes of a few of our study participants that speak to the broad trends and patterns we have picked up from our on-going analysis of the research data. The focus is on the qualitative data; the findings have been analyzed and presented under some main themes/sub-headings that reflect the significance of traditional medicine as a facet of Indigenous ways of knowing. We should also point out that, for qualitative studies, it is equally important to cover material more in-depth, even when using a small sample (see Lichtman, 2006).

a. *The Study of Plant Medicine as Indigenous Knowledge: Content, Method, and Source*

The knowledge of Indigenous plant medicine is often stored in peoples' heads, written documents, material objects, everyday routine social practice, cultural artifacts, folkloric productions, societal values and morals. The methods for studying such knowledges include listening and talking to people, interviewing herbalists as practitioners, and observing their medicinal practices daily; further, through apprenticeship, children learn from their parents/elders as herbalists. Such knowledge strengthens personal relationships and reinforces the bond between persons, communities, and ecosystems. It is knowledge embedded in sacred traditions and practices, and persons who know these traditions are responsible for teaching the 'morals' and 'ethics' of herbal medicine to younger practitioners. The latter are given responsibility for this specialized knowledge and its dissemination. In many cases, knowledge of herbal medicine becomes Indigenous knowledge as an extended kinship passes on its teachings and social practices from generation to generation. In defining plant medicinal practice as Indigenous knowledge, we must be careful not to reduce such knowledge to simply the practical, mundane, everyday, or routine knowledge. Such knowledge exhibits a great degree of sophistication, complexity, and abstract and conceptual thinking and knowing.

Mr. T. is a 29 year-old student 'traditional medicine practitioner' who has now completed his first degree at a local university. He enthuses about learning traditional medicine when very young from his grandparents:

> Whenever I brought the herbs, [my grandfather] would ask me to take a critical look at the herbs, he in turn [then would tell], this is what we use this herb for. Should somebody come to you with this kind of complaint, this is what you do. My younger and elder brothers were not interested in these things so I developed an interest in them. Added to this, there was a time I had a big sore on my leg and I suffered. But it was through the use of herbs that I got healed. So I started using them.

The intergenerational transmission of such knowledge that Mr. T. speaks about is important. It serves to maintain continuity of knowledge in a given community. By treating a sore on his foot with traditional herbs, he came to appreciate the potency of traditional medicine and has since been a practitioner and advocate. Since childhood he has been "very curious and asked my grandfather a lot of questions on how things happen." He acknowledges that initially things had been done by 'trial and error':

> I also did a lot of trial and error at the beginning to get medication for some ailments. Then after I started schooling, there were occasions in which I studied the causes of some ailments before, and the understanding I got from knowing about the cause of ailments, etc., I also tried to develop something from it.

His curiosity fed on the passion for traditional medicine and his knowledge of such traditional science increased with the years, like all forms of knowledge practice. There is a depth of knowledge possessed by local herbalists. For possessing such knowledge, herbalists are generally well known and respected in their communities. In interviews, herbalists would often show us plant varieties collected and available in the household, used for treatment of common ailments. The narration of the everyday activities of their profession usually demonstrates a combination of social and scientific knowledge and the importance of the social implications of traditional plant medicinal practices. Many herbalists would agree that Indigenous knowledge is a traditional science with its own corpus of rules of conduct and etiquette to be followed. Among the herbalists interviewed were specialists in the treatment of major ailments including headache, migraines, madness, fever, rheumatism, fibroids, snake bite, dog bite, cat bite, mouse bite, fracture and bone setting, circumcision, stomach pains, breast cancer, chest pains, boils and piles, waist pains, knee problems, urinary retention, guinea worm, fever/malaria/typhoid fever, hernia, etc.

Many of the herbalists encountered in our Ghanaian research have been practicing for over 55 years and this length of time has come with expertise of plant pharmacology. In our conversations, respondents would point out that with each passing day they learn something new in their profession. This speaks to the dynamism of plant medicinal knowledge. Traditional herbalists also generally see the acquisition of such knowledge as God's gift and they point to the power of intergenerational transmission of knowledge (e.g., father to son) and the imperative of continuing such family tradition in order to retain the viability of such Indigenous knowledge. Some traditional herbalists seek to protect their knowledge and would acknowledge a degree of secrecy in their profession.

Knowledge of the seasonality of plants is critical to successful harvesting and treatment of the sick. For example, knowledge of when to harvest plants, including time of day, etc. may affect the plant's vital nutrients essential for particular treatments. Similarly, knowledge of human physiology is critical.

b. *Education and Integration of Knowledges: Traditional Medicine and Orthodox Medicine*

In their responses to interview questions, a number of local subjects acknowledged the competition between Western/orthodox medicine and traditional medicine. They see this as something worthy of attention as it robs the citizen of adequate health care. Education is key here both in terms of making the vital connections but also in providing the sites, spaces, and moments to make such connections possible. For example, most traditional herbalists noted the urgency and the need to teach youth about the existence of such knowledge as well as the need to collaborate with medical doctors in Western clinics/hospitals. All herbalists interviewed agreed teaching such knowledge to youth would be a benefit to the community, provided there are quasi-formal training procedures and some agreements of who teaches, how, and what. One issue generally shared is that there are well-respected ethics of the profession that need to be followed in the teaching of plant medicine as science knowledge. Integration of practice and theory is most effective in the pursuit of the education of traditional plant medicine in schools. The synergy between herbal practitioners and classroom educators is critical. We need educators well vested in the science of herbal medicine, its efficacy, and relevance for community health development. But such teachings about local community health cannot be compartmentalized. There must be an attempt to provide a bridge between Western science knowledge and local knowledge; the interface of herbal medicine and Western medical practice is significant.

Kweku is a lecturer at a local university. His words point to the connections between different health care systems. The educator brings a historical dimension to his analysis. He makes some critical observations about the connection between traditional medicine and orthodox medicine. Basically, he sees the former as foremost a medical practice for Indigenous communities and believes the advent of orthodox medicine should not necessarily have led to a devaluation of traditional medicine. Kweku holds the latter in high esteem:

> Before the Westerners came to Africa, we were solving a lot of these problems. There were so many diseases we were dealing with effectively. So I would say that orthodox medicine should have rather been supplementary to what we already have. The new thing should have rather come and help, rather than turning the table so that what was there is rather relegated to the background and the new thing becomes the ultimate. That is unfortunate. It should have been complementary, not supplementary....Why should it be supplementary? Before the Whites brought orthodox medicine, we had something already. So what is there should be there, then we add. But the way we are behaving, we seem to be clearing the table, so that we bring the new one and it is as if it were driving away the original thing. But the two must be together. Now it has come to a situation where it seems as if we are destroying what we had before. The two must work together. Because there are some people for whom orthodox medicine would not work. My wife, for example, because of her upbringing, does not trust traditional medicine. But it works for her whenever she takes it.

He shows displeasure with how traditional and Indigenous knowings have been devalued with the advent of Western thought and knowledge systems. Rather than supplementing what we know with new knowledge, we have allowed new knowledge to make secondary our traditionally held practices, some of which have worked for communities over time. This does not mean we remain uncritical of such traditional knowledge. Rather, it means we appreciate our knowledge and see how we can bridge any divide and strengthen human existence. The two health delivery systems, traditional and orthodox medicines, must coordinate efforts in illness prevention and treatment. But traditional medicine must not be secondary or necessarily supplementary to orthodox medicine. It must be viewed and respected in its own right.

When asked about any distinctions between traditional and plant medicine, the student practitioner, Mr. T., brings a depth of knowledge and critical perspective to the discussion. He does not make any distinctions between herbal medicine and traditional medicine but acknowledges the place of the spiritual in traditional medical practice as a holistic approach to health care. As he says:

> They are the same, only that if you look at traditional medicine, the man goes to look for herbs, plant roots, etc., he brings them home to come and burn them. In herbal medicine, the man uses herbs. In traditional medicine, the man also goes to the bush to bring things to come and combine. The only slight difference is that in traditional medicine, they try to bring in some spiritual things.

It appears then that teaching about traditional medicine will embrace more than having herbal medical knowledge. Traditional medicine speaks of the society-nature-culture nexus in a way that heralds the physical and metaphysical connections. There are religious, spiritual, and mythical dimensions to traditional medicine that any education about integrating knowledge systems has to contend with, yet the place of religion, spirituality, and myths/mythologies in plant medicinal practice is not something readily conceded to by many local herbalists. They insist there is nothing 'supernatural' about their practice. Yet some practice can be shrouded in some secrecy of knowledge and the unwillingness to pass on the details of their knowledge confirms this aspect. We cannot simply attribute concerns of intellectual property rights to the careful guarding of their knowledge by some practitioners.

Kweku maintains he has been "a big enthusiast [of] plant medicine and traditional healing" for some time now. In our interview with this affable educator, we got a sense of his deep knowledge of the uses, effectiveness, and philosophical underpinnings of traditional medicine. As the interview lasted longer than usual, we took the opportunity to explore in depth some of our key research questions. When asked about any difference between traditional healing and plant medicine, he aptly comments:

> Plant medicine uses all types of plants to deal with health problems. Traditional healing may not use plants at all. It may use minerals and other things which orthodox medicine may not connect with healing....[Thus] [t]raditional healing is bigger and more holistic. But invariably traditional healers will include plants in the remedies.

Thus, plant medicine is simply plants whereas traditional medicine brings a whole repertoire of traditional health knowledge into focus. Kweku's narrative points to the holistic and comprehensive nature of traditional medicine.

Kweku adds to our understanding of the spiritual and social dimensions of health and what it means to engage in traditional medical practice. He concedes to the spiritual and mythical aspects of traditional medicine and asserts that it is not superstition but observation and verification of the happenings of the social and natural worlds. He disagrees with those who say that traditional medicine is based on superstition. It is, according to him, scientific knowledge based on experimentation and verification of facts and he insists orthodox medicine has borrowed a lot from traditional medicine. He asserts:

> Traditional medicine is not superstition, because it is based on plants....We know that orthodox medicine borrows a lot from plants. Let's take the man who brought inoculation/vaccination to a scientific level. He learned from traditional healers. He knew that when cowpox is used to infect an individual, that person is able to resist smallpox. That thing did not come from the lab. It was the practice of cow hands that, when they had children, they infected them with cowpox and when they suffer from cowpox, which is milder, small pox was not able to affect them. Even traditionally, there are certain incisions. We prepared certain carbons and we used such carbons to prevent certain diseases. Well we are veering toward preventive medicine. What I am saying is that traditional medicine is not superstitious because it works. If it does not work, then you can say it is superstition, but it works. Look at bone setting for example, and you are put in POP; the POP does not work as fast as if I bind you with certain plants. It works, so you can't tell me that it is superstitious.

In effect, Kweku is asking how something that has been proven to work can be superstition. Traditional medicine is based on careful observation of local environments and knowledge of what works and what does not work.

d. The Environment

Throughout, our study discussions with local subjects and herbalists revealed the importance of the surrounding environment and how it was the main source of plants. The discussions also highlighted the extent to which knowledge of the environment matched knowledge of the uses of segments of plants and herbs. Herbalists would generally assert that many leaves are medicinal plants. Given that the surrounding environments are crucial to their practice, herbalists expressed deep concern about the impact of contemporary developments on local environments, including farming, firewood harvesting, and charcoal burning. It was asserted by many that they would support setting aside parts of the environment as restricted areas, to aid traditional herbal practice. However, others noted that even within communities in which some areas are traditionally restricted, these areas are now being encroached upon. Therefore, they would welcome official help in this endeavour. It is evident that the success of traditional medicinal practice rests on safeguarding the natural environment. The need to pay attention to this issue was salient for most local herbalists.

The knowledge from the local herbalists that many leaves are medicinal was powerfully expressed to pinpoint the need for more research on still unidentified plant medicinal sources in local communities. There can be no adequate study (teaching and learning) of traditional plant medicine without an appreciation of how local communities understand and use their environments. It is worthwhile to quote Kweku's words at length, as they impinge on understandings of Indigeneity and traditional sustainable ecological development. Without a doubt, the local ecological base is relevant for the survival of traditional medicine. There are local taboos and cultural practices intended to maintain the viability of local environments. These traditions have been powerful sources of knowledge that have helped guide human conduct and social practice and maintain environments for local populations and generations unborn:

> Look. Let me tell you, before the Europeans came, there were big forests which were preserved without forest guards, forests which were preserved. The elders will first meet and say this particular forest is a sacred forest. Don't put any wood, whether dead or alive, from this forest into fire. The tree may die but leave it like that there

dead. Do not use any part of the trees. The forests were preserved. They did not use a guard to guard them. Today we have forest guards, incidentally some of the forest guards could be....to fell the trees. Because they know that it is human beings who will see them with their eyes before they are punished. But our people say it is the divinities; they will tell you it is Nana Densu, Nana Prah, Nana so and so which is watching. Whether you see it or not, it is there watching you. So the forests were preserved. The moment foreign religions came and we said oh those things are useless, look at what [has happened to] the forest, they are gone. This is the way I look at it. So we can explain it to the student....it may not be physical that this is what it is but it is physical. The result, because once you preserve the trees then you have vegetation covering the soil and therefore there will be rain. Because the tree will help [with] evaporation. The moisture will evaporate into the sky and go and form clouds, the clouds will condense and fall as rain. So far as we are concerned, it is the divinities that are doing that.

Taboos and cultural norms have a place in maintaining the survival of local communities. If, as researchers and educators, we are interested in teaching about local science and Indigenous knowledge, the protection of environments, the place of local culture and traditions and understanding of health and social well-being in science education cannot be underestimated. Teaching traditional medicine is teaching about Indigenous science, local geography, human ecology, notions of spirituality and political economy. An approach to Indigenous health science is a holistic way of teaching and learning about communities and their histories. Traditional medicine raises key questions about education. The teaching of health science in schools through traditional medicine and its practices can go a long way in arresting national development challenges.

e. Gender and Herbal Knowledge

Gender is always an important consideration when dealing with everyday human realities and social practices. Gender matters in the understanding of human life. There are very few female traditional medicine practitioners. There is a strong belief that female herbalists cannot cure some diseases. The gendered nature of the profession, however, can be attributed to the training received by the practitioner and the practice of continuing an established tradition rooted in the intergenerational transmission of knowledge. Still, the gender dimension of herbal medicine practice is a largely underexplored area in traditional plant medicine. Questions of 'whose knowledge' are demarcated along lines of gender, age, ethnicity, and class. Local knowledge, unfortunately, conceptualizes gender simply as male/female custodians of knowledge. The questions of power and how intergenerational communication of such knowledge reinforces traditional gender boundaries and hierarchies need to be fully explored. For example, what does it mean to affirm the patriarchal practice that female herbalists cannot treat certain ailments?

Kweku, the university teacher, brings a gendered dimension to the discussion of traditional medicine. When asked about how gender factors into the discussion of traditional medicine, he notes:

> If you go to my area, both men and women are practitioners. Do people go to men the same way as they would to women practitioners? It depends. If it comes to gynaecological problems, most women would want to go to women practitioners rather than men practitioners. They happen to be the midwives, the traditional midwives, so they go to them for pregnancy, lack of pregnancy.

Women are an embodiment of some forms of knowledge about traditional medicine and medical practice. We need to document what the genders know and why and how such knowledge is recognized in a given community as far as local health care, prevention, and cure are concerned. There are implications for teaching science education in schools, colleges, and universities. Thus, a gendered aspect of the study of traditional medicine in terms of who is doing what, how matters of health are viewed by practitioners and users, and the relevance of such considerations as care, comfort, and understanding, are critical issues.

f) The Protection of Indigenous Knowledge: Appropriation, Marketization, and Commodification of Herbal Medical Knowledge

All forms of Indigenous knowledges present challenges in terms of the perception, appropriation, systemization, and accreditation of knowledge. The capture of plant medicinal knowledge has raised questions regarding the commodification, propertization, and protection of Indigenous knowledge. To understand the geographies of appropriation of Indigenous knowledge we must raise questions regarding the asymmetrical power relations between local herbalists and established state, government, and non-governmental bodies and companies who enter communities in pursuit of such local knowledges. In fact, the question of intellectual property rights is real for most traditional herbalists. They are quick to insist on the distinction between teaching about the existence of their knowledge for the promotion of health development and knowing the actual formulae for their practice. This requires formal training and protection of the knowledge from abuse and appropriation without due credit given them. Connected to the foregoing point is the growing commodification of such traditional knowledge and the fear that most customary safeguards protecting such knowledge will be lost, including their efficacy due to individual greed and motivation for profit rather than community health safeguarding, which is a cornerstone of such traditional practice.

How do we educate others about the responsibilities to our knowledges? Student practitioner, Mr. T., in his wisdom, calls for collaborations among all health practitioners and users. He argues that such collaborations will work if practitioners are imbued with a sense of social responsibility and shirk any attempts to simply make monetary gains from their profession. He tells a story of greediness that points to some of the pitfalls of the health care system and the significant role of public education not just to users, but among practitioners as well:

> I have noticed that herbalists are greedy. In the north it is not like that, but at the south it is more pronounced. An example was when a medical doctor from Swedru came to me with people with stroke, he was asking me to give him the plants I used, but I refused and rather opted to treat the people. Will you believe that? He collected money from the people but did not give it to me. Another, a Pastor, came from Tema and was more interested in getting samples from me than coming to learn.

The traditional health profession will survive if we seek to learn the service rather than see it simply as a quick way to make money. Those who learn grow in their knowledge and are able to help the community. When asked if he thinks it is possible to teach our children about the uses and effectiveness of traditional medicine, Mr. T. is very emphatic, yet his answer is problematic. He shows a limited understanding of the spiritual as distinct from 'religion.' For many in the local community, religion is the basis of their spirituality and this understanding is relevant for acknowledging the place of the spiritual in local/traditional health promotion:

> ...[Nodding, yes]....it is very important, sir. You asked about a healthy community; this goes to back my answers. If we all know what to do and are well in terms of health, money spent on treatment will be used for development. I will suggest that, the idea of bringing religion into herbal medicine, should not be encouraged.

> If you do that, it will not work. A woman came to me and asked if I used some spirits in preparing my medications, I told her no, and that pastors even come to me for treatment. I told her my medicine does not go against religion.

g. Traditional Knowledge, Local Health, Spirituality, and Community Well-Being

In examining the practices of traditional herbalists and the knowings of local users of traditional medicine, one can discern a connection as well as a distinction between the ability to diagnose and treat local health ailments. While the connection is there for a successful practice of plant/herbal medicine, diagnosing an ailment does not necessarily translate to successful treatment. This is where the broader social/community implications of illness and treatment become critical. This was demonstrated in the in-depth interviews with local herbalists and users whose narration of herbal practice and treatment show a fit between plant and body physiology and the social implications of everyday herbal practice in local communities.

In many local communities, speaking about the health of a person or group always evokes feelings of community well-being. When the student practitioner, Mr. T., is asked about what it means to speak of a 'healthy community,' he offers this interesting response:

> When we talk of a community being healthy, a community is simply a group of people living together and doing all things in common. They have the habit of sharing knowledge. Everybody is open to one another. If someone has a problem you are ready to offer services to those people and in that respect nothing is hidden. In those days sometimes some of the herbalists used to be a bit greedy. Excuse me for saying this. What they knew, they would never share; so in that respect you see that others are enjoying whilst others are suffering. Where we have that kind of cordial relationship, then community becomes more decent and everybody is happy and healthy. There is no sickness and other things.

The above narrative speaks to the essence of seeing health knowledge as 'community knowledge.' The health of every person in the community speaks about the health of the larger community. The work of traditional medical practitioners has been to heal not just the individual, but the entire community. The work has entailed sharing information and traditional medical knowledge. This has not always been easy. Mr. T. laments the greediness that has seeped through the work of some herbalists and the implications it has for working to promote community health. He also shares some knowledge on sickness and who is a sick person:

> Normally a sick person is when you have unknown conditions in the body and you are not familiar with those conditions and you feel like you are in a different environment than the usual one.

In other words, sickness is living in an unfamiliar environment. It affects not just the physical body, but the entire socio-cultural realm of the person and her or his surroundings. This perspective is informative in adding to a conception of health that goes beyond the body and the individual to a larger community and social well-being. Obviously there are lessons here for how we should come to appreciate traditional medicine and the treatment and prevention of sickness and illness. It calls for a holistic approach to knowing and understanding 'health.'

The observation of the larger social-cultural and physical realms in which traditional medicine is practiced and understood brings to the fore critical questions about the place of the spiritual in illness treatment, prevention and cure. In discussing traditional medicine, Mr. T. appreciates the deep and mystical content that cannot be easily dismissed as 'unscientific.' Practitioners are often conflicted about the claims of the sick concerning the spiritual dimensions of the disease and the 'scientific' approach that seeks to dismiss such claims. He acknowledges that:

> Certain times the thing happens and actually is beyond the compass of your knowledge. Anything we do not understand, we say it is spiritual to some extent, you see. Anything we cannot clearly define, we say it is spiritual. That is it. People come to me and say my sickness is spiritual. When I get such a person, I encourage them to discard that knowledge as I have no eyes to see beyond what is physical.

Saying a practitioner cannot "see beyond what is physical" does not negate the presence of the spiritual. It is merely an affirmation of the empirical reality. A holistic approach to traditional medicine acknowledges this fact. Other respondents' words shed light on the link between 'health' and 'sickness.' In response to what we mean when we say a person is sick, Kweku, for example, observed:

> In traditional healing, a person is not sick only in the body. The bodily sickness is only a manifestation of what is happening in the

spirit world or in the soul. So the person falls sick spiritually before the disease or ill health or illness manifests itself. This is where the traditional healer would deal with the problem using plants as well as other materials or sometimes totally intangible things.

A sick person is not healthy socially, spiritually, mentally, and physically. Sickness requires that treatment take into account the emotional, psychological, spiritual and physical well-being of the sick. The connection between sickness and health is easily drawn. Kweku's words are very informative about who is a healthy person:

> A healthy person is one who is physically, mentally and spiritually sound, and you must also have a general sense of well-being. So it is not only sickness; like when you are sick and you are feeling pains physically, that is not the only sickness you have. And we even believe traditionally that even before ill health manifests itself physically, you have been spiritually sick. This is why even being worried, mentally, you can become sick. You may not be physically sick, you may not have an infection, yet you may be sick.

Having a general sense of well-being means appreciating one's inner and outer environments, as well as living in peace and harmony with oneself. The individual fully functions as a member of the community. Kweku's analysis of traditional medicine offers significant insights regarding the philosophical underpinnings of traditional medicine as Indigenous knowledge and Indigenous health practices:

> The traditional medicine practitioner does not look at your body as body alone, but he believes that behind or beside the body there is something else, so when he is treating you, for instance, they give you plant materials to crush in water and bath, even sometimes before they give you the treatment they give you plant material to crush in water and bathe with it. They are trying to purify you mentally, spiritually before they give you the physical treatment.

Treating the sick and the ill means going beyond the physical manifestations of the illness to get to the soul and mind. Kweku's words show the importance of understanding traditional medicine as 'Indigenous knowledge.' Such knowledge is not simply based on careful observation of surrounding social and physical environments. It is also about how local communities make sense of their worlds and a people's place in a given space. More importantly, such Indigenous knowings centre broader questions of society, spirituality, physicality of the environment, and material matters.

Discussion

We devote this final section of our chapter on the social implications of research in the area of local cultural resource knowing and the 'why?' issue of Indigeneity. It goes without saying that local subjects see the need to sustain local environments in order to contribute to the achievement of sustainable health care development. For our part as researchers, we share the need to learn, and perhaps document the knowledge and use of traditional plant medicine by local communities through sustained field research. We need to understand how and why local subjects use their environments to promote local health and well-being. We must also understand the limits of their knowledge and the potential for growth in social and health development. For science educators, we have a responsibility to develop appropriate instructional and pedagogical approaches to the teaching of traditional medicine. This is one way to ensure their sustainability and to make such knowledge available on a wider scale to the local populations. This is more than imperative in the climate of rising health care costs, when national governments under stringent budgetary conditions are finding appropriate ways to meet local needs using available local resources and cultural knowledge (Asabere-Ameyaw, Dei, & Raheem, 2009). This is 'development from within' rather than an overreliance on external help, creating conditions that cannot be sustained over the years.

Within local communities, the ways such traditional medicinal knowledge is transferred, including intergenerational communication, point to significant age, class, and cultural dimensions. Working with local community users of plant medicine and traditional herbalists, we can help uncover the intergenerational, ethnic, social class, and gender dimensions of such knowledge systems and what this means for education and health care promotion, as well as for national development. Research information would also be helpful in the resolution of perceived tensions between Indigenous/traditional medicine and Western/modern medicine, and assist health workers and policy makers in health and national development issues. A specific academic preoccupation is how to introduce these knowledges into the school and community science curriculum and how the work of Indigenous herbalists and health care workers can be coordinated for effective community health science education. The ways local populations reach a synthesis of traditional science (as in Indigenous medicine) and Western science (as in modern medical practice) and the implications of such knowledge in the teaching of school and community science in schools is worthy of academic investigation.

As argued in Dei (2010), culture is seen as critical to knowledge production. In fact, cultural paradigms shape knowledge. The advancement of any one cultural perspective cannot be universally applied and/or seen as superior to other perspectives. This is the basis of the critique advanced by Indigenous knowledges regarding the ways in which hegemonic knowledges (e.g., Western Eurocentric ways of knowing) often masquerade as superior and 'all knowing.' Indigenous knowledges also affirm that there are cultural, physical, and metaphysical continuities as well as discontinuities in a people's experiences. Knowledge does not necessarily leave the body with a re-location. Knowledge can reside in cultural memory and can be called upon to deal with contemporary pressing problems in different contexts. The belief is that all knowledges are shared and accumulated across time and space.

A culturally-grounded perspective helps centre Indigenous peoples' worldviews. It also helps local peoples resist the dominant perspectives that downplay knowledges located in the everyday understanding of the people's social and material reality. When reclaimed and affirmed, Indigeneity and Indigenous knowings provide intellectual agency to marginalized, colonized peoples who then become subjects of their own histories, stories, and experiences. The Indigenous philosophical tradition provides a space for local peoples to interpret their own experiences on their own terms and understandings, rather than being forced to do so through dominant paradigms. The politics of Indigenous knowledge production is to (re)construct an Indigenous identity rooted in place, culture, and history.

Indigenous knowledges cannot be romanticized, however, as they are also embedded in power relations. There is always the difficult question as to who can claim 'Indigeneity' and Indigenous knowledge. The claiming of Indigenous knowledge is not about denying others their knowledge. Given that Indigeneity and Indigenous knowledge are connected to, not fossilized in, time and place, there is not an easy answer to the question. Historically, all groups can claim an Indigenous past and history insofar as it is outside the realm of colonial domination and the colonizing experience. The time and space dimensions to Indigenous knowledge merely speak to the contextual basis of knowing and the fact that all knowledge is first and foremost local and needs to be situated in appropriate cultural and political contexts (see also Dei, 2009).

The Indigenous landscape makes a claim to Indigeneity, which must be understood in terms of the society, culture, and nature nexus. Such Indigeneity is about a spiritual and spiritualized view of human existence (Asabere-Ameyaw, Dei, & Raheem, 2009). Indigeneity cautions that the material and non-material aspects of life cannot be dichotomized and neither can we evade the power issues of knowledge making, validation and dissemination. Given that knowledge 'borrows' and learns from other ways of knowing, Indigeneity is about resistance to domination and colonization, and a welcoming of new members into existing communities. Indigeneity is not simply about rights (e.g., who has rights to a place) but more about our individual and collective responsibilities to ensure the existence of a sustaining community. The issue of responsibility means owning up to the knowledge we produce and allowing such knowledge to compel the action that brings about social transformation and change.

We conclude our essay by reiterating that traditional medicine as health science, when taught in schools, must take into account local understandings of the workings of culture, society, and nature. Such teachings must affirm the emotional and spiritual well-being of the individual, and of the social group as the bedrock of any health development process. Our study findings point to benefits for educators, health care practitioners, and policy makers. Without a doubt, traditional plant medicine constitutes an Indigenous science dealing with cultural norms and practices, as well as ways of knowing about health, disease, prevention, and cure. Such knowledge shows dynamism, reflecting a continual process and renewal on the part of traditional herbal practitioners and users of plant medicine. Traditional medicine is also important for future research to explore other uses of plants in communities that are yet to be identified, and whether or not some of the medicinal plants identified in the existing local literature and texts also have other uses besides those currently known.

NOTES

1. All names are pseudonyms in order to protect confidentiality and to maintain anonymity of local respondents.

ACKNOWLEDGEMENTS

We would like to thank the following:

Dr. Anthony Normeshie, traditional medicine practitioner, Health for All Herbal Clinic, Owuram, Ghana, for data collected from his clinic.

Isaac Darko, Department of Sociology of Equity Studies, Ontario Institute for Studies in Education, University of Toronto, for graduate assistance with the literature review.

References

Acheampong, E. Q. (1989). *Conventional medical practice and research into Indigenous herbal medicine.* Paper presented at the inaugural lecture, University of Ghana, Accra, Ghana.

Addae-Mensah, I. (1989). *Herbal medicine—Does it have a future in Ghana?* Paper presented at a public lecture, University of Ghana, Accra, Ghana.

Anamuah-Mensah, J., & Asabere-Ameyaw, A. (Eds.) (2002). *Plant medicine: A report on plant medicine seminar: Its development and implications for science education.* Winneba, Ghana: SACOST production.

Anfom, E. E. (1989). Traditional medicine in Ghana. *J. B. Danquah memorial lectures, V 1*(17 series), 1-13.

Arcury, A. T., Grzywacz, G. J., Bell, R. A., Neiberg, R. H., Lang, W., & Quandt, S. A. (2007). Herbal remedy use as health self-management among older adults.

Journal of Gerontology Social Sciences, 62B(2):142-149.

Asabere-Ameyaw, A., & Anamuah-Mensah, J. (2006). Taboo systems and rituals: A simple technology for environmental resource management—the case of the Dagaaba and Mamprusis of Ghana. *Journal of Development Alternatives and Area Studies, 25*(1/2), 104-115.

Asabere-Ameyaw, A., Dei, J. F. S., & Raheem, K. (2009). Examination of traditional medicine and herbal pharmacology and the implications for teaching and education: A Ghanaian case study. *Alberta Journal of Educational Research, 55*(3), 298-318.

Barimah, K., & Teijlingen, E. R. (2008). The use of traditional medicine by Ghanaians in Canada. *BMC Complementary and Alternative Medicine, 8*(30), 1-10.

Bodeker, G. (2001). Lessons on integration from the developing world's experience. *BMJ, 322*, 164-167.

Blumenthal, M. (1999). Harvard study estimates consumers spend $5.1 billion on herbal products? *Herbalgram, 45*, 68.

Calixto, J. B. (2000). Efficacy, safety, quality control, marketing and regulatory guidelines for herbal medicines (Phytotherapeutic agents). *Brazilian Journal of Medical and Biological Research, 33*(2), 179-189.

Chao, M. T., & Wade, M. C. (2008). Socioeconomic factors and women's use of complementary alternative medicine in four ethnic groups. *Ethnicity and Disease, 18*, 65-71. Chinese Health Newspaper (in Chinese), 9th. Jan. 1996.

Darko, I. N. (2009). *Ghanaian Indigenous herbal practices: The use of herbs.* Toronto:University of Toronto.

Dei, G. J. S. (2009). *Teaching Africa: Towards a transgressive pedagogy.* New York: Springer Publishing.

______. (Ed.). (forthcoming). *Indigenous philosophies and critical education.* New York: Peter Lang Publishing.

Elujoba, A. A. (2003). Medicinal properties of plants with oral health implication. In *Proceedings of the 2nd Dr. David Barmes' Memorial Public IIealth Symposium.* Jos, Nigeria: Regional Center for Oral Health Research and Training for Africa & WHO Regional Office, Brazzaville.

Elujoba, A. A., Odeleye, O. M., & Ogunyemi, C. M. (2005). Traditional medical development for medical and dental primary health care delivery system in Africa. *African Journal of Traditional, Complementary, and Alternative Medicine, 2*(1), 46-61.

Erah, P. O. (2008). Traditional or orthodox medicine in Africa: A new look. *International Journal of Health Research, 1*(4), 175-176.

Ernst, E. (1999). Second thoughts about safety of St. John's Wort (Hypericum perforatum L.). *Lancet, 354*, 2014-2015.

Ernst, E., & Fugh-Berman, A. (2002). Complementary and alternative medicine: What is it all about? *Occupational Environmental Medicine, 59*, 140-144.Foote, N. (1999). Traditional medicine in contemporary Ghanaian society: Practices, problems, and future. *Drug Information Journal, 33*, 309-313.

Gunasena, H. P. M., & Hughes, A. (2000). *Food for the future 1 Tamarind (Tanarindas indica L.).* Southampton, UK: International Centre for Underutilized Crops.

Grunwald, J. (1995). The European phytomedicine market: Figures, trends, analysis. *Herbalgram, 34*, 60-65.

Haq, I. (2004). Safety of medicinal plants. *Pakistan Journal of Medical Research, 43*(4), 160-165.

Iwu, M. W., Duncan, A. R., & Okunji, C. O. (1999). New antimicrobials of plant origin. In J. Janick (Ed.), *Perspectives on new crops and new uses.* Alexandria, VA: ASHS Press, 457-462.

Kuo, M. G., Hawley, T. S., Weiss, L. T., Balkrishnan, R., & Volk, J. R. (2004). Factors associated with herbal use among urban multiethnic primary care patients: A cross-sectional survey. *BMC Complementary and Alternative Medicine, 4*(18), 1-9.

Lichtman, M. (2006). *Qualitative research in education: A user's guide.* Sage Publishers.

Makhubu, L. (2006). Traditional medicine: Swaziland. *African Journal of Traditional, Complementary and Alternative Medicine.*

McGee, H. (1998). In victu veritas. *Nature, 392*, 649-650.

Odugbemi, T. (Ed.). (2008). *A Textbook of Medicinal Plants from Nigeria.* Nigeria: University of Lagos Press.

Okigbo, R. N., & Mmeka, E. C. (2006). An appraisal of phytomedicine in Africa. *KMITL Science and Technology Journal, 6*(2).

Ryder, P. T., Wolpert, B., Orwig, D., Carter-Pokras, O., & Black, S. A. (2008). Complementary and alternative medicine use among older urban African Americans: Individual and neighborhood associations. *Journal of the National Medical Association, 100*(10), 1186-1192.

Smitherman, C. L., Janisse, J., & Mathur, A. (2005). Pediatrics. *Journal of the American Academy of Pediatrics, 115*(3), 297-304.

The State Administration of Traditional Chinese Medicine of the People's Republic of China. (1997). *Anthology of policies, laws and regulations of the People's Republic of China on traditional Chinese medicine.* Shangdong: Shangdong University.

Straits Times. (2000, November 14). Kuala Lumpur, Malaysia.

World Health Organization. (1978). The promotion and development of traditional medicine. *Technical Report Series 622.*

_____. (2001). Legal status of traditional medicines and complementary/ alternative medicine: A worldwide review. WHO Publishing.

_____. (2003). *Traditional medicine.* Retrieved from <http://www. rootandbranchom.com/docs/WHO%20_%20Traditional%20medicine. pdf>

Chapter Three

CONCEPTUALISING ILLNESS FROM AN ISLAMIC PERSPECTIVE

Sumaya Laher

Abstract

Islam is one of the major religions on the African continent. Hence, no book on traditional healing and healing practices in Africa would be complete without a chapter on illness from an Islamic perspective. This chapter presents an understanding of physical, psychological, and spiritual illness in Islam. Where possible, parallels are drawn to illustrate similarities between Islamic beliefs and traditional African and Asian beliefs. The information in the chapter is based on Western and Islamic literature, interviews with Muslim volunteer counsellors, interviews with Muslim Faith healers, and the author's personal experience.

Introduction

Ratele, Duncan, Hook, Mkhize, Kiguwa, and Collins (2004) argue that modern psychology is a Western product that does not necessarily work in developing societies like South Africa as it imposes an understanding of people and behaviour that is grounded in conceptual categories and theories developed in the West. Meyer, Moore, and Viljoen (2002) add to this notion, stating that ignoring the cultural context and belief system of African people has caused a lot of pain as a consequence of misdiagnosis and the application of inappropriate therapeutic techniques. They cite the example of schizophrenia, which is frequently misdiagnosed among African patients. Ill-informed psychologists and psychiatrists have diagnosed paranoid delusions and auditory hallucinations in patients who believed they were bewitched or that ancestors had spoken to them. Thus, Mkhize (2004) argues for indigenisation—an attempt to blend imported theoretical and methodological frameworks with the unique elements of the culture in question. In line with this quest for indigenisation, this chapter presents an understanding of physical, psychological, and spiritual illness as it is conceptualised in Islam. Islam is one of the major religions on the African continent; 43.3% of the people in Africa are Muslim (Kettani, 2010). Where possible, parallels will be drawn to illustrate similarities between Islamic beliefs and African and Asian beliefs.

Understanding Illness in Islam

In Islam, the person is understood as being composed of four interacting parts, namely, mind (*aql*), body (*qalb*), self (*nafs*), and soul/ spirit (*ruh*). All four parts interact continuously with each other to maintain a harmonious balance in the body. Disease occurs when this balance is interrupted for some reason. The person functions within a natural environment that consists of tangible and rationally explained beings, and a supernatural environment, within which intangible or unseen forces function. It is within this natural environment that the balance between the four interacting parts may be disturbed, resulting in physical, psychological, and/or spiritual illnesses that may impact one or more parts of the individual. Thus, scholars of Islam recognize that illness is caused by spiritual conditions as well as by physiological conditions. Islamic understandings of physical and psychological illnesses conform to illnesses as described in the DSM-IV-TR (2004) and the ICD-10 (WHO, 2011), which is not surprising considering that much of modern medicine has its roots in the works of Islamic scholars like Avicenna, Averroes, and Rhazes. However, the major difference lies in the inclusion of spiritual illnesses within the taxonomy of illness in Islam.

Islamic schools of psychology, along with African and Asian approaches, understand illness in terms of its prescription to a spirituality principle. In certain African cultures, the person is conceived of as four layers. The first layer represents the body, the second represents a vitality principle often linked to physiological functioning, the third represents another vitality principle akin to psychological functioning, and the final, inner layer, is the spiritual principle. These concentric layers of personality are in constant relationship with the environment, and any disruption in these layers produces illness (Sow, 1980). Paranjpe (1998, 2010) describes a similar model of the person in Indian culture. Five concentric layers are identified, namely, the body, the 'breath of life' or physiological processes, the 'mind' or sensory function co-ordinator, the intellect and cognitive aspects of an individual including self-image, and the 'jiva,' or seat of experience of bliss.

Understanding Spiritual Illness in Islam

Spiritual illnesses in Islam can be split into two broad categories: *sihr* (black magic) and *nazr* (ill will).

Black Magic

In Islam, magic, sorcery, and witchcraft all fall under the term 'sihr.' Sihr, according to Abdussalam-Bali (2004), is defined as an act that brings one closer to the devil. The Muslim belief in the existence of this act is precipitated not only by cultural affiliations, but also by the religious book of Islam, the Quran. Evidence from the Holy Quran says, "Suleiman (Solomon) did not disbelieve, but the devils disbelieved teaching men magic" (Abdussalam-Bali, 2004, p. 21). It is further stated in the Quran that "I take refuge with the Lord of the daybreak from the evil of what He has created, from the evil of darkness when it gathers, from the evil of the women who blow on knots, from the evil of an envier when he envies" (Abdussalam-Bali, 2004, p. 22).

Black magic is achieved via the use of plants or through the help of *jinn*. This concurs with the understanding of voodoo presented by Morrison and Thornton (1999). According to them, voodoo is defined as "a system of magic, divination, herbalism, and conjuring involving root doctors and herbalists....Mythical possession is a common part of the rituals in which laos (spirits) enter into people" (p. 446).

In black magic, the medicinal properties of plants are abused by individuals to induce harmful symptoms in other individuals. Plant extracts are placed in the food or rubbed onto the clothing of those who are to be harmed with the intention of causing erratic behaviour, fear, delusions, hallucinations, fever, epileptic fits, excessive weight gain, infertility, miscarriages, physical illness, and in the most extreme cases, death. Interviews with Muslim faith healers suggest that this is a common method used by individuals with enmity toward another person, often arising from occupational functioning, social or relationship issues, rivalry or social standing. One of the faith healers interviewed mentioned the case of a lady who could not become pregnant for 18 years. The woman and her husband had sought a variety of medical opinions from general practitioners and fertility specialists. There was no apparent medical reason for not conceiving. Eventually the couple came to see the faith healer who diagnosed a case of severe sihr. A family member with animosity toward the husband's family was using black magic to ensure that the lady never conceived. However, the faith healer indicated that faith healers (particularly those involved in curing) never reveal the identity of the person responsible for the sihr. They simply provide treatment. The lady in this case was given herbal treatments to remove the effects of any toxins from the body. The lady was also given amulets to place in her house and to wear so as to prevent any further sihr from affecting her. She needed to perform certain prayers and burn *lobaan* in her house. Five months after continuing with the faith healers' treatments, the lady conceived. Throughout the pregnancy the lady was treated by both the faith healer and a gynaecologist.

In addition to the hallucinatory properties that can be found in plants, it is believed that jinn can send black magic. In Islam, jinn are a separate race that can appear in different forms and are only visible to one who has the power to contact the spiritual realm or one who obtains control of the jinn. The power of contacting the unseen is something which may be inherited but can also be learned. Once this power or control is established, an individual will have the ability to use it either for good (to cure people from their spiritual afflictions) or for bad (to harm those who are the targets of jealousy). Thus, the person who has malevolence as a motivator can utilize the power of the jinn to harm others, while the witchdoctor or faith healer will focus on curing the ailments and defeating the spells of the evil witch.

Just as there are individuals who use their abilities for good or to cause harm, there are also good and evil jinn. One sometimes sees good jinn aligning themselves with faith healers to counteract the effect of evil jinn who align themselves with sorcerers or witches wishing to cause harm. It is also possible that a person may be possessed by good or evil jinn. Evil jinn are usually sent by those wanting to cause harm but possession by good jinn usually occurs in cases where jinn are attracted to certain humans because of their spiritual or other qualities. The beneficial or harmful effects of jinn determine whether they are good or evil. Thus, it is believed that if a possessed individual is displaying religious qualities, then it is a good jinn, whereas, if the individual displays qualities that are against the doctrines of religion, it is an evil jinn or an evil spirit that has possessed the body.

Evil jinn, like evil sorcerers, are usually regarded as those that have aligned themselves with the devil. Coker (2004) adds to this by stating that when the jinn are evil, they may be referred to as devils or evil spirits, often interchangeably. On this basis, one can say that the terms demon, evil spirit, and jinn all depict the same process (i.e., the possession of an individual by an unseen spirit). Thus, the terminology used to describe a religious/cultural diagnosis will depend largely upon the culture or religion to which the diagnosis applies. For example, in Islam, it is common to hear of a jinn possession, whereas in the Christian faith, the terms evil spirit or spirit possession are used.

Symptoms of possession include unexplained sadness or anger, bad dreams, fever, epileptic fits, excessive weight gain, infertility and miscarriages, physical illness, accidents, and in the most extreme cases, death. Victims of possession may show supernatural strength or agility. Jinn possession also manifests itself in bizarre, multiple behaviours and odd movements that may fall under psychotic or non-psychotic disorders. Some victims may arch their spines, while others may roll on the ground; the tone of voice of the inflicted may change, the individual may use the plural 'we' on rare occasions, or speak a foreign language. Some of the other features include eye rolling, screaming, gagging, odd smells, and a cold feeling in the room (Abdussalam-Bali, 2004; Hussain & Cochrane, 2004; Karim et al., 2004; Stafford, 2005). It is also believed that more than one jinn can possess the body of the inflicted, demonstrating behaviour characteristic of dissociative identity disorder.

Many cases of jinn possession have recently been reported by various authors. Among the most cited cases are those of Dein, Alexander, and Napier (2008), who reported on jinn possession among East London Bangladeshis. They report on the case of Rashida, a 56-year-old woman who suffered from chest pains. Despite seeking consultations from general practitioners and a hospital consultant, her condition did not improve. She sought treatment from a faith healer who diagnosed jinn possession and read verses of the Quran to exorcise the jinn. Rashida recovered shortly thereafter. They also cite the case of Nirban's sister-in-law, who was experiencing strange things in her house. Her doorbell would ring continuously but no one would be at the door, her baby cried uncontrollably, and the entire family experienced sleep problems. Nirban put his sister-in-law in touch with a faith healer, but later that day Nirban's 15-year-old son collapsed in the bath. Nirban called the faith healer, who recited verses over the boy to revive him. According to the faith healer, the same malevolent jinn who was responsible for the events at his sister-in-law's house had caused his son to have the accident as a warning to Nirban not to get involved in assisting his sister-in-law. Cases such as those of Nirban and others, as reported in Dein et al. (2008), provide evidence in the argument for the existence of jinn or spirits. In the case of Rashida, however, even though evidence points to possession, Dein et al. (2008) make the point that a lot of Rashida's narrative centred on a discussion of racism and deprivation, leading them to question whether the condition of spirit possession may be linked to the powerlessness these communities face.

Ill Will

In addition to witchcraft/black magic, the Quran also identifies the ill will or jealous intentions of others as a source of illness. This is termed 'nazr' in Islam. The best description of ill will comes from a faith healer who said, "Each person within his eyes has something which he is not aware of. If he is somebody of a jealous nature, he will radiate evil. If he is a good hearted person, he will radiate good, so by him looking jealously at somebody, it can just make him sick, maybe you know, and he ... err, he might not even realize that he's doing it, but he can make the person sick" (M1, personal communication, 2008). Whereas sihr is usually premeditated and intentional, nazr is quite often unintentional. It can be caused by any human being. To have an evil eye one does not require training or need to undergo various tests, as is typical of witchcraft or jinn control.

Symptoms of ill will tend to be similar to those of black magic but are often not as severe. The victims present with lethargy, loss of appetite, nausea, fever, bowel problems, disturbed sleep patterns, bad luck, and misfortune. Unlike black magic, where the effects are continuous and become more severe with time, the bad luck and misfortune of nazr wear off after a period of time—usually once the inflicted person loses contact with the jealous individual.

Cases of nazr are quite common among children. With babies, uncontrollable crying without an obvious medical cause is often understood as nazr. After treatment, which can be done by anyone, there is usually an improvement in crying, and within a day or two most cases disappear. When this is not successful, the infant is taken to a faith healer, who will usually recite verses of the Quran over the child. An amulet may be given for the child to wear, and water, over which verses of the Quran have been read, will be given for the child to drink.

Treatment of Mental and Spiritual Illness

In Islam, believers often simply refer to 'the will of Allah' and accept that their illnesses are a test from the Almighty. This is even more so for psychological or spiritual illnesses. Based on this belief, many will not seek any form of help. However, the Prophet Muhammad (peace be upon him) is reported to have said, "Utilize medicine O servants of God; verily God has not sent down a sickness except that a cure has also been sent down for it. He who has knowledge of it knows it; he who does not will not." This suggests that not only is one encouraged to use known methods and medicines, but one should also be open to all those which can and will be discovered through research and experimentation.

While Islam advocates the use of current medical and psychological treatments, it also advocates additional treatments based on natural and herbal remedies. Treatments used, specifically the use of natural products, originate from Islamic (*Unani*) medicine, which has its roots in treatments prescribed in the teachings of the Prophet Muhammed (p.b.u.h.) in the book *Tibb-an-Nabawi*. *Tibb-an-Nabawi* refers to the specific words and actions of the Prophet Mohamed (p.b.u.h) with regard to disease, treatment of disease, and care of patients. *Tibb-an-Nabawi* integrates body, mind, matter and soul.

Islamic traditional healing practices cover a wide range of remedies. Treatments for medical conditions include herbal remedies, massage therapy, and cupping. Treatments for mental and spiritual illnesses may include herbal remedies, massage therapy, *taa'weez* (amulet with Quranic verses), the administration of water over which verses of the Quran are read, and special *zikr* and *duas* (prayers). In the case of mental illnesses, treatment might also include burning lobaan or other natural substances.

It is further mentioned that recitation of the Quran and other spiritual practices such as daily prayer can be effective in the treatment and healing of patients. The Muslim prayer consists of contact prayer (*salaah*), remembrance of Allah (*zikr*), and recitation of the Holy Quran. These forms of prayer elicit a physiologic relaxation response that serves as a buffer against the adverse effects of stress. The relaxation response also results in lowered blood pressure, heart rate, breathing, and metabolic rate, which yield many long-term benefits in both physical health and mental well-being (Sayed, 2003).

When it comes to spiritual illnesses, the physical and psychological symptoms may be temporarily alleviated through treatment by a doctor or psychologist, but the actual spiritual illness will only be cured once the black magic or ill will is removed. This can only be done by a faith healer. Faith healers can be considered those individuals who have attained a comprehensive understanding of, and practice from within, a particular religious or cultural viewpoint (Al-Habeeb, 2004), allowing them to effectively render assistance to community members who are afflicted by a religious-cultural diagnosis (Khan, 2002). As elaborated by the African Regional Office Experts Group (WHO, 2000, as cited in Eldam, 2003, p. 47) a traditional healer is "a person who is recognized by the community in which he lives as competent to provide health care by using vegetable, animal, and mineral substances and certain other methods based on the social, cultural, and religious background as well as on the knowledge, attitudes, and beliefs that are prevalent in the community regarding physical, mental, and social well-being and the causation of disease and disability." Different forms of traditional healers exist, ranging from bonesetters, traditional midwives, herbalists, and religious healers like shamans, priests, and moulanas.

In the Islamic faith, traditional healers (e.g., moulanas, *sheikhs*, or *matawaas*) are the mediums through which mental illness is dealt with, as they are considered well equipped to drive the evil spirit or the evil eye away (Sayed, 2003). Exorcists in the Islamic faith recite specific verses from the Quran and splash water on the affected parts of the person (Khan, 2002). The recitation of Quranic verses also assists in differential diagnosis. Should a person be suffering from a purely medical or psychological illness, the faith healer will be able to determine this at the onset of the healing process when specific verses are recited. These verses are read and then blown onto the client and/or into natural products (e.g., water, honey, sugar, salt, olive oil) that the person is to ingest or cook with. Further, the verses of the Quran are written on a piece of paper to be kept with the person at all times (a taweez/protective amulet). It is believed that this will either cleanse the inflicted person from the inside out, or form a protection for that person from the effects of black magic and/or nazr.

Further elaboration of the impact of spiritual practices on the precipitation of and the curing of spiritual illness was obtained from a faith healer who reported that "our deen (religion) has taught us that if a person...reads namaaz regularly and properly, reads Quran then Insha'Allah (with the will of God) firstly he will be less susceptible to err in these type of things, also his cure will be faster, and if a person is far away from deen, does not perform salaah, or lead an Islamic lifestyle, then they may be more susceptible" to spiritual illnesses (M5, personal communication, 2008). Thus, it can be said that a spiritual illness will have spiritually inclined cures in the form of spiritual practices. It is important to note that even though spiritual practices are regarded as vital in the treatment of mental illness, they do not make one immune to the effects of black magic and ill will. They only make one spiritually stronger.

Finally, an essential element in the treatment of spiritual illnesses is belief—belief in the Almighty and in the fact that through the grace of the Almighty, the spiritual element causing the illness will be removed. One does not have to follow Islam or any of the other religions in particular, but a firm belief in a higher power needs to be present.

Conclusion

From the discussion presented in this chapter, it is evident that an understanding of diverse belief systems is imperative if one is to holistically and effectively prescribe treatments to individuals from non-Western cultures. Although the DSM-IV-TR (2004) states that cultural considerations in the evaluation and treatment of individuals are important, and although Western investigators have come across startling Eastern conclusions concerning mental processes and ways of promoting psychological well-being, there exists a tendency for traditional healing to be dismissed as mere superstition (Sheikh & Furnham, 1996). Likewise, there are many modern psychiatrists, psychologists, and general practitioners who believe in the existence of supernatural spirits, yet would not make a spiritual diagnosis or diagnosis by religious variables (Al-Habeeb, 2004; Bulbulia & Laher, in press). With this said, it can be ascertained that even though Western empiricism has opened its doors to the possibility of alternate aetiologies, the treatments and ultimate explanations of illnesses are seen within the framework of the Western viewpoint, a viewpoint that only considers objectively observable and measurable phenomena. Given the diverse nature inherent in the South African and African contexts, this Western viewpoint needs to re-align itself with the various culturally inclined taxonomies that exist (Ally & Laher, 2008).

References

Abdussalam-Bali, W. (2004). *Sword against black magic and evil magicians*. India: Al-Firdous Books.

Al-Habeeb, T. A. (2004). Pilot study of faith healers views on the evil eye, jinn possession, and magic in Saudi Arabia. *Mental Health and Addiction*. Retrieved from http://www.ecommunity-journal.com/pdf/c01a70.pdf

Ally, Y., & Laher, S. (2008). South African Muslim faith healers' perceptions of mental illness: Understanding, aetiology and treatment. *Journal of Religion and Health, 47,* 45-56.

American Psychiatric Association. (2004). *Diagnostic and statistical manual of mental disorders* (4th ed.). Washington, DC: American Psychiatric Association.

Coker, M. E. (2004). The construction of religious and cultural meaning in Egyptian psychiatric patient charts. *Journal of Mental Health, Religion & Culture, 7*(4), 323-347.

Eldam, A. E. (2003). *Tendency of patients towards medical treatment and traditional healing in Sudan.* Unpublished doctoral dissertation, Germany, University of Oldenburg.

Kettani, H. (2010). Muslim population in Africa: 1950-2020. *International Journal of Environmental Science and Development, 1*, 136-142.

Khan, F. (2002). Spirituality, religious wisdom and the care of the patient. *Yale Journal for Humanities in Medicine.* Retrieved from http://yjhm.yale.edu/archives/spirit2003/dignity/scallahan2.htm

Meyer, W., Moore, C., & Viljoen, H. (2002). *Personology: From individual to ecosystem.* Cape Town: Heinemann Publishers.

Mkhize, N. (2004). Psychology: An African perspective. In D. Hook (Ed.), *Critical Psychology* (pp. 24-52). Cape Town: UCT press.

Morrison, E. F., & Thornton, K. A. (1999). Influence of southern spiritual beliefs on perceptions of mental illness. *Issues in mental health nursing, 20*, 443-458.

Paranjpe, A. C. (1998). *Self and identity in modern psychology and Indian thought.* New York: Plenum.

Paranjpe, A. C. (2010). Theories of self and cognition. *Psychology and Developing Societies, 22*, 5-48.

Ratele, K., Duncan, R., Hook, D., Mkhize, N., Kiguwa, P., & Collins, A. (2004). *Self, community & psychology.* Cape Town: UCT press.

Sayed, M. A. (2003). Conceptualization of mental illness within Arab cultures: Meeting challenges in cross-cultural settings. *Social Behaviour and Personality, 31*, 333.

Sheikh, S., & Furnham, A. (2000). A cross-cultural study of mental health beliefs and attitudes towards seeking professional help. *Social psychology and psychiatric epidemiology, 35*(7), 326-334.

Sow, A. I. (1980). *Anthropological structures of madness in Black Africa.* New York: International Universities Press.

Stafford, B. (2005). The growing evidence for 'demonic possessions': What should psychiatry's response be? *Journal of Religion and Health, 44*, 13-30.

Chapter Four
CAPTURE THE SPIRIT TO BECOME A TRUE AFRICAN MEDICAL PRACTIONER

Professor Meki Nzewi, University of Pretoria

Abstract

The Indigenous African medical practice is holistic, and combines two cardinal principles of wellness—health care (public health) and health cure (individual health)—that prioritize preventive health management. The science of healing relies on interstructuring and interaction between the four cardinal curative agencies that operate in concert: spirituality, community, musical arts, and medicine. Indigenous medical practice in Africa entails the rehabilitation of psychical health, community health, physiological health, and impaired life force. An average member of a cultural group grows up acquiring knowledge of basic health cure—common curative herbs/elements for treating minor ailments—as well as actively partaking in healing musical arts activities. Knowledge of diagnostic and curative procedures/materials for serious sicknesses requires a period of training and ritual induction. The process of qualifying as a specialist traditional doctor invariably culminates in undertaking a binding, mystical or 'blood' oath that compels the 'divine' doctor to be a conscientious practitioner. Contravention of the life-saver oath is known to incur severe psychosomatic affliction. Ill health in Indigenous African cultures is known to have tangible and intangible, but palpable, causes. Thus, the curative science and practice in Indigenous Africa embraces intangible connections along with tangible resources. This contribution draws from research interactions with healing practices in West and South Africa.

Position

Autochthonous African culture groups are differentiated by their cultural knowledge rationalizations and cultural knowledge manifestations, as derived from a common underlying philosophy, theoretical logic, and principles of practice that engender humanity conscience. The Indigenous culture groups that inhabit Africa south of the Sahara desert, while cherishing ethnic autonomy in cultural lore, have been moving, intermixing, and combining knowledge practices over millennia before the traumatic intrusion of inhumane Arabic and European forces. The studies that inform this discussion are derived primarily from years of research interaction with traditional health practitioners in Nigeria and South Africa, as well as Indigenous ideologies about wellness, illness, and healing from spiritual, medicinal, and musical arts perspectives.

The following axioms, rationalizations, and mores concerning health position the transaction of health care and health cure practices in traditional Africa:

- Science, evidenced from Indigenous medical practices, is fundamentally the practical exploration of intuition in the process of which tests validate effective outcomes that become widely applied. Traditional healing commands exploring the causes of health impairment and the tangible ecological (pharmaceutical) resources as well as the potent (immaterial) energies that produce replicable and updateable solutions. Traditional healers are thus creative/scientific intellectuals, a number of whom are mystics and competent musicians.
- Ill health could manifest as mental impairment (psychosomatic/stress), physiological infection, and organ/tissue/system malfunction/failure or injury, which invariably triggers some degree of psycho-physiological disquietude. Treating the mind then becomes central to healing. A healthy mind makes for a healthy body, unless external harmful agents intrude and induce ill health.
- Ill health generates multi-dimensional disequilibrium—social, spiritual, economic, etc. Hence even if not infected, the entire psyche and physiology become misaligned.
- Ill health could be self-generated, transmitted by others, congenital, the product of misfortune, a supernatural sign, or caused by a polluted environment.
- Ill health could be any deviation from the norm that traumatizes a group's ethos or psyche; otherwise, the norm could be negotiated within tolerable boundaries.
- Ill health could be avoided, contained, or countered.
- Ill health occasions communal concern, rallies communal empathy; wellness could be accelerated by communal support.
- Healing is a fundamentally holistic procedure—from the total person to the specific ailing part—but the mind is the first port of call in health management.

- Healing as a process of restoring the abnormal/dysfunctional is structured and systematic. It involves the identification of cause and effect (diagnostic), stabilizing the disturbed psychology of the sufferer (humanistic), contextualizing the community (empathy), harnessing any intangible corrective potencies (meta-cure), administering healing activities/substances (material cure), and rehabilitation.
- Physical and emotional isolation of the mentally or physically impaired, including the aged, could induce a psyche of abnormality and societal rejection. Social integration in the family, as much as communal performing arts activity, manages syndromes of abnormality. The sick patient is not a thing but an afflicted, sensitive human subject.

Types of Healing

The Indigenous worldview and concept of health and healing are not rationalized and experienced in the narrow sense of remedying a diseased part. Rather, they command a holistic (Makgopa, 2004, p. 52) practice of systematically obviating and restoring good health. Traditional African cultures thus emphasize two primary principles of societal health management: the preventive and the curative. Preventive health practice is given serious attention and coerces mass, proactive conformity with established traditional practices; curative remedying of impaired mental or physiological disorder often entails both tangible and intangible means.

Indigenous health management systems correlate spiritual, environmental, community, medicinal, and rehabilitative measures to engender human and ecological wellness. Healing in traditional Africa often commands a ritual theatre that commonly involves musical arts activities. Accordingly, Mufamadi (2004) articulates that in Africa, "sickness is perceived as a religious matter" and "healing takes place in the context of religion" (p. 59). She credits Dawes and Honwana (1996) as observing that: "Health is defined by the harmonious relationship between the individual and the natural environment, as well as with the deceased ancestors and with other community members." Mufamadi further states that: "The principle among Africans is that, 'if part of me is sick, then the whole of me is sick'" (p. 59). This is the critical difference between the conventional perceptions of medical rescue of the sick as curing, and the traditional perception as healing. Makgopa (2004, p. 52) quotes Felhaber and Mayeng (1997, p. 35), who discuss traditional treatment of sickness as being "holistic in nature because of its comprehensive approach. It is holistic because it cannot be reduced to a single dimension of treatment or remedy. The purpose of traditional treatment is aimed not only at curing the disease, but also at healing the patient."

Through systematic cultural education, often anchored on belief-coerced compliance, an average member of an African community observes personal and environmental hygiene, ensuring that their body and spirit as well as their surroundings are looked after. They also know the common herbs for administering first aid and the medication for minor ailments. Babies and children acquire basic immunity by playing with earth and natural elements, creating little danger of contact with synthetic pollutions. The recognized specialists are ritually imbued with uncommon spiritual personas. They undergo rigorous training to acquire their godly temperaments and specialist healing knowledge, knowledge that includes medicines prepared with natural curative materials (vegetable, animal, mineral, and elements); musical arts healing that is underpinned by the science of musical structures, choreographic idioms, instrument technology, and transcendental theatre; and the mystical process of restoring an unsound mind or group psyche to normalcy using potent formulae, active conjuration, or any other meta-scientific harnessing of intangible healing energy.

Spiritual Health

A proactive, religious disposition once permeated the Indigenous worldview, a worldview currently devastated. Spirit emanations and ancestral consciousness mediated the totality of existence, including living nobly after death. Spirit actors were a virtual reality that induced noble conscience, and deterred noxious aspirations and actions. As such, supra-human agency was invoked and applied to ensure the general wellness of individuals, the community, and the ecosystem. Spirit essences were routinely interacted with in everyday living and imagination through rituals/rites, invocations, proverbs, aphorisms, obligations, communions, token offerings, dramatic enactments such as spirit-manifest theatre (Nzewi, 2007, pp. 119-154), folktales, object lessons, place names, and praise names. African traditional religious doctrines infused benevolent spirituality in the conduct of private and public life, humane policy systems, and social conscience. Specialist Indigenous health practitioners were revered and trusted as spirit agents.

Consciousness of supernatural interventions, mainly instilled through folktales and rituals, saturated the traditional African worldview and experience—the spirits inspire and oversee, while humans rationalize and conduct the affairs of life. The maxim, "a person who dares to wrestle a spirit [contest spiritual injunctions] is inevitably floored," is an example of the type of thinking that enabled spiritual management of conformity within societal norms and ethical conduct.

Environmental Health

An Indigenous axiom postulates that a healthy living environment is an enemy of sickness. Historically, the sanitation of dwellings, community meeting places, economic sites, religious grounds, and communal water sources was socially-politically organized and enforced. Priest-doctors in some culture groups performed annual rites for purging the collective ills of the community, and occasional ritual healing of the community space, especially during times of particularly virulent diseases.

Knowledge of Medicine

Traditional medical treatment in Africa is a science that commands knowledge of the pharmaceutical properties of the natural world, the potency of such properties, and the types of ailments a plant/animal/mineral/elemental extract could cure, contain, or exacerbate. Quite often, meta-scientific diagnostic probing enables a determination of the nature of sicknesses, and the appropriate healing interventions. Extraordinarily imbued traditional medical practitioners aver that medicinal plants do 'reveal' their healing or poisonous potencies. They possess the extra-sensory capability to detect medicinal potencies communicated para-linguistically by plants and other natural forms.

Musical arts complements material medicine in Indigenous healing. Musical sound in Indigenous worldview and life is regarded as a force agent, a transcendental medium of communication between humans and supernatural beings, as well as natural objects. Whatever was communicated musically, in old African imagination, carried divine authority and could not be violated, neither could the spirit voice (musician) be harmed. A traditional musician, by the same divine mandate, could not lie when communicating musically. Hence some extraordinarily adept healers and specialist musicians were revered as spirit agents in performance contexts, irrespective of social status or material means.

Knowledge of the phenomenal bond in old Africa between humans, the supernatural, and the natural (plant) world is preserved and transmitted through folk tales. For instance, some species of mushroom are edible, and others are poisonous. In an Igbo, Nigeria, folk tale, a particular species of mushroom communicated to a cure-searching healer through super-sensory song emissions that the mushroom was a 'king' (*eze*) among mushrooms because of its potencies, including the ability to talk. It commanded the researching herbal doctor to uproot it for ingestible-medical purposes.

The African ecosystem boasts an abundance of medicinal plants and minerals that have enabled a thriving civilization in health cure and health care to develop through millennia of research, experimentation, testing, and advancement. Gelfand, Mavi, Drummond, and Ndemera (1985), for instance, conducted an extensive study of traditional medical practice in Zimbabwe. Their statistical documentation of pharmacopeia resources and practices, which they also compared to other regions/countries in Africa, is exemplary. The study identifies 5,000 species of flowering plants and ferns in Zimbabwean vegetation, out of which 500 that are used for medical purposes have Indigenous names. Such names and terminologies evidence scientifically and theoretically valid healing knowledge rationalized in traditional Africa. The researchers studied 250 medical practitioners (the N'nanga) who helped them identify a range of Indigenously known and named health conditions that traditional healers deal with. The health conditions identified include infections, organ malfunction, pains, mental disorder, injurious inflictions by devious human elements, supernatural afflictions/inflictions, preventive treatments, epidemics and charms, and the health disorders of domestic animals. The study has tables that list the 500 plants, the parts that are used, and the details of medicinal use and application. Two or more different medicinal plants could be used for similar cures, while a plant could be used for different health conditions. It further lists how the use of specific plants for healing purposes in Zimbabwe compare to other African regions/countries. Fifty-one plants are used for similar cures in Zimbabwe and other regions/areas of Africa. Poisonous plants identified by the healers are listed. The documentation also lists animals, birds, and insects used for medicinal preparations. Magwa, Cooposamy, and Mayekiso (2004, p. 49) additionally report that, "with South Africa's remarkable biodiversity and cultural diversity, it is not surprising to find that approximately 3000 plant species are used as complementary medicines, and that their use exceeds that of orthodox medicines." The two sample studies cited establish that the science of pharmacopeia and a systematic knowledge of sicknesses, as well as the associated curative and preventive measures, have always governed health practices in traditional African cultures.

Becoming a Healer: Selection, Training, Ritual/Supernatural Induction

Selection

In Indigenous imagination, a person who effectively restores ill health or rectifies an impaired body organ/part is a life-saver. Such a person has a closer affinity than normal to the Supreme Creator, and is revered for it. To become a healer in traditional Africa is primarily a subliminal calling, and most traditional healers are supernaturally selected through visitation, commonly by the ancestral spirits of deceased healers of a generation or lineage.

Visitation is experienced in dreams, as well as in certain persistent sicknesses, misfortunes, or mental dissociations that defy normal explanation or remedy and denote a person whom ancestral or other supernatural forces are impelling to become a healer (see abridged sample recruitment experience in the appendix). Divination will reveal such a condition. The afflicted can then comply or continue to suffer. In most cases, they are visited by ancestral personages that were healers in life and are projecting signs and afflictions on the healer-to-be, denoting a consanguineous healer-successor relationship. Necessary rites are performed to acknowledge the tutelary ancestral spirit(s). A period of training with an established healer will then commence. Eight traditional healers (*sangoma/inyanga*) and trainees were surveyed in a healing dance project in Pretoria, South Africa. Their briefs on electing to become healers are published in the brochure of a DVD on the Sangoma dance aesthetic, *Choreographing Spirituality* (Nzewi, 2005). All testify that they opted for the profession as a result of dreams, sicknesses, supra-normal encounters, or some combination of the three.

Training

The pupil healer lives with the mentor for a period of time, acquiring skill in divining, diagnosing sicknesses, pharmaceutics, intangible and tangible healing procedures. The pupil serves the specialist, learns the virtue of humility, such as lying down in respect of older healers/spirits, and inculcates the humble disposition that marks spiritually imbued traditional healers and priests. S/he participates in all healing theatre staged in the clinic of the trainer, and could undergo involuntary states of altered consciousness when his/her own spirit patron, identified during divination, rides his/her psyche in such contexts (Nzewi, 2007). Invocatory music and dance activity restores normal consciousness with or without medical treatment. The pupil learns how to identify healing plants, minerals and elements, as well as how to prepare and administer them. Cleansing rites, which may entail water and fresh animal blood oaths, are administered to the trainee at stages of acquiring the knowledge and discipline of healing. Blood, particularly human blood, is sacrosanct in African traditional imagination. Hence blood is the most sacred substance when ritually applied to seal oaths or bind obligations in the human or supernatural realms. To let or shed blood wantonly is an abomination, and has traumatized African religious sensibility and consciousness since the Arabic/European intrusions that desecrated the blood of African populations.

The induction rite that marks the completion of a healer's training is normally a meta-drama of capturing the essence of the healing deity, a deity called Agwu among the Igbo. As the Agwu spirit becomes ingrained in the healer's psychic perceptions and consciousness, the healer is imbued with an abiding godly conscience. The spiritualizing drama of chasing-the-spirit transpires in an open space. In an Igbo, Nigeria case study, the climax of the induction rite additionally requires the emerging healer to undergo the divine oath of swallowing the fresh heart of a ram (Nzewi, 2006, p. 97). This blood oath sanctifies the healer, empowers her/him to heal, and demands that the healer never knowingly dispense harmful medicine or neglect an ailing life. To perjure the oath incurs psychosomatic affliction—the raw heart of the ram will metaphysically choke her/him to agonizing death. Other cultures require the pupil-healer to undergo the divine oath of spiritual purgation-cum-sanctification by drinking and vomiting the fresh blood of a preferred animal. Upon successfully capturing the spirit, a ceremony follows wherein the healer is escorted home by practicing and training healers and well-wishers, to establish his/her own healing practice with a stock of drugs and materials. The homecoming ceremony stages prescribed rites of purification, installation, and offerings conducted with special healers' musical arts theatre and feasting to welcome the community as audience and witness. A capable, godly healer emerges and is introduced to the society at large, establishing his/her own clinic complete with consulting/healing sanctum, empowering insignia, and pharmacy.

Testimony

The following is a sample account on how a traditional healer is super-normally selected, and thereafter inducted (cited from Nzewi, 2006, p. 98):

> *My name is Ntombi Mawela. I was born November 8, 1965 [in Pretoria, South Africa]...I started school in 1973...In 1980 I attended Flavius Mareka High School for my Standard 6 and 7...*

and when I was in Standard 8, I started to get sick. I did not know what the problem was with me. When I went to school I started thinking many things and could not concentrate on my schoolwork. I was wondering what was happening to me because for many years I had no problem with my mind or body. Also, when I tried to read books my eyes started paining me...My teacher noticed what was happening to me and asked me what the problem was. I answered that I did not know, that maybe something unknown was coming to disturb me. He said to me that I am an intelligent person and good in my school work, so he did not understand what the problem could be. He asked me to go home and come back to school whenever I felt better.

When I got home I felt better, but back at school I was still not feeling well. Sometimes I felt dizzy and started to cry because I did not know what was happening to me. Then I was sleeping at night and dreamt that I saw my ancestors, who came to me and said:

'You do not want to hear us. We come to you every day, and you ignore us. We will take you away to stay with us because you do not remember us. Go and prepare our homemade beer, and put snuff to show us that you have not forgotten us, that you still remember that you have ancestors.'

When I woke up in the morning I was crying, but did what they asked me to do. One night they visited me again in my dream and said:

'You can go for training to do our job.'

I got up again and cried that night. In the morning I went to Hammerskraal, and found a woman healer who saw me and smiled, and asked me why I was crying. I gave no answer because I was upset. The woman took me into her house, brought out bones, and threw them. Then she told me the bones said that my ancestors were angry and that I must inherit and continue their healing job, or they were going to kill me. I was scared about what could happen to me if I refused to do their job because I was still very young.

In 1990 I consulted an Inyanga about my training. He welcomed me to train with him. But I had told nobody where I was. I told him that I had no money to pay him. He said that I should not worry, that I would pay him when I finished my course.

The following day they started to play the drums for me. I was afraid because I did not know what to expect. As they beat the drums, something began to change in my body's feeling. My mind changed, and my legs became tired. When the drum beating finished, he said that the following day we must go to the mountain to do something, which we must not do at his home. When we got to the mountain he said that...nobody could just come to me to say: 'I am in your body to do this or that.' When we say that there is an ancestor, the ancestor is my grandparents and my parents, and I must do what they were doing when they were alive, and I must respect them as spirits...

He gave me medicine, lay me down, and put a shobo (healers' symbol) by my feet. When they beat the drum, my heart beat faster. I closed my eyes and could see a big hole, the inside of which was dark. There came a bad smell inside my nose. Cramps attacked my legs. When all this was happening I could hear people talking around me but I could not talk or relate to them because I must show respect for the spirits—I was with the ancestors. Only a Sangoma/Inyanga would know what happens in such situations. My trainer taught me that when my ancestors come out I should ask them their names, where they have come from, and what they want. And when I do, my voice will change, and I must do what they command me to do.

In 1991, the ceremony for me to dance outside was performed. I danced the whole night until morning, and it was raining. I had to dance. That day my legs were paining, and I was tired. When I talked, my voice sounded different. During the break people ate. After that the drums were beaten, and I danced.

My second ceremony was for sniffing the shoba and running to find my mfihlo (healing spirit). First a goat was killed, and the blood was given to me to drink. I drank a medicine (muti), then drank the blood and vomited it. Then he came to me and told me that they will put something (my mfihlo) in another house, and I must run, and run, and sniff my shoba until I located it through spiritual guidance. When I was running, my face changed and I cried because I was tired of running and dancing. But I finally located my mfihlo. He next taught me how to divine for somebody by looking at her/him without throwing the bones (Nzewi, 2006, p. 98).

The Healer

The typical healer in traditional Africa is imbued with a godly conscience and communes with enabling spirits. S/he has empirical knowledge of the pharmacological constituents of ecological resources and grounded knowledge of human/animal anatomy, and is capable of diagnosing and treating sicknesses. S/he is also able to interpret divination objects and harness intangible realities to sustain human and environmental well-being. There are cultural peculiarities about becoming a healer in African societies, but the principles of practice, as well as the sanctity framing the discipline, are fairly common. Some exceptionally capable healers are known and consulted across cultural boundaries. Generally, strict codes of ethical conduct enforced by supra-human forces enshrine the practices of managing human and ecological health. Prescription of medicine is not ad hoc, and the healing procedure recognizes the intangible dimension of community empathy that rehabilitates the affected into group psyche.

Ego indulgence and obsession with wealth are antithetical to the Indigenous conscience of the healing profession. The code of practice requires a client who comes for consultation to present a prescribed customary offering to 'awaken' the potency of a healing or divination atmosphere and properties. The offering is a respectful tribute to the healer on behalf of the intangible forces aiding his/her practice. The traditional healer's commission by divine injunction is to save, not to profit, from ill health or misfortune. The healer does not therefore bargain a fee as a condition for divining or healing. Rather, the patient has a responsibility for procuring the essential material objects needed for treatment beyond the standard stock a healer uses. When a healing is effected, cultural mores expect the healed to pay whatever she/he can afford to compensate the restorer of her/his health. Thus some proficient healers could attract impressive material wealth donated by beneficiaries. But ordinarily a healer's material wealth does not come from fees demanded for a cure, as bargaining for a fee corrupts the conscience of the profession, and a healer is free to engage in other subsistence occupations such as farming.

A traditional person who acquires basic or specialized knowledge of pharmacology knows which drugs can cure or harm. There are occasional instances of charlatans who set up bogus practices, or of imbued and adequately trained healers who perjure their divine, life-saving oath. Such practitioners could deliberately collude with nefarious clients to harm or poison fellow humans. Such a rare (in traditional societies) diabolical practitioner, when identified, could be sanctioned with mass social and ritual isolation. S/he inevitably suffers psychosomatic affliction and "bad" death. Hence, in the Igbo society, a distinction is made between the doctor who has swallowed the heart of a ram to become a sanctified healer of divine integrity, and "a *dibia* (doctor)-with-a-heart-of-stone" (Nzewi, 2006, p. 98) who consciously perjures the healing oath and contravenes the code of ethical conduct.

The Musical Arts in Traditional Healing

The Indigenous African musical arts, as a singular construct, unify the theoretical and experiential peculiarities of music, dance, mystical drama, and material art. The somatic ambience of mass dancing experiences provides overall body-mind therapy for community participants. The raw harmonies generated by various musical instruments transmit healing energy that vibrates, thereby subtly massaging sensitive organs and tissues, boosting their functional fitness. Hence drums and bells made of natural materials (wood, cast iron, earth, etc.) are preferred in music-healing practices. Formulaic incantations that process divination are also musically delivered.

Healing intentions inform the structural, formal, and staging configurations of musical arts types featured in the healing and management of congenital psychological disorders, as well as in priming the mind and body for specialized activities. Health science informs the theory of repetition, cyclic thematic development, mood-form, metaphysical dramatic actions, and choreographic idioms and formations (Nzewi, 2005).

Mass musical arts were occasionally staged in traditional Africa to regenerate group psyche or purge collective ills. The musical arts processed the spiritual-physical healing of the community, as well as the individual. By rallying the community to a healing ceremony, they are acting as essential companion souls that inspirit the sick, causing the sick to feel alive.

Music is a spirit agent in its own capacity. In traditional Africa, relating or communing with intangible forces in the cosmos, effective as well as affective, generally commands a musical medium. In a healing or invocation ceremony, musical arts activities induce a state of substituted consciousness in the susceptible, usually healers or trainees. An ancestral personage then takes over the mind and body of the healer-medium, who begins to portray strange actions, including delivering significant communications in an altered spirit-voice. The possession phenomenon can be calm or rigorous: The Sangoma's body will suddenly rigidify, eyes staring without blinking; or the body will erupt in tremors accompanied by guttural wailing and utterances emitted in an altered voice—the voice of the visiting ancestor spirit. The Sangoma personifying the spirit will next engage in initial pacification dialogue (with verbal and finger signs) with a senior Sangoma nearby (Nzewi, 2005, p. 9).

Over the years, the musical arts have facilitated the psychological management of life, society and sickness in Indigenous cultures. Every member of a traditional community, from childhood through old age, was coerced to actively participate in many of the musical arts activities that imperceptibly but routinely engineered psycho-physiological well-being as a basic preventive health ideology. Hence music was mind wellness, dance was body wellness, drama was spiritual wellness, and all co-acting together was designed as the performance of holistic health care for all.

The Contemporary Practice

Traditional African healing science has become an endangered knowledge type. Its empirical efficacy, developed over millennia, has been put on the defensive by modern scholarship sophistry. Indigenous knowledge has been severely intimidated, patronized, and disparaged by researchers, hegemonic knowledge theorists, and flippant modern religious preachers who are too arrogant to perceive its prodigious merits. Prejudice and intolerance have led to traditional healers being spitefully referenced as 'witch doctors,' even in some well-meaning literature about African knowledge. The idea of a witch doctor is Eurocultural, and very remote from the philosophy and epistemology of traditional Africa's divinely ordered health practice. The modern medical sector globally witnesses capitalist exploitation and other deleterious practices that were rare and abhorred in traditional African societies. Sometimes the same elite modern practitioners and researchers who denigrate Indigenous health systems collude to expropriate, re-process, and commercialize the original inventions of traditional medical practitioners.

Some contemporary traditional doctors in Africa have become so overwhelmed by the prejudices and unmerited aspersions on their characters that a number of them abuse their oaths as conscientious life-savers. They succumb to the modern spiritual decadence of greed, popularized by exogenous ideologies and lifestyles, in the hopes that the healers will attract modern respectability. The once noble and priestly profession has become severely undermined, and there are now instances of exploiting their clients and other deleterious practices.

Supernatural selection of traditional healers still occurs in Africa. Some indigenes, however, ignore the signs, and prefer to suffer rather than be seen obeying viable cultural norms. Others obey, undergo the routine training, and thereafter renege on the divine oath for materialistic preoccupations. Nevertheless, genuine traditional healers and healing can be found in urban settings. It is not unusual to find contemporary elites with all of the modern privileges who resort to traditional healing for rescue, especially when failed by modern medical/hospital systems, or when a health/life problem defies the corrective sophistications of modern medicine.

In spite of doctors swearing the Hippocratic oath, the divine human touch is greatly lacking as the practice increasingly becomes a capitalist commodity enterprise. A patient gets non-empathically treated as a 'thing' that generates wealth for health practitioners through fees for consultations, tests, and the purchase of drugs, whether or not the patient is actually cured after. Holistic healing of the sick person is not much of an issue in modern medical practice, where the training and procedures aim narrowly at using machine diagnosis and detection in an impersonal manner. The traditional principle of empathetically healing the soul, thereby rehabilitating a troubled fellow human spirit, is very much lacking. The primary distinction between modern curing and traditional healing in the management of ill health is that the modern micro-perception of life, sickness, and cure targets rectifying the specific manifestation of ill health facilitated by technology and synthetic drugs, while the traditional holistic view of life and healing targets the specific ailment in the context of the total, connected mind and body. Every sickness conflicts the mind, whether or not the mind itself is the particular sick organ.

The aim of this discourse has been to explore the normative scientific and meta-scientific integrity underpinning the research-informed, conscientious, and effective medical knowledge system of Indigenous Africa. The diagnostic, pharmaceutical, and treatment praxes have continued to be developed, systematically practiced, advanced, and transmitted through training and memory. The nature, procedure, and products may not appear to be sophisticated by modern perceptions; however, the philosophy, theory, and procedure of the contemporaneously valid and viable Indigenous medical knowledge systems deserve respect, proactive recognition, institutionalization, and promotion in the modern milieu. This discourse is not intended to provide narratives about the sick who fail to recover despite normative medical intervention. Death continues to occur in both systems. The advocacy here is that the Indigenous and the modern health care systems both have merits, and need to complement each other in the best interests of humanity everywhere.

References

Gelfand M., Mavi, S., Drummond, R. B., & Ndemera, B. (1985). *The traditional medical practitioner in Zimbabwe.* Gweru: Mambo press.

Felhaber, T. & Mayeng, I. (1997). *South African traditional healer's primary health care handbook.* Cape Town: Kagiso.

Makgopa, M. (2004). Indigenous healing system: an oral transmission. In M. Masoga & A. Musyoki (Eds.), *Building on the Indigenous – an African perspective* (49-50). Pretoria: National Research Foundation.

Magwa, M. L., Cooposamy, M. R., & Mayekiso, B. (2004). A comparison of the relationship between modern/Western and South African Indigenous approaches to medicinal plant utilisation. In M. Masoga & A. Musyoki (Eds.), *Building on the Indigenous—an African perspective* (51-57). Pretoria: National Research Foundation.

Mufamadi, J. (2004). Diagnosing and treating mental illness in South Africa: cultural considerations. In M. Masoga & A. Musyoki (Eds.), *Building on the Indigenous – an African perspective* (58-62). Pretoria: National Research foundation.

Nzewi, M. (2005). African musical arts creativity and performance: The science of the sound. *Nigerian Music Review*, 6, 1-7.

_____. (2005). Sangoma dance aesthetic: choreographing spirituality. (DVD booklet.) Pretoria: CIIMDA.

_____. (2006). *Okeke: music, myth and life: an African story.* Pretoria: Unisa.

_____. (2007). Backdrop to music and healing in Indigenous African society. In M. Nzewi & O. Nzewi. *A contemporary study of musical arts informed by African Indigenous knowledge systems. Volume Four – Illuminations, reflections and explorations* (pp. 286-289). Pretoria: CIIMDA series.

_____. (2007). The force that rides the sound. In L. Bresler (Ed.), *International handbook of research in arts education* (pp. 1443-1448). Dordrecht: Springer.

Chapter Five

FOOD AS MEDICINE: THE CHANGE IN INDIGENOUS DIET AND THE CONTINUOUS INCREASE IN THE DEVELOPMENT OF NON-COMMUNICABLE DISEASES AMONG THE INDIGENOUS PEOPLE

Mary Ashiedu, PhD Student, University of Toronto

This paper is dedicated to all those suffering from a disease in one form or another and who could have found some relief through nutrition if only that help was available.

"Diet is the essential key to all successful healing"
The Way of Herbs by, Michael Tierra, C.A., N.D.

Abstract

Among the Indigenous people of sub-Saharan Africa, colonialism, migration, globalization, and urbanization have brought about a nutritional shift from the ancestral diet toward a Westernized diet. This move has contributed to an increase in the incidence of non-communicable diseases. Heart disease, obesity, diabetes, and dental disease are some of the diseases that have been linked to nutrition. This argument is echoed by Cohen and Armelagos (1984) as they contend that "as humans migrated over the globe and cultures changed nutrition increasingly diverged from the ancestral pattern. Genetic evolution was unable to keep pace, and, consequently, various pathologies developed" (as cited by Eaton, Konner, & Cordain, 2010, p.1). Migration and urbanization made access to fresh local foods more difficult to attain. Moreover, the present fast-paced lifestyle and the proliferation of fast foods, along with the high cost of a balanced diet, have also contributed to the nutrition transition. Blue collar and white collar jobs have taken the place of farming and gardening. To make it possible for people to avail themselves of the obvious benefits of a balanced diet, the foods should be available, accessible, and affordable. Also, adequate information about the nutritional value of foods and a continuous research on them is important. In particular, the health benefits of coconut oil should form part of this research.

Introduction

This paper will focus on the African Indigenous diet. It is no secret that the introduction of European influence in Africa has had a detrimental impact on Indigenous knowledge. This is unfortunate for a continent whose culture of healing and nutrition is rooted in Indigenous knowledge. The paper will highlight the continuous shift toward a Westernized diet and its health consequences. It will also highlight research already carried out with regard to Indigenous foods, as well as the dietary habits responsible for various illnesses. Fortunately, we are in an era of increased global consciousness about health and well-being, coupled with a renewed interest in natural foods. It is therefore hoped that there will be a renewed interest in Indigenous food culture, especially since the current trend in pathology traces non-communicable diseases to a deviation from ancestral nutrition to modern diet.

Research has also determined that "nearly all the genes and epigenetic regulatory mechanisms we carry today were originally selected for behaviourally modern humans who appeared in Africa between 100,000 and 50,000 years ago" (Eaton, Konner, & Cordain, 2010, p.1). It is also noteworthy that Mazess, 1966; Ströhle, Hahn, & Sebastian, 2010, as cited by Eaton et al. 2010, (P. 1) reported that the "striking prevalence of osteoporosis in Inuit skeletal remains from the early contact period was because plant foods are necessarily scarce in circumpolar environments". In order to take full advantage of a nutritious diet, we have to be mindful of many things, including the type of food, where it came from, the method of preparation and storage, daily nutritional requirements, and the best time of consumption. In the light of the above, what are some of the available Indigenous foods and what are their nutritional benefits? How readily accessible are they?

Locating Myself

As an African who has had the opportunity to live in both the rural and urban areas of Nigeria, my relationship with Indigenous plants started as a young girl. Interacting with nature was a way of life and we did not really think much of it. Unfortunately, some of the food items we benefited from are almost at the brink of extinction. Some of the fruits we ate grew in the wild; some of the vegetables were perennial and they grew in the compound. It was commonplace to go into the backyard and harvest some leafy vegetables for cooking. Some of those same leaves were also dispensed as medicinal herbs when necessary. Notable among these was *aluluisi* (*ocimum gratissimum).* We simply washed a handful of *aluluisi* leaves with water, put them in a bowl, crushed them in the palm of our hands by rubbing them together, and then drank the dark brown extract. Another leaf we used in this way was *onugbu,* which also goes by the common name of bitter leaf (*veronia amygdalina*). A lot of the food crops and fruits were either produced by the family or bought from the local market. These included a variety of yams, cassava products, mushrooms, very large escargots, palm nut products, pineapples, oranges, mangoes, guava, *udala* (*chrysophyllum albidum*), pear (*ube*), and many others. Some of these products grew in the compound or on the family's farm. There were hardly any imported foods in the area at the time. There was imported canned corn beef and canned tomato paste, and these were used only occasionally. At that time, Asian rice was preferred to African rice due to its appearance and the fact that it was more expensive made it more desirable.

Purpose

My appreciation of the Indigenous way of life has increased with the passage of time. However, so much still needs to be done, especially with the positioning of our values and the need for proper documentation of our Indigenous knowledge systems. My aim, therefore, is to research our traditional foods before urbanization, globalization, and the subsequent nutritional transition toward a Westernized diet are complete. Some of the food crops mentioned in this paper are also found outside the continent of Africa under different local names. This paper will therefore serve as a reawakening of our sense of values, as we become more conscious about our identity, we want to know as much as possible about who we are, including information about our ancestral food habits. I would also like to highlight the need for a detailed online database of Indigenous African food habits, nutrient compositions, daily requirements, and suggested methods of preparation. This database will hopefully encourage more consumption of these foods and subsequently reduce the incidence of non-communicable diseases and malnutrition among children, expectant mothers, and the elderly. According to the Child Survival, Protection and Development (CSPD) in Nigeria, as reported by UNICEF in 1995 and cited by Hart, Azubuike, Barimalaa, and Achinewhu (2005, p. 9):

> In spite of the reasonable intake of vegetables ..., reports indicate that in Nigeria, vitamin A deficiency in mothers and children is about 11-35% in the north and middle belt and 5-30% in the south, and anemia is responsible for 10% of maternal mortality while the prevalence of endemic goiter is 13-37% with a national average of 20%.

Constraints

It was difficult and sometimes impossible to locate research and the botanical names of some of the plants and food crops. In some cases, there were no pictures or illustrations of the items. This is probably due to the fact that a lot of the plants and foods have not been explored. While it was easier to find Asian and Mediterranean herbs and food pyramids, I could not find any food pyramid that focused on foods from Africa. There were also instances of conflicting reports on some African foods, particularly coconut oil and palm oil.

Indigenous Framework

This paper explores the topic of food as medicine through the lens of an Indigenous framework, highlighting African Indigenous food habits with particular regard to the nutritional benefits for the maintenance of optimum health. The Indigenous people mostly depended on local foods for nourishment. Ailments were often treated with the same plants used in food preparation. The use of Indigenous plants in healing is particularly helpful since a lot of Indigenous areas are not well equipped with bio-medical facilities. The relational nature of Indigenous epistemology dictates that there is a time and method acceptable for food handling. This explains the reason behind the various ceremonies surrounding harvesting and eating farm produce. For instance, in the northern part of Delta State of Nigeria, new yams cannot be eaten until after the New Yam ceremony has been performed. This also guarantees that the yams reach maturity before they are eaten.

Lack of Diversity in Our Local Food Stores

With the increase in immigration and urbanization, the high cost of biomedicine, and a growing awareness of the nutritious value of Indigenous foods, the need to reflect diversity in our local food stores cannot be overemphasized. Outside the continent of Africa, some Indigenous foods can mostly be purchased in specialized stores. On the other hand, there are big chain grocery stores in every neighbourhood with shelves full of processed foods. As a result of their proximity and convenience, these stores become a first choice for grocery shopping. It is therefore not surprising to discover that "in contemporary affluent nations, complex degenerative diseases such as atherosclerosis, numerous cancers, and hypertension reflect discordance between ancient genes and current diets, whereas the 'epidemics' of obesity and diabetes can be largely attributed to our unholy (and unpaleolithic) alliance of sedentism and hypernutrition" (Eaton, Cordain, & Sparling, 2009, as cited by Eaton et al., 2010, p.1). As long as people continue to buy whatever is on the shelf, the stores will continue to stock their shelves for profit. However, if people demand healthier natural foods and provide the stores with the details of the items, including where to find them, seasonal availability, and nutritional value, the stores will find a way to stock the items. It is therefore the main responsibility of the consumer to continue to advocate for healthy alternatives at the grocery store. For example, Nigeria is the world's largest producer of yams, cocoyams, and cassavas, yet one can hardly see a healthy display of any of these products on the grocery shelves.

Inadequate Nutritional Information about Indigenous Food

Many people in Africa have lost the knowledge of the practical uses of our Indigenous plants. This loss of knowledge has contributed to an unnecessary nutritional imbalance. For example, in my town we have a common plant called *nti oke* (rat's ears —*portulaca oleracea*). The name has to do with the shape of the leaves. Professor Louis Grivetti 1976, as cited by Lipski, 2010, p. 6, observed that the knowledge of over 200 Indigenous plants helped the Kswana people of Botswana to thrive, while 2 million West Africans perished in the draught of 1965-1973 due to their modernized way of life and inability to recognize and use the available natural resources. Non-communicable illnesses sometimes arise not just because of inadequate food supply, but also as a result of inadequate information about the uses of the available resources. This includes methods of preparation and storage, the amount of micronutrients contained in the food, the best time for consumption, and the right amount needed for optimum health. It is important to know which foods are best eaten raw or steamed and the best ways to safeguard the enzymes, vitamins, and minerals. The availability of detailed information will make it easier to make wiser food choices and most likely discourage the shift toward a Westernized diet. For example, the increasing choice of rice and wheat over millet and sorghum does not demonstrate a wise food choice, as noted by the samples interviewed by Raschke, Oltersdorf, Elmadfa, Wahlqvist, Kouris-Blazos, and Cheema (2007):

> The traditional African diet is superior to the increasingly prevalent and insidious *Westernized* diet, citing 'nutrient density and diversity,' 'low saturated fat' and 'no preservatives' as key determinants of health. Moreover, the Indigenous African experts interviewed noted reduced millet and sorghum consumption and increased wheat and rice consumption as primary staple foods within their regions of origin. Empirical investigations

> have demonstrated the superior nutritional indices of millet and sorghum as compared to rice and wheat. (p. 11)

In addition to the above, it will help to suggest multiple ways of using a particular food item. For example, hulled millet can be cooked just the same way as rice. It is also important to have information on gluten and non-glutinous foods. This will be especially helpful to people suffering from allergies and celiac disease. Such gluten free crops include *acha* (*fonio, digitaria exilis*), cassava, teff, sorghum, millet, soy, potatoes and cocoyam (*taro, eddo, dasheen*), and African rice (*oryza glaberrima*).

Apart from being gluten-free, millet is highly nutritious:

> Millet is nearly 15 percent protein and contains high levels of fibre, the B-complex vitamins (including niacin, thiamine and riboflavin), the essential amino acid methionine, and lecithin. It also has high levels of magnesium, phosphorus, zinc, copper and potassium, and it is considered to have the highest level of iron of any of the cereals. There is evidence that the seeds are rich in phytic acid, which is thought to lower cholesterol, and phytate, which is associated with a reduction in the risk of cancer. The grain's alkaline pH makes it an easy grain to digest. The pH stays high after cooking, an important consideration for wheat-intolerant consumers. The grain also contains relatively high levels of oil (4.2 percent), which is 50 percent polyunsaturated. (Vinning & McMahon, 2006, p. 26)

In spite of all the nutritional benefits that have been highlighted about millet, Vinning and McMahon (2006) noted that:

> one potential difficulty lies in the fact that millet hulls and seeds contain small amounts of substances that limit the thyroid gland's uptake of iodine. Whether these substances are solely responsible for the relatively high incidence of goiter in millet-consuming communities or whether other dietary deficiencies are involved is yet to be clarified. Another area of uncertainty is whether cooking plays a part in destroying these thyroid function inhibitors. (p. 26)

Indigenous Foods Before Colonialism and Globalization

As we discuss healthy eating within the sphere of Indigenous knowledge, it is worthwhile to look into what constituted Indigenous nutrition before colonialism and globalization. Before colonialism, food sources were localized. There were no industrial additives or frequent reports of chronic diseases. According to Lipski, "Indigenous people have patterns of illness very different from Western civilization; yet, they rapidly develop diseases once exposed to Western foods and lifestyles. Food and medicine were interwoven" (2010, p. 1). The staple foods included tubers and roots such as yams, potatoes, and cassavas; leafy green vegetables, grains such as millet, sorghum, African rice, *acha* (*fonio*), spices, free range animals such goats and chickens, wildlife, and oils such as palm oil. These are wholesome foods with obvious health benefits. In the various regions of Africa, food was preserved by drying it under the sun, or smoked on a shelf above the cooking area, and food processing was mostly done by fermentation. We still make cereals from maize, sorghum, and millet through fermentation. The end product is called *akamu*, *ogi*, or *pap*. Eaton and Konner (1985), as cited by Raschke et al. (2007), "investigated dietary shifts over several millennia in Africa and concluded that the human diet was far superior with the hunting and gathering subsistence of Palaeolithic times as compared to the present-day diet largely based on processed and manufactured foods" (p. 5). Detailed information is shown on Table 4. The impact of the ancestral diet is further elaborated by Eaton et al. (2010):

> In East Africa, late Palaeolithic plant-to-animal energy intake ratios would have approximated 50:50, and diet-dependent net endogenous acid production (NEAP) would have been alkaline—the norm for human biochemistry, physiology, and bone health. In contrast, for traditional Inuit HGs, whose subsistence derived overwhelmingly from aquatic and animal sources, NEAP would have been acidic, contributing to their osteoporosis. (p. 1)

Unfortunately, due to neglect, very little is known about several African plants that are underexploited. Among these is African rice (*oryza glaberrima*).

> The African species of rice *oryza glaberrima*) was cultivated long before Europeans arrived in the continent. Native to sub-Saharan Africa, *O. glaberrima* is thought to have been domesticated from the wild ancestor *oryza barthii* (formerly known as *oryza brevilugata*) by peoples living in the floodplains at the bend of the Niger River some 2,000–3,000 years ago....At the present time, *O. glaberrima* is being replaced everywhere in West Africa by the Asian species, introduced into the continent by the Portuguese as early as the middle of the 16th century. (Portères, 1962, as cited by Linares, 2002, p. 1)

Another neglected food crop is *acha (fonio, digitaria exilis* and *digitaria iburua*). One excuse people from my place give for not cooking *acha* is that the grains are so tiny that it is extremely labour intensive to get impurities such as sand out of it. However, *acha* is very nutritious and it is doubtful that the Indigenous people know the full extent of the nutritional value. In fact, *acha* has become extremely scarce and is hardly found in the local market.

Table 1: The production of some important cereal grains in Africa

Grain	World Production	African Production	Major producing countries in descending order
Sorghum	58,700	23,282	USA, Nigeria, India, Mexico
Millets (total)	29,295	9557	India, Nigeria, China, Niger
Pearl Millet	13,351	7,330	Nigeria, Niger, Burkina Faso
Finger Millet	3,763	855	India, China, Uganda, Nepal
Teff	Very low	1,063	Ethiopia, South Africa, Australia
Fonio (Acha)	309	309	Mali, Burkina Faso, Guinea, Nigeria

Table 2 Nutritional comparisons

Nutritional comparisons	Ancestral	Contemporary Western
Total energy intake	More	Less
Caloric concentration	Very little	Much
Dietary bulk	More	Less
Total carbohydrate intake	Less	More
Added sugar and refined carbohydrate	Very little	Much more
Glycemic load	Relatively low	High
Fruit and vegetables	Twice as much	Half as much
Antioxidant capacity	Greater	Lesser
Fiber	More	Less
Soluble/insoluble	Closer to equal	Far more insoluble
Protein intake	More	Less
Total fat intake	Equivalent	Equivalent
Serum cholesterol–raising fat	Less	More
Total polyunsaturated fat	More	Less
Long-chain essential fatty acids	More	Less
Cholesterol intake	More	Less
Micronutrient intake	More	Less
Electrolytes	Much more potassium	More sodium
Acid-base effect (NEAP) (net endogenous acid production.)	Alkaline	Acidic
"Dairy" products	Mother's milk only	Considerable
Cereal grains	Very little	A great deal more
Free water intake	More	Less

Source: Eaton, S.B, Konner, M.J, & Cordain, L., 2010.

Indigenous Foods as a Resistance to Globalization

The African Indigenous food habits before colonialism and globalization were simple and wholesome. Processed and unhealthy food habits have been introduced to the Indigenous areas as a result of colonialism, globalization, urbanization, and Westernization. This is not necessarily for the benefit of the people. Indeed, this phenomenon was succinctly described by Susan George (1976) as cited by Raschke and Cheema 2007, p. 663 as "a source of profits, a tool of economic and political control; a means of ensuring effective dominance over the world at large and especially over the 'wretched of the earth' ". Unfortunately, the introduction of foreign food habits has resulted in the decreased production of Indigenous foods, leading to a health situation made worse by the increase in non-communicable diseases. Raschke, Oltersdorf, Elmadfa, Wahlqvist, Kouris-Blazos, and Cheema, (2007) added that:

> amongst the difficulties facing the Indigenous people of Africa today is the deleterious shift from traditional food habits to the processed and packaged food products of Western-owned corporations...This *nutrition transition* has been implicated in the rise of type 2 diabetes, cardio vascular diseases, hypertension, obesity, cancer, and related non-communicable diseases (NCDs) throughout Africa (p. 5).

There is an urgent need to return to the African Indigenous healing foods. The consequences of a Westernized diet continues to be detrimental to the health of the people, since the "consumption of these food products results in elevated intake of saturated fat, trans-fatty acids, food preservatives, reduced intake of dietary fibre, vital nutrients and phytochemicals when compared to basic dietary guidelines" (Shetty, 1995; Drewnowski & Popkin, 1997; Walker & Segal, 1997, as cited by Raschke et al., 2007, p. 1). This has contributed to poor quality of life and an increase in diseases such as "type 2 diabetes, cardiovascular disease, hypertension, obesity, cancer, and non-communicable diseases throughout Africa" (World Health Organization, 2002, Popkin, 2001, 2002, as cited by Raschke et al., 2007, p. 5). "84% of those interviewed" by Raschke et al. (2007) "believed that the traditional African foods were healthier than the Westernized diet" (p. 9). In addition to that, Voster, Bourne, Venter, and Oosthuizen (1999) and the WHO (2005) contend that "transition in dietary practices has resulted in the increased consumption of refined flour, cheap vegetable fats, refined sugars and food additives such as monosodium glutamate, all of which are known to hasten the development of the major non-communicable diseases—e.g., obesity, diabetes, cardiovascular disease" (as cited by Raschke and Cheema, 2007, p. 662).

In his own contribution, Burkitt (1973) argued that:

> the prevalence of these diseases in populations of developing countries appears to relate to the extent of their departure

> from traditional patterns of life. In Africa and Asia most if not all these diseases first appear or become common in the upper Socio-economic groups and in urbanized communities.... the first change in traditional food is usually the addition of sugar. This is followed by substituting white bread for part of the less processed cereals customarily eaten....obesity is...the commonest form of malnutrition...and is known to be associated with many diseases. (pp. 275-277)

The typical traditional cereal in Nigeria is *pap* (*akamu, ogi*), made from fermented maize, sorghum, or millet. Spices and ground nut paste are sometimes added to pap and it is usually made with hot water. It can be taken any time of the day but especially in the morning. It is for all age groups. These days, packaged, Western-oriented, industrial-produced cereals are widely advertised and sold in the commercial centers, and are replacing the homemade variety.

In addition to the above, a study of Indigenous people from different parts of the world, including Africa, indicated that those who ate an Indigenous diet were of "superb health," while those who ate a modernized diet had changes in salivary PH and other oral health problems; children conceived on a Western diet had changes in facial features, physical deformities, and club foot (Price, 1978, as cited by Lipski, 2010, p. 2). Moreover, Denis Burkitt, who spent 24 years in Uganda, reported that of 52 hospitals surveyed in Africa, 44 of the hospitals had never seen a case of colon cancer, heart disease, diverticulitis, or appendicitis. He added that Africans ate about 50 grams of fibre daily, in comparison to about 14 to 15 grams daily for Americans today (Kennedy, 2004, as cited by Lipski, 2010, p. 1). Given the available research, a rejection of the Westernized diet will most likely lead to better health. There is enough information to suggest that the epidemic of chronic diseases plaguing Africa is a result of deviation from the Indigenous diet that was most suited to the people's genetic makeup. According to the WHO,

> 23% of all deaths in Africa are due to chronic disease...and an estimated 28 million people will die in the next 10 years due to these conditions. The major causes are linked to poverty, globalization, the adoption of Western dietary patterns, facilitated by advertising for the consumption of unhealthy foods and lack of physical activity. (UNSCN, 2006, p. 5)

Furthermore, Dr. Albert Schweitzer, a frontier doctor, gave the following account about his trip to Africa:

> On my arrival in Gabon in 1913, I was astonished to encounter no case of cancer . . . I cannot, of course, say positively that there was no cancer at all, ... I can only say that if any cases existed they must have been quite rare. . . . In the course of the years, we have seen cases of cancer in growing numbers in our region. My observations incline me to attribute this to the fact that the natives were living more and more after the manner of the whites. (Berglas, 1957, as cited by Lipski, 2010, p. 1)

Another troubling aspect of Westernized diet is that it adversely affects the very core of our being. Many years ago when I had the opportunity to spend some time in a rural area in Nigeria, the people looked healthier than the people I see in urban areas today. There were absolutely no weight problems. Everybody looked lean and healthy. The people had excellent oral health as well. We used different types of chewing sticks, and as children, took a great pride in our oral health and frequently compared the whiteness of our teeth.

Lack of Data on African Foods

As I searched for data on African foods and plants, I realized that there is an urgent need for a central or regional online database for African foods and plants. It is also important for the database to have open access for the general public. This will encourage more research and promote worldwide knowledge of African Indigenous knowledge systems. Raschke et al. (2007) noted in their research that "knowledge is necessary to gain an understanding of how traditional dietary patterns could potentially reverse current non-communicable disease trends and improve the health status of Indigenous populations throughout Africa, and perhaps abroad" (p. 6). They also observed that of the nine database collections identified, "none of them were specifically designed to raise awareness of traditional African food habits" (p. 3). The authors went on to add that:

> Approximately 82% of those interviewed believed that there was currently a gap in online collections focused on presenting information on traditional African food habits. 92% indicated their preparedness to make use of a novel, online collection of data on traditional African food habits. The findings revealed a critical need to collate and present data on traditional African food

habits...that could be used to stimulate education and research of food habits and their health implications. (p. 3)

Table 3: The major online collections of African food habits

Database (time series)	**Available data related to African food habits**
AJOL 31 1998 – present	Database of 230 African-published journals
IPGRI-online publications catalogue/ database 32 1977 – present	Publications on indigenous/traditional food systems and documentation about indigenous species/foods for all of Africa
FAOSTAT 24 1961 – present	Food balance sheets for all African countries, including information on: -Domestic supply -Domestic utilization -Per capita supply
*AFROFOODS** 25 1952 – 1999 (*one of INFOODS (International Network of Food Data Systems) regional data centers;	Food composition table for various African countries
SAFOODS 26 Published in 1991	Energy, macronutrient composition of different foods consumed by people in South Africa
SEPASAL 27 since 1981	Information on more than 6300 useful *wild* and semidomesticated plants of tropical and subtropical dry lands including Africa (scientific name, plant family, geographical distribution, ecology, use of plants, properties and chemical analysis)
PROTABASE 28 initiated in 2000	Review articles for nearly 400 African plant species (botanical names and botanical descriptions, including a plant's useful properties, cultivation and potential as a crop)
NewCROP 30 since 1995	Crop database on scientific crop profiles including African species (crops by name, uses including food use, geography, commodity, cultural practices, nutritional value)
Famine Food Database 29 since 1995	Information on African crops (scientific name, plant family, vernacular, geographical distribution, ecology, use and preparation of plants)

Source: Raschke, V.,Oltersdorf, U., Elmadfa, I., Wahlqvist, M.L.,Kouris-Blazos, A. and Cheema B.S.B. (2007)

It must however, be pointed out that Raschke et al. (2007), reported that there is an existing database from East Africa which contains "traditional foods and food habits of various ethnic groups located throughout Kenya, Tanzania, and Uganda from the 1930s to the 1960s" (p. 6).

It is hoped that the establishment of an open online database would encourage more research into African Indigenous food habits with the ultimate goal of discovering additional health benefits and the best methods of preparation in order to achieve these benefits. Africa has a wide range of food crops, however, Smith, Eyzaguirre, Matig, and Johns (UNSCN, 2006) noted that "one of the main causes of the poor results often reported with food-based interventions is the lack of knowledge, not only of available foods but [also] of their nutritional and health attributes" (p. 25). The authors added that there is enough information to justify the diversification of Indigenous diets.

Loss of Indigenous Plants

Without a reliable and well-equipped database of African foods and plants, it is only a matter of time before African plants become completely lost. A lot of them are either extinct or near extinction (see, for example, Africa's lost plants: http://pdf.usaid.gov/pdf_docs/PNABX951.pdf). Some are harvested in the wild and when they run out, new ones are not cultivated. It is recorded that seventy-eight percent of people interviewed by Raschke et al. (2007) "believed that knowledge of traditional African food habits is being lost due to lack of promotion, documentation, and research of Indigenous foods in Africa (56%), Westernization/globalization and/or colonization (35%), ignorance and stigma of traditional food (5%), and international food aid programs (5%)" (p. 10). The authors went on to add that:

> The faster people adopt new food patterns, the less likely traditional food knowledge will be passed on to the next generation. In general, the loss of traditional food habits results in a decrease in culture-specific food activities, a decrease in dietary diversity and, if history and current trends are of any indication, abysmal reductions in economic circumstances, health status, quality of life, and cultural integrity. (Kuhnlein & Receveur, 1996, as cited by Raschke et al., 2007, p. 6)

Some of the fruits that we ate when I was young are not readily available anymore. In fact, I have no idea what their botanical names might be. They did not come up when I researched them using the local names. The names are *udala enwe* (different from the common *chrysophyllum albidum*), *anene, ugwa,* and *ugege.* With the exception of the ugege tree, the others grew in the wild. More efforts obviously need to be made to re-establish the disappearing fruit trees and plants. Two other disappearing fruit-yielding trees are the pepper fruit (*dennettia tripetala*), locally called *mmimi* or pepper fruit, and the African oil bean tree (*pentaclethera macrophylla*). The pepper fruit tree is culturally believed to take so long to mature that whoever plants it will not live to see the fruits. As such, people are not usually motivated to plant it. The oil bean tree bears very long, flat pods. When the pod is dry, it produces a loud sound as it cracks open and releases the large beans. The beans are usually a lucky find since no one can tell exactly where they will land when the pods explode. They are used to prepare a local delicacy. The explosion of the oil bean pod gave rise to a saying in my town that "when the oil bean claps its hands it lets go of its children." This proverb is used when somebody passes away and leaves a family behind.

Coconut Oil

As a demonstration of the fact that food should serve as medicine and not cause illness, I feel that it is important to discuss coconut oil. The most widely used oils in Nigeria are palm oil, palm kernel oil, groundnut oil, and coconut oil. We also have a variety of imported 'vegetable' oils, but I cannot say for sure what they actually contain. Palm kernel oil is mostly used on the skin and for soap making. As children we made these ourselves. The family produced palm oil, and as result, there were always palm kernels around. Our neighbour, on the other hand, produced coconut oil.

> In the past four decades misinformation and disinformation provided by certain politically biased agricultural groups and repeated in professional and lay press have lead people to believe that all saturated fats are unhealthy. Saturated fatty acids... comprise three subgroups; short- (C2-C6), medium- (C8-C12) and long- (C14-C24) chain fatty acids. The medium chain fats are found exclusively in Lauric Oils.... Studies showing harmful

> effects of so-called "tropical oils" were generally carried out in the absence of essential fatty acids in the diet. In 1987, a 50-year review showed the anticancer effects of coconut oil. In chemically induced cancers of the colon and breast, coconut oil was by far more protective than unsaturated oils. For example: 32% of corn oil users got colon cancer whereas only 3% of coconut oil eaters got the cancer. (Kabara, n. d., pp. 1- 2)

The use of coconut oil by Dr. Newport in 2008, in the treatment of her husband, Steve who developed Alzheimer's at the age of 58 further illustrates the nutritional potency of the oil. Dr. Newport (2008), "found out that coconut oil is about 60% medium chain fatty acids (MCFA), contains no cholesterol and also contains omega-6 fatty acids some other short and long chain fatty acids of up to 18 carbon chains" (p. 2). She also noted that MCT oils are digested differently. Instead of being stored as fats, they are converted to ketone bodies for energy, (p. 1). Dr. Newport added 35 milligrams of 100% "virgin" coconut oil to Steve's breakfast and after sixty days,

> He walks into the kitchen every morning alert and happy, talkative, making jokes. His gait is still a little weird. His tremor is no longer very noticeable. He is able to concentrate on things that he wants to do around the house and in the yard and stay on task, whereas before coconut oil he was easily distractible and rarely accomplished anything unless I supervised him directly. (Newport., 2008, p. 2)

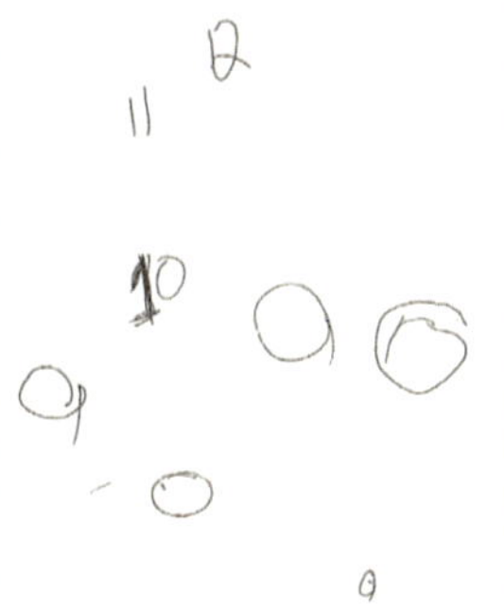	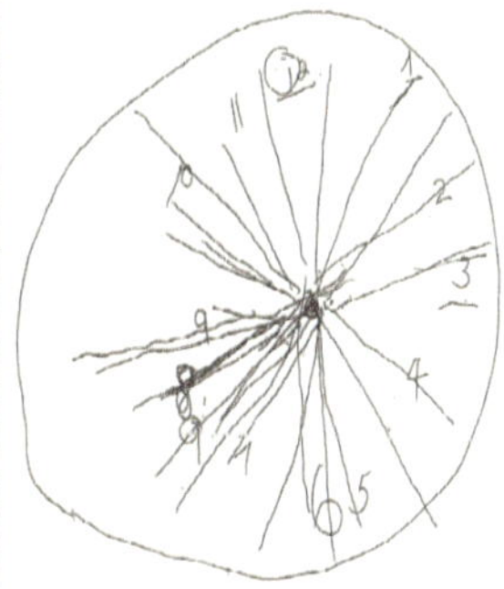	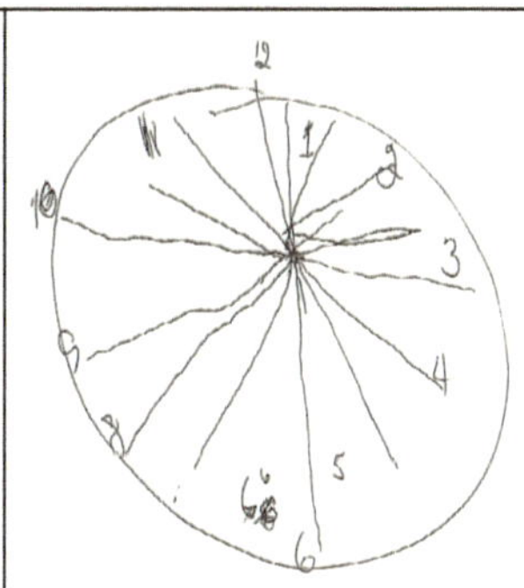
Clock #1 - drawn by Steve a day before starting coconut oil under the supervision of Dr. Margarita Nunez as "a specific test for Alzheimer's."	Clock #2 - drawn by Steve two weeks after starting coconut oil.	Clock #3 - Thirty-seven days after starting coconut oil.

Source: Newport, 2008, p. 2

Dr. Newport (2000, p. 1), noted that Alzheimer's disease usually begins about a decade before it is detected and with the brain atrophy that her husband has developed, he would never be "normal" but every drop of coconut oil used is worth it, (p. 3). She went on to advise anybody still using hydrogenated oil, or any oil with trans fat to get rid of it, and to compensate for the lack of omega-3 in coconut oil by eating relevant foods including salmon, flax seed products, walnuts, and fish oil capsules (p. 4). Interestingly, Dr. Newport (2008), noted that the articles on the possible therapeutic uses of ketone bodies are "not found in journals that the average physician would read, much less the lay public" (p 1).

Coconut oil: Good or Bad Oil?

There is a lot of confusion about the health benefits of coconut oil. Dr. Newport (2008, p. 1), argues that there is a widely held misconception that coconut oil is the 'artery clogging oil' (a term coined in the mid-1900s by the president of Proctor and Gamble, the manufac¬turer of Crisco and other hydrogenated vegetable oils). Ahrens (1957), as cited by Newport (2008, p. 2), contends that "the early studies in animals used hydrogenat¬ed coconut oil, which we now know produces the notorious trans-fats, and the essential fatty acids were excluded from the diet". Newport (2008, p. 2), added that "co¬conut and palm oils are currently added to prema¬ture and full term infant formulas, along with ARA and DHA to mimic breast milk". (p. 2). More researchers have also added their voice to the beneficial qualities of coconut oil:

> Coconut oil and certain coconut products contain approximately 50 percent lauric acid and approximately 6–7 percent capric acid...there is evidence that some monolaurin is formed with the ingestion of lauric acid. Lauric acid is the main antiviral and antibacterial substance found in human breast milk... viruses inactivated to some extent by monolaurin include HIV, measles, *Herpes simplex-1*, vesicular stomatitis, visna virus, and cytomegalovirus. (Liberman, Enig, & Preuss, 2006, p. 2)

Table 4: Lauric Acid Content of Selected Foods

Food	Grams/cup
Coconut cream, raw	37.0
Coconut cream, canned	23.3
Fresh grated coconut, packed	19.4
Fresh grated coconut, loose	11.9
Granola cereal (with coconut oil and coconut)	6.05
Coconut cream pudding	1.29
Whole milk	0.23

Source: U.S. Department of Agriculture Handbook as cited in Liberman, Enig, & Preuss, 2006, p. 2

African Indigenous Foods

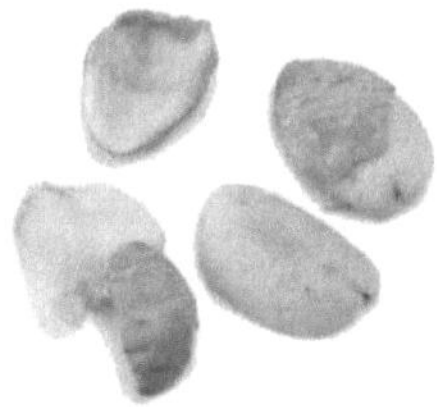 Agbono (*Invingia gabonensis*)	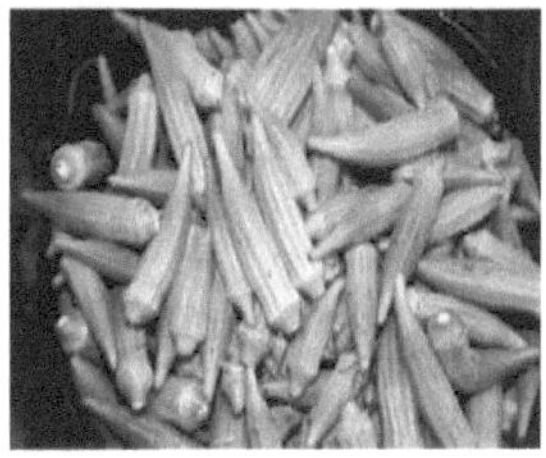 Okra pods	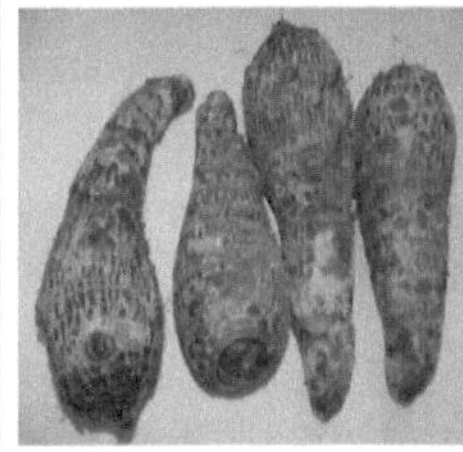 Cocoyams
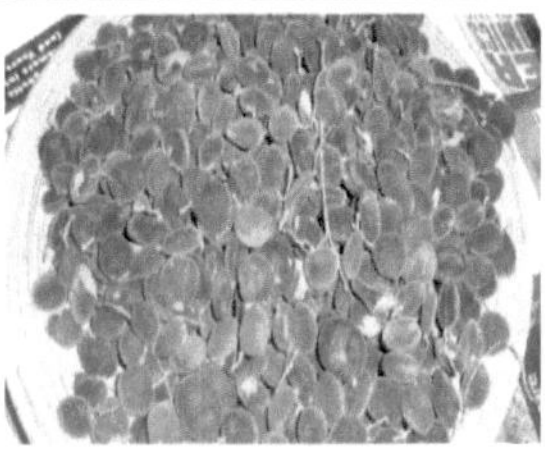 Ichekwu (*Dialium guinenses*), Black tumbler: Anti-ulcer/a source of vitamin C	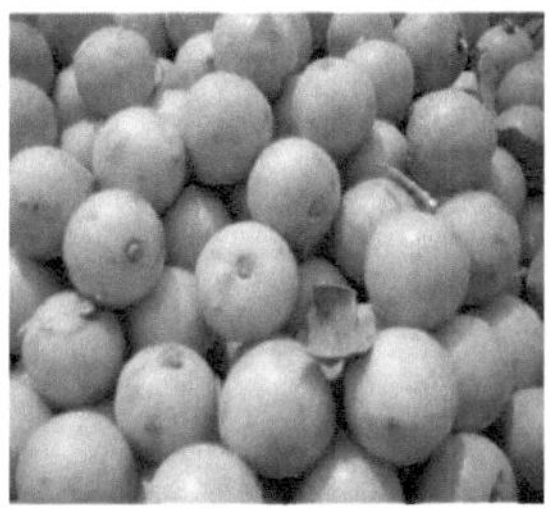 Udala (*Crysophylum Albedum*): Anti-nausea fruit	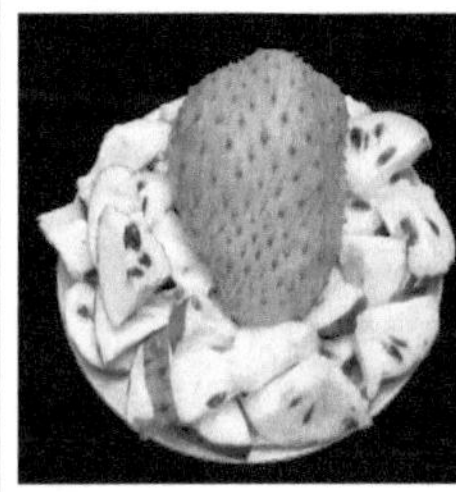 Soursop (Annona muricata): leaves usedfor relaxing nerves
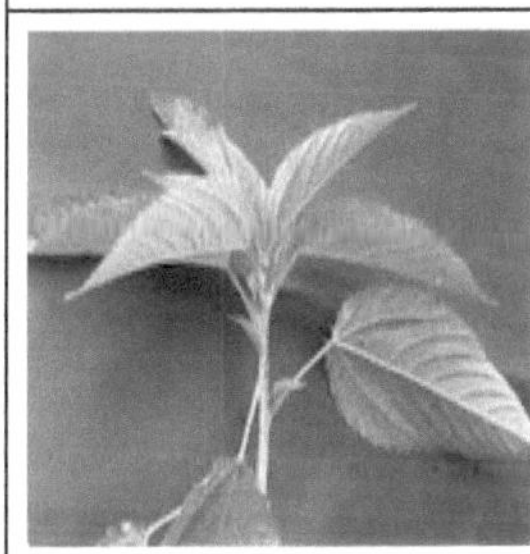 Ewedu, jute leaf.	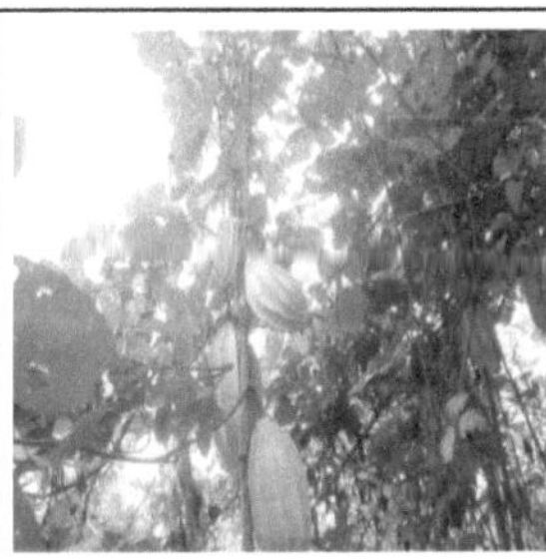 Fluted pumkin (*Telfairia Occidentalis*): Anti-anaemic (blood tonic) leaves	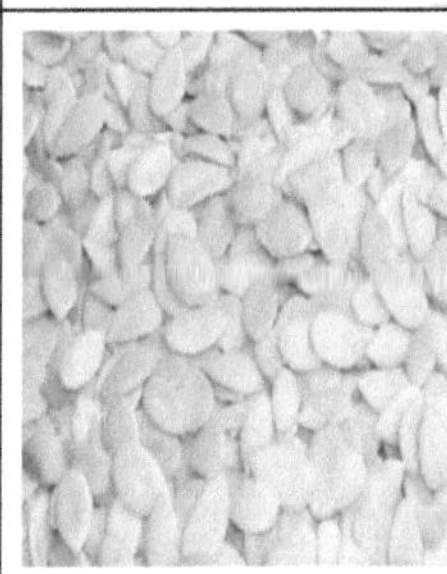 Egusi
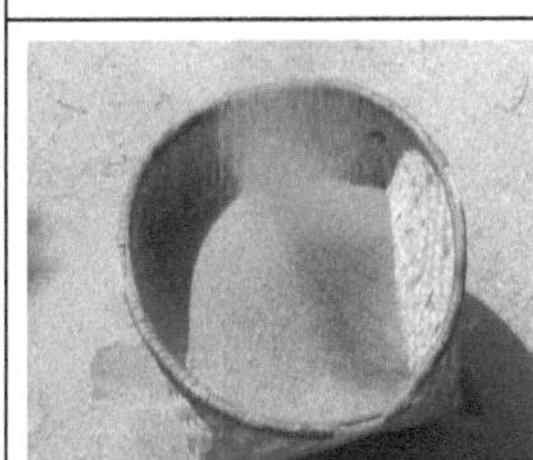 Acha (fonio)	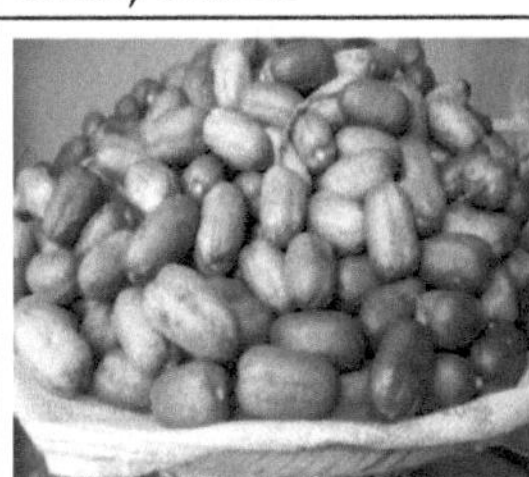 Ube (pear) (*Dascroides edulis*)	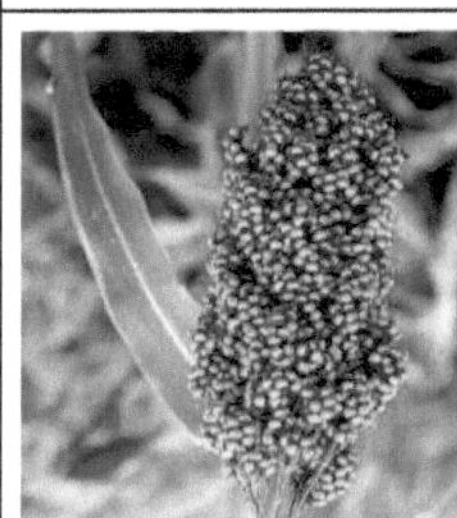 Sorghum

Discussion

The nutrition transition among the Indigenous people has been like the proverbial ill wind that does no one any good. The health news in these areas now reads more like the urban disease forum. Almost every family has one or more sufferers of diabetes, cardiovascular disease, hypertension, osteoporosis, arthritis, obesity, dental disease, and cancer. To make matters worse, biomedical health care facilities are grossly inadequate in these areas. For many years, these diseases have been mainly characterized as the developed world's 'diseases of affluence' (Thiam, Samba, & Wanga, 2006, p. 8). How then did the 'diseases of affluence' become the scourge of Indigenous people? Who and what was responsible for the nutrition transition and the incidence of chronic diseases plaguing the Indigenous population? Even though African nations are supposed to be independent, much of their thinking is still governed by colonial mentalities. The governments of the day and policy makers have succumbed to the lure of globalization and Westernized ideals, to the detriment of their people. Indigenous knowledge is being eroded and replaced with Western values and lifestyles without consideration for its consequences and resultant chronic diseases.

It is important to begin to re-educate the masses about the importance of the Indigenous diet to our health. It is equally important to provide information about the available resources because a lot of nutritious vegetables are still treated as weeds and people do not want to eat them because they don't know if they are poisonous. Some foods are simply attributed to certain ethnic groups and are not eaten by others in order to maintain an ethnic divide. Some of the neglected vegetables are actually more nutritious than the ones we value. People need to have adequate information about their food so they can make informed choices. There is therefore an urgent need to retrace our steps to our Indigenous healing foods and curtail the devastation and turmoil that is threatening the fate of the continent of Africa. Food aid donors need to re-evaluate the types of food sent to Africa. Food donation needs to be relevant to the genetic makeup of the consumers. Instead of sending Western style foods to the Indigenous people, equally nutritious foods could be purchased from neighbouring areas with similar biodiversity. Another option is to bring in farming equipment and help produce the foods locally.

Conclusion

In order for food to adequately serve as medicine by providing the needed health benefits to the body, it is important to have good knowledge of what is available and the best way to obtain the optimum value from it. It is important to maintain a policy of defiance in the face of globalization and reject the unhealthy Western diet as well as the unhealthy franchise establishments in Indigenous areas. In addition, there is an urgent need for the decolonization of the mind in order to develop or re-develop an appreciation for our Indigenous knowledge systems. Various governments' ministries of agriculture and health have the obligation to promote nutritious Indigenous foods both at home and abroad. Food aid providers from the Western countries need to take into account the local nutritional needs of the people and make their donations accordingly. The food could be sourced from neighbouring countries with similar agricultural and nutritional needs. The nutritional transition in Africa and its characteristic health problems prompted Raschke et al. (2007), to warn that "staple foods in Africa are shifting toward an unfavourable direction" (p. 11). UNSCN (2006) added that "to tackle this double burden of under and over nutrition, it is necessary to increase awareness among policy makers through advocacy and implement integrated programs... at all levels including schools and communities" (p. 5).

Additional Information on Indigenous Vegetables in Nigeria
Azu-igwe (hogweed, *Boerhavia diffusa*)[i]

Nutrient	Nutrient Composition/100g (edible portion)
Moisture, g	65.9
Energy, Kcal	117
Protein, g	8.6
Fat, g	0.2
Carbohydrate, g	20.2
Fiber g	0.4
Ash, g	2.4
Vitamin A, RE-µg	18
Vitamin A, RAE-µg	9.0
Retinol, µg	-
β carotene, µg	109
Total carotene, µg	-
Thiamine, mg	0.21
Riboflavin, mg	0.31
Niacin, mg	0.41
Folic acid, µg	7.0
Vitamin C, mg	5.49
Calcium, mg	193
Phosphorus, mg	686
Iron, mg	6.1
Zinc, mg	5.2

I decided to include the above vegetable (azu-igwe) because I was surprised to find it when I was researching for this paper. I was very familiar with this vegetable as a child because it grew around the house, and though we were aware it was edible, we never ate it. The plant was not respected. It might have made a difference if we had known the nutritional value. This further validates the need to make information about Indigenous food plants widely available.

---

i Uses: *Used for egusi soup. Roots chewed for stomach pain.* Source of nutrient data: *Analyzed at the Federal University of Technology, Akure and the University of Nigeria (Crop Science Laboratories)*

Okazi, *Gnetum africanum*[i]

Nutrient	Nutrient Composition/100g (edible portion)
Moisture, g	56.7
Energy, Kcal	210
Protein, g	18.0
Fat, g	4.8
Carbohydrate, g	23.6
Fiber g	0.6
Ash, g	2.7
Vitamin A, RE-µg	65
Vitamin A, RAE-µg	32.5
Retinol, µg	-
β carotene, µg	387
Total carotene, µg	-
Thiamine, mg	0.15
Riboflavin, mg	0.02
Niacin, mg	0.30
Folic acid, µg	13
Vitamin C, mg	0.52
Calcium, mg	597
Phosphorus, mg	473
Iron, mg	18.6
Zinc, mg	3.3

This vegetable is very popular in the Eastern part of Nigeria but it is hardly grown anywhere else.

i Uses: *for soups and for traditional salad.* Source of nutrient data: *Analyzed at the Federal University of Technology, Akure and the University of Nigeria (Crop Science Laboratories)*

Ujuju Leaves, *Myrianthus arboreus*[i]

Nutrient	Nutrient Composition/100g (edible portion)
Moisture, g	58.1
Energy, Kcal	159
Protein, g	8.3
Fat, g	1.2
Carbohydrate, g	28.8
Fiber g	0.5
Ash, g	4.4
Vitamin A, RE-µg	16
Vitamin A, RAE-µg	8
Retinol, µg	-
β carotene, µg	96
Total carotene, µg	-
Thiamine, mg	0.23
Riboflavin, mg	0.36
Niacin, mg	0.54
Folic acid, µg	8.0
Vitamin C, mg	7.71
Calcium, mg	7.9
Phosphorus, mg	420
Iron, mg	3.7
Zinc, mg	2.0

This is a well-loved vegetable in the southern part of Nigeria but because it is not actively cultivated, it is becoming harder to come by.

i Uses: *Soups.* Source of nutrient data: *Analyzed at the Federal University of Technology, Akure and the University of Nigeria (Crop Science Laboratories)*

Aluluisi, *Ocimum gratissimum*[i]

Nutrient	**Nutrient Composition/100g (edible portion)**
Moisture, g	16.8
Energy, Kcal	119
Protein, g	4.6
Fat, g	1.2
Carbohydrate, g	22.4
Fiber g	0.2
Ash, g	3.4
Vitamin A, RE-µg	56
Vitamin A, RAE-µg	28
Retinol, µg	-
β carotene, µg	333
Total carotene, µg	-
Thiamine, mg	0.09
Riboflavin, mg	0.77
Niacin, mg	1.0
Folic acid, µg	3.0
Vitamin C, mg	14.98
Calcium, mg	1028
Phosphorus, mg	529
Iron, mg	14.0
Zinc, mg	5.0

i Uses: *Soups and drink extract from crushed leaves. University of Technology, Akure and the University of Nigeria (Crop Science Laboratories)*

Uziza, Black Pepper Leaves (*Piper guineense*)

Nutrient	**Nutrient Composition/100g (edible portion)**
Moisture, g	67.6
Energy, Kcal	114
Protein, g	16.9
Fat, g	1.3
Carbohydrate, g	8.7
Fiber g	1.2
Ash, g	2.4
Vitamin A, RE-µg	-
Vitamin A, RAE-µg	-
Retinol, µg	-
β carotene, µg	-
Total carotene, µg	-
Thiamine, mg	-
Riboflavin, mg	-
Niacin, mg	-
Folic acid, µg	-
Vitamin C, mg	-
Calcium, mg	759
Phosphorus, mg	403
Iron, mg	19.8
Zinc, mg	3.6

i Uses: for boiling meat and flavouring soups. Source of nutrient data: Analyzed at the Federal University of Technology, Akure and the University of Nigeria (Crop Science Laboratories)

Oha, Cam Wood, *Plerocarpus soyavxii*

Nutrient	Nutrient Composition/100g (edible portion)
Moisture, g	56.3
Energy, Kcal	144
Protein, g	3.5
Fat, g	0.8
Carbohydrate, g	30.8
Fiber g	0.5
Ash, g	3.8
Vitamin A, RE-µg	28.3
Vitamin A, RAE-µg	14.2
Retinol, µg	-
β carotene, µg	170
Total carotene, µg	-
Thiamine, mg	0.29
Riboflavin, mg	0.19
Niacin, mg	1.14
Folic acid, µg	1.0
Vitamin C, mg	1.57
Calcium, mg	12
Phosphorus, mg	289
Iron, mg	20.5
Zinc, mg	2.1

i Uses: soups. Source of nutrient data: Analyzed at the Federal University of Technology, Akure and the University of Nigeria (Crop Science Laboratories

Nti Oke, *Portulaca oleracea*[i]

Nutrient	Nutrient Composition/100g (edible portion)
Moisture, g	56.7
Energy, Kcal	163
Protein, g	22.7
Fat, g	0.1
Carbohydrate, g	17.9
Fiber g	0.1
Ash, g	1.4
Vitamin A, RE-µg	31
Vitamin A, RAE-µg	15.5
Retinol, µg	-
β carotene, µg	187
Total carotene, µg	-
Thiamine, mg	0.39
Riboflavin, mg	0.12
Niacin, mg	0.87
Folic acid, µg	13
Vitamin C, mg	16.63
Calcium, mg	264
Phosphorus, mg	353
Iron, mg	24.1
Zinc, mg	3.3

i Uses: for increasing appetite, mixed with other vegetables for malaria. Source of nutrient data: Analyzed at the Federal University of Technology, Akure and the University of Nigeria (Crop Science Laboratories).

Gbologi, Water Leaf (*Talinum triangulare*)[i]

Nutrient	Nutrient Composition/100g (edible portion)
Moisture, g	90.2
Energy, Kcal	52
Protein, g	2.4
Fat, g	0.8
Carbohydrate, g	8.8
Fiber g	1.6
Ash, g	1.8
Vitamin A, RE-µg	44
Vitamin A, RAE-µg	22
Retinol, µg	-
β carotene, µg	264
Total carotene, µg	-
Thiamine, mg	0.24
Riboflavin, mg	0
Niacin, mg	3.8
Folic acid, µg	7.0
Vitamin C, mg	0.46
Calcium, mg	299
Phosphorus, mg	430
Iron, mg	5.3
Zinc, mg	4.7

i *Uses: with other vegetables for soups and stews.* Source of nutrient data: Analyzed at the Federal University of Technology, Akure and the University of Nigeria (Crop Science Laboratories)

Upulutu, Senna Leaves, *Scientific name*[i]

Nutrient	**Nutrient Composition/100g (edible portion)**
Moisture, g	58.4
Energy, Kcal	159
Protein, g	6.8
Fat, g	0.6
Carbohydrate, g	31.5
Fiber g	0.1
Ash, g	1.8
Vitamin A, RE-µg	52
Vitamin A, RAE-µg	26
Retinol, µg	-
β carotene, µg	310
Total carotene, µg	-
Thiamine, mg	0.45
Riboflavin, mg	0.58
Niacin, mg	0.54
Folic acid, µg	15
Vitamin C, mg	7.74
Calcium, mg	755
Phosphorus, mg	739
Iron, mg	14.8
Zinc, mg	3.7

i Uses: for soups and as a laxative. Analyzed at the Federal University of Technology, Akure and the University of Nigeria (Crop Science Laboratories).

Ugu, Fluted Pumpkin, *Telferia occidentalis*[i]

Nutrient	Nutrient Composition/100g (edible portion)
Moisture, g	60.3
Energy, Kcal	81
Protein, g	4.8
Fat, g	2.6
Carbohydrate, g	9.6
Fiber g	0.4
Ash, g	0.6
Vitamin A, RE-µg	30
Vitamin A, RAE-µg	15
Retinol, µg	-
β carotene, µg	179
Total carotene, µg	-
Thiamine, mg	0.37
Riboflavin, mg	0.77
Niacin, mg	0.67
Folic acid, µg	12
Vitamin C, mg	0.64
Calcium, mg	171
Phosphorus, mg	626
Iron, mg	3.7
Zinc, mg	1.4

i Uses: for soups and other dishes. Source of nutrient data: Analyzed at the Federal University of Technology, Akure and the University of Nigeria (Crop Science Laboratories).

Onugbu, Bitter Leaf, *Veronia amygdalina*[i]

Nutrient	Nutrient Composition/100g (edible portion)
Moisture, g	62.1
Energy, Kcal	154
Protein, g	14.6
Fat, g	2.1
Carbohydrate, g	19.2
Fiber g	0.2
Ash, g	1.6
Vitamin A, RE-µg	31
Vitamin A, RAE-µg	16
Retinol, µg	-
β carotene, µg	187
Total carotene, µg	-
Thiamine, mg	0.13
Riboflavin, mg	0.21
Niacin, mg	0.23
Folic acid, µg	4
Vitamin C, mg	3.30
Calcium, mg	734
Phosphorus, mg	603
Iron, mg	8.9
Zinc, mg	5.7

Source: www.mcgill.ca/files/cine/Igbo_Vegetables_and_Mushrooms_6June07.pdf

i *Uses: Soups.* Source of nutrient data: Analyzed at the Federal University of Technology, Akure and the University of Nigeria (Crop Science Laboratories).

References

Burkitt, D. P. (1973). Some diseases characteristic of modern Western civilization. *British Medical Journal, 1*, 274-278. Retrieved from http://www.ncbi.nlm.nih.gov/pmc/articles/PMC1588096/pdf/brmedj01541-0038.pdf

Eaton, S. B., Konner, M. J., & Cordain, L. (2010). Dict-dependent acid load, paleolithic nutrition, and evolutionary health promotion. *The American Journal of Clinical Nutrition, 91*, 295-297. Retrieved from http://inferno.typepad.com/files/editorial-paleolithic-diet.pdf

Hart, A. D., Azubuike, C. U., Barimalaa, I. S., & Achinewhu, S. C. (2005). Vegetable consumption pattern of households in selected areas of the old rivers state in Nigeria. *African Journal of Food Agriculture and Nutritional Development, 5*(1), 1-19.

Kabara, J. J. (n. d.). Health oils from the tree of life (nutritional and health aspects of coconut oil). Retrieved from http://www.apccsec.org/document/Kabara.pdf

Lieberman, S., Enig, M. G., & Preuss, H. G. (2006). A Review of Monolaurin and Lauric Acid Natural Virucidal and Bactericidal Agents. *ALTERNATIVE & COMPLEMENTARY THERAPIES*, Retrieved from http://www.scribd.com/doc/97180874/Natural-Bactericidal

Linares, O. F. (2002). African rice (*Oryza glaberrima*): History and future potential. *Smithsonian Tropical Research Institute, Box 2072, Balboa-Ancon, Republic of Panama, 99*(25). Retrieved from www.pnas.org\cgi\doi\10.1073\pnas.252604599

Lipski, E. (2010). Traditional non-Western diets. *American Society for ParenteralandEnteralNutrition, NutritioninClinicalPractice, 25*(6). Retrieved from http://online.sagepub.com doi: 10.1177/0884533610385821

Mcgill University Files. (2007). Igbo vegetables and mushrooms. Retrieved from http://www.mcgill.ca/files/cine/Igbo_Vegetables_and_Mushrooms_6June07.pdf

Newport (M.D), M. (2008). WHAT IF THERE WAS A CURE FOR ALZHEIMER'S DISEASE AND NO ONE KNEW? A Case Study by Dr. Mary Newport. Retrieved from http://www.coconutketones.com/whatifcure.pdf

Raschke, V., & Cheema, B. (2007). Colonisation, the new world order, and the eradication of traditional food habits in East Africa: Historical perspective on the nutrition transition. Public Health Nutrition, 7(11), doi: 10.1017/S1368980007001140

Raschke, V., Oltersdorf, U., Elmadfa, I., Wahlqvist, M. L., Kouris-Blazos, A., & Cheema, B.S.B. (2007). The need for an online collection of traditional African food habits. *African Journal of Food, Agriculture and Development, 1*(7), Retrieved from http://www.ajfand.net/Volume7/No1/Verena2330.pdf

Smith, I. F., Eyzaguirre, P. B., Matig, O. E., & Johns, T. (2006). Managing biodiversity for food and nutrition security in West Africa: Building on Indigenous knowledge for more sustainable livelihoods. *United Nations System, 33*. Retrieved from http://www.unscn.org/layout/modules/resources/files/scnnews33.pdf

Taylor, J. R. N., & Emmambux, M. N. (n.d.). Traditional African cereal grains: Overview. Dept. of Food Science, University of Pretoria, South Africa. Retrieved from http://www.sik.se/traditionalgrains/review/Oral%20presentation%20PDF%20files/Taylor.pdf

Thiam, I., Samba, K., & Lwanga, D. (2006). Diet related chronic disease in the West Africa region. *United Nations System, UNSCN, 33*. Retrieved from http://www.unscn.org/layout/modules/resources/files/scnnews33.pdf

United Nations System. (2006). Diet-related chronic diseases and the double burden of malnutrition in West Africa. *United Nations System, Standing Committee on Nutrition, 33*. Retrieved from http://www.unscn.org/layout/modules/resources/files/scnnews33.pdf

Vegetables and mushrooms. (2007). Community Food System Data Table #1, Retrieved from http://www.mcgill.ca/files/cine/Igbo_Vegetables_and_Mushrooms_6June07.pdf

Vinning, G., & McMahon, G. (2006). Gluten-free grains a demand-and-supply analysis of prospects for the Australian health grains industry. Rural Industrial Research and Development Corporation, RIRDC publication No. 05/011 (RIRDC project No. AMR-10A). Retrieved from https://rirdc.infoservices.com.au/downloads/05-011

Chapter Six

THE TRAGEDY OF MODERNITY: TRADITIONAL HEALERS OF KAKAMEGA FOREST IN A BRAND NEW ORDER

Tom Mongare Ndege
George Brown College, Canada
and
Joash Abere Migosi
South East University, Kenya

Abstract

In this chapter, modern and Indigenous medical practices are subjected to competitive assessment. This comparison is underpinned by the realization that the dynamics in the attitudes toward traditional medicine in Africa remain largely unexplored. Limited access to modern medicine coupled with traditional spiritualistic understandings akin to Indigenous African knowledge enhance rather than undermine the need for an in-depth study of the place of herbal medicine in modern African societies. The paper uses Kakamega Forest, a conserved equatorial forest in Kenya, to study the views of traditional healers and patients on how the simultaneous representation of modernity and Indigeneity impacts the choice, use, benefit, and sustainability of traditional healing. In the process, the realities that confront healers in a fluid quasi-modern environment are analyzed and presented. Data is drawn from four traditional healers who describe their trade within the confines of the Indigenous and post-independence period. Additional information is collected from forest conservators in Kakamega. We employ the metaphor of "the tragedy of modernity" to categorize and discuss the data along with both its positive and negative aspects. The results show that the colonial epistemologies that classify Indigenous knowledge as superstition have adverse impacts on the use of traditional resources and may be of little benefit to communities that depend on them. Policy implications of these findings are discussed.

Introduction

There is an increasing rally for Indigenous knowledge as an alternative episteme in research on communities emerging out of a colonial experience (Dei, 2011). Though an earnest application of Indigeneity to education is fairly recent, the practical use of Indigenous ideas is a long-trodden path. Literature is replete with the use of traditional songs, dances, food, and forms of language to confront novel challenges and create new experiences. Nowhere is this more established than in the science of treating people and animals. Ironically, scientific practice has made little admission of the role of traditional healers in the creation, transformation, transmission, or conservation of knowledge, creating a glaring asymmetry in the power and resources associated with these processes. This is most atrocious in colonized societies where the maxim of "civilization" continues to provide a convenient rationale for colonial occupation of the mind and concomitant subjugation (Hodge, Limb, & Cross, 2009).

Kenya is a country that went through one of the most brutal colonial experiences, depleting both human and natural resources. The post-colonial government that was established in 1963 perpetuated rather than exterminated colonial practices. As a result, the country inherited, in its entirety, the colonial education system that propagated unveiled contempt for Indigenous practices. Indigenous healing practices were not only regarded as primitive but also associated with ungodliness and savagery. Though this severely undermined traditional healing, it did not entirely destroy it. There is ample evidence that traditional healing survived the onslaught of modernity through the resilience of the people, rather than through government policy regulation.

The stability of herbal healing within the African context is not a constant but rather an organic process that has continued to evolve according to the specific local and national circumstances. The complexity of the changes confronting traditional healing in Africa may thus not be adequately satisfied by a general or generic case, but rather by critical assessment of the circumstances and conditions that define the healing practices. Orthodox literature studies the application of traditional healing within the confines of linearized conceptualization that concerns itself with factors often called the social determinants of health—attitudes, level of income, settlement, and employment. While this is an important conceptualization, it belies the varied institutional frames that define traditional healing. Admittedly, appreciation of the social determinants of health alone may not account for the resilience of communities that continue to sustain herbal medicine. This paper not only focuses on the social determinants but also goes beyond them by incorporating institutional and cultural systems that define the spirituality of herbal medicine.

The value of herbal medicine in Africa cannot be overemphasized. In societies where diseases are increasingly taking an epidemic proportion amidst huge levels of poverty, modern medicine is often out of reach for the majority. The result is an increasing dependence on herbal solutions for a vast majority of the population. According to a recent World Health Organization report, for example, 80 percent of the population in African countries relies on herbal rather than Western medicine to address their medical needs.

Ironically, this high dependence on traditional healing has not translated to enhanced positions for the traditional healers. On the contrary, the place of these healers is increasingly marginalized, with severe impacts on the quality of healers and the services they provide. The increasing marginality of healers and lack of government regulations into the trade portend significant risks to the health of a large segment of the population in countries such as Kenya, where the erosion of skill levels among healers may not trigger compensating effects on the demand end. Earlier efforts have sought to enhance healers' status through integration of traditional medicine with Eurocentric medicine. As shown by Wane (2011), for example, such efforts are not well received by the Western-trained medical class:

> The herbolists clearly articulate their frustration with how their practices are viewed despite the fact that different herbs are known to cure incurable diseases in Kenya. The Western-trained doctors in Kenya have indicated that there is very little room for negotiating with Indigenous healers who are not adequately trained because it will contaminate their Western model that has given them a certain privilege in society. (p. 235)

Clearly, society may not effectively engender traditional healing practices without first promoting education of what is traditionally considered legitimate practice in the health sector. Substantial reconstruction and the deconstruction of knowledge in medicine are required and entail achieving learning outcomes that promote appropriate practices in diagnosing and treating ailments as well as engendering social and institutional changes necessary for their adoption.

For a long time, materials used to produce healing substances were derived from forests. In Kenya, these forests are increasingly threatened by farming practices, and the destruction of the environment, which characterizes African countries, may, however, be traced to colonial times. The genesis of this is the commercial interests that were the primary motivation of colonial activity. Mercantile trade that evolved after colonialism promoted rapacious depletion of forests, shrines, and other traditional healing sites that put traditional healing in significant danger of extinction. The only solace was in conservation projects that promoted Western leisure interests such as Kakamega Forest in Western Kenya. Because of their simultaneous satisfaction of colonial and Indigenous interests, these have come to represent a hotspot of cultural conflict (McGeoch et al., 2008). The linkages between natural forests and traditional healing practices cannot be overemphasized, especially in poor countries, where significant segments of the population continue to subsist on natural resources (Ndege et al, 2011).

This chapter seeks to offer a fresh assessment of the linkage between nature and traditional healing in three ways: 1) Examining the current literature on the use of Indigenous knowledge in developed countries; 2) Exploring the medicinal herbs' potential for promoting enhanced well-being in poor countries; 3) Discussing the philosophical underpinnings of using African herbal healing practices as legitimate ways of knowing.

Current studies on Indigenous healing have generated significant data that inform education concerning Indigenous people and their worldview. There is far less focus on Indigenous African practices. This is surprising given the increasing need to provide equality in educational experiences across the globe. The need for wider representation of the African Indigenous experience is therefore significant. Increasing globalization underscores rather than diminishes this need. Though Africans have similarities in their culture, a lot of studies opine that there are also areas of significant variations. Kenya provides a convenient setting for a study on African Indigenous healing because of the predominance of morbidity in its population. Inadequacy of formal hospital facilities and high price of medicines drive a great proportion of the population to the herbal sector (Wane, 2011). The matter is strengthened rather than weakened by the emergence of new ailments such as HIV/AIDS and concomitant morbidity in the population. The rise in the need for herbal medicine is limited by a declining natural resource base that often compounds the crisis of inadequate medical services. This chapter seeks to assess the most appropriate navigation strategy that would ensure effective collaboration between traditional social resources with natural resource management to catapult poor communities from dire levels of need to more socially desirable conditions.

Recent physical science studies indicate that medicinal herbs have an immense potential for promoting enhanced well-being in poor countries (McGeoch et al., 2008). These studies are, however, limited by virtue of the fact that they are often not integrated into modern solutions to medical problems in poor countries. Inadequacies in medical policy as well as the orientations of medical professionals militate against more effective integration of herbal healing in the health systems of poor countries (Simuyu et al., 2010; Wane, 2011). This is surprising, given that developing health innovation often motivates various scientific studies. Admittedly, overcoming the barriers that undermine the succession of herbal healing from the cradle to the globe would provide the most critical milestone for integrating traditional medicine. A retinue of factors account for a state of affairs where African herbal healing, unlike Chinese or Indian herbal healing, continues to stagnate in the cradle. Most important among these, perhaps, are the cultural limitations associated with a brutal colonial experience that confines the African mind. Clearly, African scientists have not appeared to free themselves from the strangling effects of this experience. According to a recent study, for example, one reason why scientific technologies stagnate in Africa "is the cultural mindset of scientists and domestic and international policy-makers" (Simiyu et al., 2010) who fail to synthesize their works with problems facing these countries. There is a corpus of literature on the efforts being made to translate Western oriented research into marketable products. Comparatively, there is far less focus on the practice of herbal medicine and its implications on education. This chapter seeks to review the role of education in the modernity tragedy that has come to characterize herbal education in Kenya.

Finally, the philosophical arguments on the use of African herbs for healing purposes advance the notion of a holistic approach (Hodge et al., 2009; Langwick, 2007; Spangenberg, 2003; Wane, 2011), rather than the piecemeal provision of health, among the African population. Western mental health is perhaps the most instructive example for how inappropriate assumptions and treatment are likely to engender ineffectiveness. According to Spangenberg (2003), for example, mental health as a therapy

> entails numerous assumptions about the nature of reality. Included among these is the assumption that "good mental health" is an end worth pursuing; various assumptions about what constitutes good mental health and dysfunctional; and the assumption that the discussions and exploration of the problem, benefit those who suffer, problems can be isolated and solutions

> targeted to localized problems, outcomes in a specific area can be monitored and measured, and secular licensed professionals are best suited to guide people through the healing process. (pp. 212-213)

Traditional healing is a complete antithesis of this practice, with its focus on the harmonization of body, mind, and spirit. Extant literature on traditional healing underscores the need "to tailor conventional psychotherapies for the benefit of people immersed in beliefs, practices, and worldviews that diverge substantially from those of the Western middle class" (Gone, 2010, p. 168). The integration of traditional healing into the conventional rigmarole is clearly compounded by the differences and similarities between traditional healing and Western healing practices. However, a synthesis of ideas about what traditional healing may offer modernity in the African context has hardly been explored. Education is perhaps the foremost vehicle for initiating the entry of traditional healing discourse into the understanding of the nuances that characterize this synthesis. Yet, as currently practiced in many countries, education is hardly informed by traditional healing in its efforts to satisfy the need of African communities. A number of factors may account for this, the primary of which is the perpetration of colonial education theories and practices that engender negation of Indigenous ways of knowing. In this chapter, we focus on the possible curriculum and pedagogical changes that may enhance education's impact on worldviews that promote persistent application of colonial epistemological orientation.

This chapter is organized in six sections. Section one provides a brief overview of Indigenous healing practices in Africa. Section two focuses on literature and the theoretical underpinnings of the chapter. Section three reviews Indigenous healing in Africa. Section four provides the methods of the study. Section five presents and discusses the data. A final and sixth section summarizes the key arguments and suggests the way forward.

Literature and Theoretical Framework

There is a corpus of literature that underscores the need to apply Indigenous practices in the development of an appropriate episteme for Africans (Dei, 2011; Gone, 2010; Wane, 2011). This literature is deeply embedded in Indigenous methods of knowing that are clearly distinct from modern, Western-oriented practices in a variety of ways. Gone, for example, outlines three significant ways in which traditional healing can be distinguished from modern professional curative practices: (a) secular versus sacred differences; (b) rational versus mystical approach; and (c) technical versus relational aspects.

(a) Secular versus sacred differences.

Modern treatment is guided by secular perspectives that assume therapeutic knowledge is dependent on "naturalistic understandings and materialistic explanations of human experience" (p. 204). In contrast, traditional healing is essentially based on sacred cosmological principles that emphasize a holistic and spiritual understanding of human experiences.

(b) Rational versus mystical approach.

In this respect, Western medicine purports to depend on rational approaches that are based on evidence while traditional healing seeks to advance mystical approaches. The limits of rational methods need not be overemphasized. The general consensus in literature that science that depends on collecting data, statistically analyzing results, and reporting such results, is not only fraught with error, but is also far too costly to effectively provide an answer to human health problems. On the other hand, traditional healing depends on non-human powers exercised through human healers. The animate nature of these non-human entities presupposes that healers appeal through ritualistic practices to the powers drawn from these forces. The integration of traditional healing into modern practice is thus of necessity limited by the differences in the approach to the healing process. In African communities, colonial interruptions that marginalized traditional healing significantly compound this process. Colonial education, by nature, viewed traditional practice with suspicion. Traditional healing, with its appeal to the ritualistic management of ailments, was often associated with viciousness rather than being viewed as a potentially enhancing force. Kenya adopted an education system based on Western norms—a largely Christian missionary education that belies a secular curriculum. Although, at independence, the government undertook to rid education of religious or cultural bias, in reality education was more a force in colonization than a liberator. Recently, Kenya adopted a new constitution that reclaims some of the hitherto ignored cultural rights as civil rights. Traditional healing as a practice of a large proportion of the population is an integral part of these rights. How can education be used to support a more accommodative health system by promoting integrative health regimes? In Kakamega, traditional perspectives underpin the resilience of traditional healing amidst hostile legal and institutional frameworks. We focus on the nuances that maintain traditional healing in an environment where official policy resides in denial of its existence.

(c) Technical versus relational aspects.

Modern Western healing presumes that healing is a technical process primarily entailing the action of a healer who provides prescriptions that have to be followed by the patient. In contrast, traditional healing sees healing in terms of ritualistic functions or mediation of the healers to the other-than-human person. The difficulties entailed in reconciling traditional healing to Western medicine in this respect transcend mere incorporation of traditional healing but are rather a paradigm shift that offers novel ways of seeing the world of knowledge, not from the perspective of one who knows and the other who-knows-not. Rather, knowledge becomes an interactive relational process where the gurus and the students play different but mutually interrelated functions. In Kenya, a large population seeks the services of traditional healers; Western medicine is dominant because it enjoys significant political and social influence. In this chapter, we seek to debunk the notion that Western medicine is necessarily a good or more effective way of dealing with African ailments.

In this study, an anti-colonial framework is applied to interrogate the place of traditional healing in the Kakamega Forest catchment, where poverty is endemic. The appeal to an anti-colonial theoretical framework is preferred because traditional healing is hitherto a marginalized area of knowledge. Following Gone (2010), this neglect is attributed to colonial practices that buttressed the notion that Africans had no knowledge. These practices negated the fact of traditional knowledge, including traditional healing, that was part of the African way of life since time immemorial. The neglect of traditional healing is a significant contradiction, especially when perceived within the prism of conservation practices that were part of the colonial experience, straddling sectors such as forestry and wildlife. The modern expression of this project is Kakamega Forest, where a tropical forest was conserved, but its role as a site for traditional expression severely curtailed. In this chapter, the role of this paradox in the prolific growth of street-based traditional healing is of immense interest. The failure of modernity to provide meaning to the application of forest goods and services is clearly brought into focus in this milieu.

There is a rising body of literature that reports scientifically confirmed values of forest-harvested herbs in the management of human and animal ailments (McGeoch et al., 2008). This literature is based on the erroneous assumption that the Western 'scientific' paradigm, with its emphasis on collection of data, analysis, and reporting of results, provides the only, or perhaps the most effective, means of determining truth. The reality of long held traditions that have for years depended on Indigenous knowledge systems creates severe tensions with this approach. The so-called modern systems that are propagated by Western epistemologies are at best partial, rather than whole, reflections of processes that create knowledge. The fact that even within their partial perspectives these systems confirm that Indigenous healing is efficacious, reinforces rather than undermines the value of Indigenous knowledge, especially in post-colonial Africa. The use of modern approaches is, however, clearly limited as it fails to recognize traditional approaches that have withstood the test of time. For example, whereas Western knowledge systems presuppose that value lies in the market where goods and services can be sold, traditional communitarian systems see value in terms of communal application. Underpinning this variation is the very significant ecological impact of Western orientations toward traditional healing. In this study we focus on the use of herbs in Kakamega Forest in modern times and how this has imposed heavy ecological dangers to the forest and human well-being.

The incongruence of traditional healing with modern mercantile economic systems is minor when compared with the more pervasive degradation of mental orientation, perpetrated by the education system. In general, Kenya's education system is structured to promote conformity to values established through colonial fiat. For example, up until very recently, the curriculum ignored life skills. In 2008, the government recognized the need to provide life skills in the curriculum. However, such skills continue to be oblivious to the Indigenous orientations that guide life for a vast section of the population (Kayne, 2009).

Traditional Medicine in Africa

The role of traditional medicine in the management of disease in African countries cannot be overstated. According to the World Health Organization, for example, more than 80 percent of the population in Africa depends on herbal medicine for primary health care (Sambo, 2010). Developing policies that conserve traditional healing in African countries is thus of utmost importance. African governments long recognized this need, adopting the development of local medicine as a critical strategy for realizing health at the 50th Regional World Health Conference (Sambo, 2010; World Health Organization [WHO], 2001). Subsequently, the role of traditional medicine in African health systems has risen rather than declined.

Although as a region, Africa has recognized traditional healing as an alternative to Eurocentric medicine, domestication of this resolution remains varied across sub-regions. In terms of policy, 46 African states adopted herbal medicine as an integral component of primary health in the period 2001-2010. This move paved the way for the development of the safety, efficacy, and quality of traditional medicine in these countries. Other countries adopted stronger institutional frameworks including establishing governmental ministries and departments dealing with traditional medicine. This led to the incorporation of traditional medicine when planning for national resources and investment in medicine. By 2010, for example, traditional medicine had acquired a legitimate space in government in 39 countries.

There was also a simultaneous rise in the commitment of resources in the support of research in traditional medicine. The overarching theme of this research is the need to develop a repository for the posterity of available Indigenous knowledge. In this respect, various countries and regions in Africa have adopted different approaches. The West Africa Health Organization is spearheading the endeavour to develop a pharmacopoeia on traditional medicine. The hallmark of these activities is enhanced documentation of the diverse herbal solutions for endemic ailments in Africa, including malaria, opportunistic HIV infections, diabetes, hypertension, and tuberculosis. A guiding principle is to add to the list of essential medications in the African disease management environment. A second set of endeavours are characterized by small scale activities primarily aimed at identifying and documenting the efficacy of herbal plants in Africa. National herbal medicine institutions have often served the role of regulating and certifying these activities.

Three critical threats confront the achievements made so far in institutionalizing herbal medicine in Africa. First is the predominance of Western-oriented approaches that are used to test the efficacy, safety, and value of traditional healing practices, causing traditional worldviews to be marginalized by Western worldviews. The flipside to this is that custodians of traditional practice are rapidly displaced by purveyors of Western medical practice to the detriment of genuine traditional values that were embedded in traditional medicine. Traditional practices, thus, are systematically eroded with perverse social, educational, and economic implications. Socially, traditional medicine dispensers suffer systematic losses as they are replaced by more urbane Western adherents. Educationally, the transformation from traditional to modern means of dispensing medicine engenders enhanced marginalization of African knowledge by transferring esoteric traditional knowledge to

Western sources that are elitist and bent on individualization rather than socialization of information. The process underpins unacceptable epistemic inequalities that are a culmination of the Western intellectual colonization of Africa. Economically, the uneven distributional impacts of this transformation clearly distort values of intellectual property with severe exploitative implications to communities in Africa.

Transformation of African traditional medicine is nonetheless an imperative given the changing global environment. The problem is therefore not whether or not African traditional medicine should change but what is the most optimal way of carrying out change to achieve desired results for communities that have long depended on traditional medicine to deal with their myriad problems.

The nature of African traditional medicine as a public good suggests immense complexities in its dispensation to potential users without impacting negatively on its sustainable supply. As a result, market allocation of traditional medicine, though desirable, is unviable because of the complexity of ensuring efficacy, quality, and sustainability of the resources involved. Change in traditional medicine must therefore increasingly depend on a regulatory process ensuring that traditional medicine continues to play its role as a sustainable alternative to Eurocentric medicine for poor communities. This process is of necessity policy-driven as it depends to a large extent on the establishment of institutional capacity in African countries.

The global consensus on the need to develop institutional capacities in developing countries to incorporate primary health care into conventional health systems can be traced as far back as the 1978 Alma-Atta International Conference on Primary Health Care. At the heart of this conference was the need to promote universal health in developing countries using health care levers such as traditional medicine. The declaration of the conference zeroed in on encouraging governments to include traditional medicine in "primary health care systems and recognize traditional medicine practitioners as part of the health care team in primary health care at the community level" (Kayne, 2009, p.4). Ironically, in countries in dire need of primary health care such as those in Africa, policy development on traditional medicine is incomplete, with many countries still not accepting traditional medicine practitioners as partners in primary health care.

There is a wide array of evidence that the integration of traditional medicine into primary health care is not uniform across Africa. Kayne (2009), for example, provides a global map of levels of policy development in various countries. According to this map, there are countries in

Africa such as Ghana, Tanzania, and Mozambique, where traditional medicine is adopted as a policy. There are also other countries where the legislative process to domesticate this integration remains undeveloped. In comparative terms, countries in the West and South African regions have more comprehensive primary health care policies than those in East Africa. Admittedly this regional classification may be fraught with oversimplification. However, it goes a long way to illustrate the disparities that still exist at the policy level in implementing international imperatives on primary health care systems.

Kenya's primary health care draws heavily from its colonial heritage, which emphasized the superiority of Western ways over traditional ways. Over the years, government policies have continued to emphasize the perspective promoted by Western scholars on the place of germs at the center of disease management. The primacy of this paradigm in Kenya's health care strategy is so all-encompassing that there is hardly any room for dissenting without risk of being labeled a purveyor of falsehoods. This entrenched, almost dogmatic commitment to Western perspectives is in part informed by an education that has derided traditional knowledge while failing to provide a significant application of Western learning. Admittedly, this cause-effect approach is important in explaining certain disease phenomena. It is, however, inadequate in dealing with pathological or endemic situations of ailment. Besides, dependence on Western medical solutions may be unsustainable in countries where ill health is so prevalent that imported products are beyond the social means of the country.

Privately, traditional medicine is widely preferred over Western medicine in many parts of Africa when dealing with a variety of ailments. Recent studies show that there are significant positive attitudes among Africans toward the use of traditional medicine in the areas of mental health, chronic illnesses, and common diseases such as malaria. This means that there is great potential for developing African traditional medicine for the management of primary health care. Attitudes, however, tend to vary depending on economic and social factors (Winkler, Ombey, Mathias, & Jik-Aall, 2010). Mediation of this wide array of issues suggests the need for a clear social policy that is informed by good practice globally. This paper assesses the effectiveness of primary health systems in incorporating traditional medicine in Kenya.

The Method

In this study, ethnography methods that seek information about Indigenous ways, values, norms, and traditions are used to study the interaction between these and modern conservation practices. The focal point of this study is Kakamega Forest. Kakamega Forest is the largest remnant rain forest in Kenya, with a land size of 241 square kilometers. Sixty percent of this area is made of Indigenous forest while forty percent is plantation forest. The forest conservation effort is run jointly by the Kenya Wildlife Service and the Kenya Forestry Service. Kakamega Forest is located within a densely populated region. Culturally, residents depended on forest resources to provide medicinal herbs that serve to manage a variety of ailments that confront the population.

This study examines a specific herbal plant, *Mondia whitei (Apocanaea)*, locally known as *mokobero.* According to local resident M. Whitei, it is a potent herb that serves a variety of functions including treatment for gonorrhoea, schistosomiasis, stomach disorders, and colds. It is also associated with aphrodisiac effects, enhanced milk production, and vitality. Application of mokobero as a medicinal product entails excavation of the roots and chewing the peelings of the roots. In commercial centers around Kakamega Forest, mokobero chewing is a popular pastime with vendors freely advertising its values to travelers and other potential clients. Part of the reason why mokobero is so popular is the inadequacy of Western medicine. Studies indicate that over 95 percent of the residents in poor countries depend on herbal medicine to address their ailments. Surprisingly, the herbal sector is hardly recognized in Kenya's health system. Mokobero is, thus, a plant that is severely undervalued, and its benefits are neglected by the wider society. Communally, however, the plant's benefits are underscored with significant enthusiasm among its users. Modern living has occasioned enhanced levels of illnesses that are related to diminished sexual libido, especially among men in the poverty-stricken Kakamega catchment, leading to a heightened need for social support. In this study, we seek to decipher the mindset underpinning the changing state of well-being among both men and women that encourages the harvesting of mokobero and its use in the management of ill health. This chapter also seeks to study how modern practices such as those promoted by Western medical practices impact the use of the mokobero herbal practices.

To effectively do this, the chapter draws data from participants in the mokobero-dispensing and mokobero-consuming communities. Dispensers, traders, and healers that use mokobero are compared with regard to their knowledge and perception of the value of the herbal plant.

The chapter uses the views of two herbalists drawn from the Kakamega-Kamukuywa area. This is a fairly rural area with limited open trade of mokobero. The herbalists that we report here vary between 50 to 65 years of age. We prefer this demographic because they are custodians of traditions concerning the use of herbal medicine in the community. Their views and practices are compared with two other herbalists drawn from among those that peddle the mokobero herb in the Kakamega municipal area. The study depended on reports of largely underemployed traders who sell their goods around the bus terminal at Kakamega. In the city of Kakamega, forest products such as honey, edible insects, and herbs are predominant. As a result, vendors of herbal products rarely specialize, often remaining highly versatile to benefit from any possible demand changes that may enhance their profit margin. Because of the knowledge needs of herbal medicine, however, dealers of mokobero tend to remain fairly consistent in their commitment to the promotion of the herb.

Reconnaissance visits to the area showed that mokobero captured a significant share of the available herbal products. In our count of eight traditional healing products, including healing ornaments such as horns or sticks, mokobero was of foremost significance in both availability and use. Traders in the product were of widely dispersed ages ranging from 15 to 80. This study conducted a baseline investigation to determine how demographic factors influence herbal knowledge and practice. The choice of respondents was thus guided by a confluence of age, experience, and area of operation within Kakamega. From these, the study focused on two traders of mokobero that were found to most appropriately represent modern practices. To complement the information that was collected from traditional healers that use mokobero; this study used the experiences of two conservators of Kakamega Forest who reported their experiences with traditional healers that come to the forest to collect herbs for use at local markets and in homes where treatment is sought.

The data is analyzed using a qualitative approach that seeks to decipher meaning from the statements of various actors in the herbal healing process. The analysis follows five distinct themes that are embedded in Indigenous education under the anti-colonial paradigm. These are: (1) Individualism and cooperation: Indigenous paradigms as an antithesis to modern paradigms emphasize cooperation as a critical instrument in the realization of communitarian approaches to problem solving. Modern or colonial paradigms emphasize individual assets that lead to the prolific duplication of effort in competition that is altogether harmful to each actor. In this study, we review the representation of cooperation and competition in the space that is Indigenous and also in the space that is modern (2) Learner experiences: In this respect the study assesses how herbal skills are acquired among modern young herbalists, especially the opportunities they have to gather pertinent information from their elders and how this influences their practices. (3) Spirituality: The appeals by Indigenous healing to spirituality as the basis for the claim to knowledge constitute an important departure point for understanding traditional linkages to human health. Colonial notions deride this as superstitious and unscientific. Anti-colonial theories opine that the persistence of herbal healing signifies clear non-violent resistance against colonial subjugation and marginalization of traditional ways of knowing. In the cities and other areas of dislocation where Indigenous people are located, the tension between succumbing to colonial orientations and remaining steadfast in the promotion of Indigenous knowledge often belies the decline in the spiritual determination of traditional healing. (4) Source: Indigenous education deals with antiquity. In Africa, this antiquity is linked to Egypt, the oldest civilization known in history. Asante and Abarry (1996), for example, argue that:

> One cannot have a full appreciation of the sources of African intellectual traditions without connecting Egypt to its natural relationship with the societies contiguous to it. A body of human sciences, constructed from the reasons, nuances, myths, and the inquiries of Africans, can only be imagined if we do not [sic] begin at the beginning of African classical civilizations. It is from this position that we are able to realize a body of human sciences and studies based upon thousands of history. We find in the classical civilizations of Africa the answers to some of the most persistent questions of African capability and possibility. (p. 6)

The focus on the source as a fundamental aspect of African intellectual wealth clearly transcends all genres of African learning. The theme of the source is thus central in understanding herbal healing among Africans as a distinct body of knowledge from Western or Eurocentric medicine. (5) Deciphering: The final theme is dealing with the basis upon which healing knowledge is deciphered among herbalists and clients in the catchments of Kakamega Forest. The coded nature of traditional healing provides meaning to traditional "literacy" and has a component of functional knowledge that finds expression in the healing of humans and animals.

The Findings

The results of this study showed that traditional healing was a cooperative rather than individualistic enterprise. The participants intimated that in traditional healing practices the patient and healer were enjoined in an effort to seek healing. The use of mukobero was thus not an end in itself but rather a means by which the healer sought to connect with the healed in mystical and spiritual terms to achieve "wholesomeness". One healer summarized his experience in the following terms:

> Sick people come to me all the time with problems that range from stomach complications to marital ones and I subscribe for them this herb as a concoction that enables us to seek the cause. They go back to their home only to return happier than they went. When we talk later I advise them to eat healthy and continue using the herb. (Interviewed participant)

The cyclical approach to healing in traditional Africa is perhaps the most remarkable aspect of its uniqueness. In this study we sought to identify the extent to which cyclical values are retained in modern forms of healing that use mukobero. The results that we received from respondents in Kakamega showed that, rather than depending on traditional forms of knowing, modernized traditional healing was competitive and unconcerned about maintaining an equal relationship between the afflicted and the healers. As a result, in the streets of Kakamega, street vendors approach you with roots of Mukobero that they pass on as healing material. The users are charged a fee for the herbs, which they either boil and take, or chew in their raw form. Street traditional healers believe that they contribute to the well-being of those to whom they sell their products. Most of the patients who have been taught in Eurocentric education systems that prescribe an expert-patient approach to treatment describe the immense tensions they face in administering traditional remedies to people whose minds are colonized. Makhoka, one of the vendors, for example, recounted to us his frustrations in providing this service:

> I am a high school graduate with no means for taking care of myself. My parents passed away just after I had completed by studies. I have no means of continuing with my studies as nobody is willing to support my college education. I have to seek bread and Mukobero is my only remedy. I may not know how it really works but people here really love it and that is all that matters.

There is a lot of extant literature that underscores the use of Indigenous methods as legitimate research frames. These studies see Indigenous education as the key that could unlock the potential of young people who find themselves incapable of charting their path in life because of the innumerable contradictions that exist between Western education and Indigenous knowledge. There are strong reasons to confront an education that fails to synchronize traditional ways of knowing into its epistemology. Dei (2011) reiterated this point more effectively when he contended that:

> We must engage issues of responsibility and appropriation of knowledge as essential dimensions of critical social research. As much as bringing a critical gaze, locating the self, identity and politics and affirming complicities and social responsibility are important, Indigenous research is about strengthening the capacity of local Indigenous peoples to undertake their own research. (p. 9)

In Kakamega, the youth appeared to be in a state of disconnect from the adults who saw herbal medicine as a distinct philosophy from modern medicine. The older population felt that the younger people misused cultural resources to seek personal wealth. One of them averred that:

> Forests are sacred and so are the plants and materials drawn from them but the traditional restrictions that used to control how these were used are now not respected with [the] widespread and dangerous use of mokobero.

This view is a direct indictment of the Kenyan education system that appears to consistently contradict its own goals. In 1964, Kenya adopted six educational goals that underscored the need for (1) national unity, (2) national development, (3) personal development, (4) cultural conservation, (5) cultural transformation, and (6) international awareness. However, since independence, the country's education system has taken little notice of the use of Indigenous values, traditions, taboos, ethos, and heritages to promote education. As Wane (forthcoming) has argued, it is this Indigenous knowledge that has over the years determined balance between natural and anthropological spheres of operation. Through Indigenous methods, adults passed on to their children the values of forests, animals, songs, proverbs, and other precious things that are crucial for good living in these environments. The advent of Westernization and its colonial control of the intellect, along with the moral imperatives of communities, have had an impact not only on the communities, but also on the ecosystems within which they reside. In Kakamega, rapacious harvesting of mukobero has not only been noted to severely undermine the plant, but may also be harmful to human health.

Conclusion

In this chapter, traditional healing is assessed in an environment where rapid social and economic changes significantly impact the principle of the connectedness of knowledge espoused by Indigenous philosophies. This chapter shows that without a deliberate adoption of Indigenous epistemologies in these circumstances, the natural environment may be more rapaciously used with negative implications for sustainability. Kenya's failure to embrace, in a practical sense, Indigenous knowledge as a significant social aspect of education not only enhances a colonial mindset among the youth, but also perpetuates a significantly less desirable way of using common property such as forests. The use of herbal resources then loses its sacred and communal purpose, replaced with irrational and unmitigated squandering of highly beneficial herbs, promoting private rather than social goals. Education should be the primary means by which the good practices of yesteryears are used to provide valuable lessons on how the present may enhance its benefits from available wealth. The chapter proposes that in Kakamega, the adoption of Indigenous epistemologies is more than justified by the evidence on the ground.

References

Asante, M. K & Abarry, A. S. (1996). Introduction. In M. K. Asante & A. S. Abarry (Eds.), African Intellectual Heritage: A Book of Sources. Philadelphia: Temple University Press.

Dei, G. J. (2011). Revisiting the question of the "Indigenous." In G. J. Dei (Ed.), Indigenous Philosophies and Critical Education: A reader (pp. 21-33). New York: Peter Lang.

Gone, J. P. (2010). Psychotherapy and traditional healing for American Indians: Exploring the prospects of therapeutic integration. The Counselling Pyschologist, 38(2), 166-235.

Hodge, D. R., Limb, G. E., & Cross, T. L. (2009). Moving from colonization towards balance and harmony: A native American perspective on wellness. Social Worker, 54(3), 211-219.

Kayne, S. (2009). Introduction to traditional medicine. In S. Kayne (Ed.), Traditional Medicine: Global Perspectives (pp. 1-24). New York: Pharmaceutical Press.

McGeoch, L., Gordon, I and Schmitt, J.(2008). Impacts of Land Use, Anthropological Disturbance and Harvesting on African Liana, Biological Conservation, 141(9), 2218-2229

Ndege, TM, Getenga, ZM, Nyongesa, H and Chacha, S (2011) Social Value Formation and Switching to Tithonia in Nzoia River Basin (NRB), Kenya, Global Business and Economics Anthology, 2(2), 127-136

Sambo, L. G. (2010, August). The decade of African traditional medicine: Progress so far. The African Health Monitor: African Traditional Medicine, 13, 1-14.

Simuyu, K., Daar, A.S., and Singer, P.A. (2010), Stagnant Health Technologies in Africa, Science, 330(6010), 1483-1484

Spangenberg, J. J. (2003). The cross-cultural relevance of person-centered counselling in post-apartheid South Africa. Journal of Counselling Development, 81, 48-54.

Wane, N. (2010). Traditional Healing Practices: Conversations with Herbalists in Kenya. In D Kapoor and E. Shizha (Eds) Comtemporary Asian and African Learning: Essentialism, Continuity and Change,(pp. 229-244) New York: Palgrave MacMillan

Winkler, S. A., Ombey, M., Mathias, B., & Jik-Aall, L. (2010). Attitudes towards African traditional medicine and Christian spiritual healing regarding treating epilepsy in a rural community in Tanzania. African Journal of Traditional, Complementary and Alternative Medicine, 7(2) 162-170.

World Health Organization. (2001). Promoting the role of traditional medicine in health systems: A strategy for African region, Harare, Zimbabwe. WHO Regional Office.

Chapter Seven

BRINGING TRADITIONAL HEALERS BACK INTO THE CONVERSATION

Immaculate Wamimbi Tumwine

Introduction

This chapter cites some of the literature that highlights the growing trend toward engaging traditional healers in delivering health services in Africa. The focus is on the partnership triggered by the failure of modern medicine to deliver successful solutions with respect to malaria, Human Immunodeficiency Virus (HIV)/Acquired Immune Deficiency Syndrome (AIDS), and with regard to the numerous illnesses that are widespread in rural areas. Even though some illnesses are easily treatable with modern medications, these have been largely inaccessible and unaffordable to low income rural communities. The chapter draws on documentation, including reports and articles, that focus on Uganda as a model in view of the advances that have been made in that country in forging partnerships between the modern medical establishment and traditional healers, in directing efforts to enhance communication between them, in making strides in training traditional healers, in ascribing roles to be played by traditional healers in the delivery of health services, and in successfully encouraging traditional healers to organize themselves.

It is asserted that the existence of impelling factors is key in bringing about formal acceptance of the practice and role of traditional healers. For favourable reception to take place, there has to be government recognition, acceptance and recognition by modern medicine practitioners, ascribing of roles, availing of resources for research and for training, and organization and self-management on the part of the traditional healing community.

The Literature on Changed Perception of Traditional Healing Practice

With the great advances in the discoveries of modern medicine, and with widespread use of advanced technology for disease diagnosis and treatment, one would not expect to witness the thriving of traditional healing practices. However, in Africa, not only has traditional healing survived, but the prospects have become much better in the last few decades due to the growing trend of governments and modern health establishments, including local practitioners and international agencies, engaging with traditional healers in the delivery of health services.

Much of the literature on African traditional healing practice, particularly with respect to HIV/AIDS management, is in the form of conference and research papers prepared for conferences and for international organizations such as the World Bank, World Health Organization (WHO) or the United Nations Joint Programme on HIV/AIDS (UNAIDS), which is the key coordinating body for global action on HIV. Some writers (e.g., Cohen, 1997; Devenish, 2005; Green, 1999; Helwig, 2001; Mohlala, 2001) have pointed out that, while previously, detractors of traditional healing practice unfairly portrayed all traditional healing practice as witchcraft or dismissed the practice as unscientific, the changed perception has involved a more accurate depiction and recognition of its healing, counselling, and supportive roles.

Literature on Reasons for Thriving of Traditional Healers in Africa

As to why African traditional healing practice has survived and even thrived in the face of modern medical inventions, numerous documents, for example a report from the WHO (1990), have pointed to the paucity of modern medical systems, including the lack of infrastructure and services, particularly in rural areas, as the reason for growing efforts to engage traditional healers in delivering health services. Cohen (1997), Helwig (2001), the National Council of Traditional Healers and Herbalists Associations of Uganda (NACOTHA, n.d.), WHO (2004), and King (2000) have reported that practically all African countries have many more traditional than modern medicine practitioners. Helwig (2001), for example, described how in “the Venda area of South Africa, there was one traditional practitioner for every 700-1,200 people, compared to one physician for every 17,400 people” (p. 1). On their website, the National Council of Traditional Healers and Herbalists Associations of Uganda stated that there was one traditional health practitioner for every 200-400 people, compared to one modern medicine practitioner for every 10,000 people. In its South African Country Press Release of March 30, 2004, the WHO underlined that “up to 80 percent of Africans depend on traditional medicine for their health care needs” (WHO, 2004, p.1).

Furthermore, the fact that modern pharmaceutical products are very costly and unaffordable to low income communities in Africa, and the reality that these modern treatments have not been able to cure the preponderant diseases, including HIV/AIDS, have been perhaps the most significant factors driving individuals to seek more affordable traditional medicine. WHO (2000) stated that in the poorest parts of Africa and Asia, over 50% of the population had no access to even the most basic essential drugs (p. 9).

Stanley (2004) reported that the African Union (AU) had declared 2001-2010 the Decade for African Traditional Medicine due to the recognition that traditional medicine was the most affordable and accessible health care system for the majority of people. He also reported on how the AU's goal of bringing together stakeholders was supported by the WHO and the International Development Research Centre (IDRC) (Stanley, 2004, p. 150).

An article published in *The African Executive* amply summed up the reasons for the survival of traditional healing in Africa as follows: "It is estimated that over 85 percent of sub-Saharan Africans access their health education and health care from traditional healers. Traditional practitioners who far outnumber modern health care practitioners are culturally accepted and respected, and more universally located" (Akosah-Sarpong, 2007, p. 1).

HIV/AIDS as the Compelling Force for Change in the Role of Traditional Healers in Africa

The reasons for governments seeking help from traditional healers have been enumerated in some of the literature, including Mohlala (2001) and Hoff (1992). UNAIDS described how the HIV/AIDS epidemic has propelled traditional healers into an important role in health delivery in Africa:

> In countries such as Kenya, the United Republic of Tanzania or Uganda, where resources are limited, there is a desperate need for care, support and prevention alternatives that are readily available, accessible and affordable.... Traditional medicine is one such alternative. (UNAIDS, 2002, p. 6)

Homsy, King, Balaba, and Kabatesi (2004), Stanley (2004), Devenish (2005), and Mohlala (2001) have also portrayed the advent of the incurable AIDS/HIV outbreak in the early 1980s as the compelling force for change in the role of traditional healers in Africa. In a literature review carried out for UNAIDS, King (2000) underlined the fact that the WHO had advocated the inclusion of traditional healers in National AIDS programs since the early 1990s due to the work of traditional healers in the area of sexually transmitted diseases (STDs) (p. 6). Writing about South Africa, Richter (2003) described the AIDS epidemic as constituting "a considerable part of the modernizing forces that constantly [challenged] and [changed] traditional healers' role and their practices" (p. 8). The linkage in the literature of the emergence of the AIDS epidemic with the urgent need to involve African traditional healers in HIV/AIDS programs is illustrated in reports from numerous AIDS conferences, including documentation from the *Consultation on AIDS and Traditional Medicine: Prospects for Involving Traditional Health Practitioners*, held in Botswana in July 1990. In his opening address at this Consultation, for example, Dr. G. L. Monekosso, Director, WHO Regional Office for Africa, stated:

> Given the paucity of resources available to African governments and the extremely high number of AIDS cases that I have just quoted, there is an urgent need for designing new approaches to contain further the spread of this dreaded disease. (Monekosso, 1990, p. 20)

Giving reasons for collaborations in the area of HIV/AIDS between the traditional and modern medical sectors reported in the various literature she had reviewed, King (2000) asserted that, apart from the better doctor/ patient ratio, the literature acknowledged that traditional healers provided culturally appropriate health care based within the community setting, which enhances the potential for community mobilization. According to the literature, King (2000) stated that traditional healers were also perceived as respected health care givers who were already treating large numbers of HIV/AIDS patients and who had more credibility than village health workers, especially in spiritual matters (p. 10). According to Ritcher (2003), in the case of a terminal disease like AIDS, the spiritual side is said to be very important (p. 9).

Literature on the Thriving of Traditional Healers in Uganda

Other literature, including Homsy et al. (2004), has indicated that Uganda had not only been among the first African countries to ascribe formal roles to traditional healers but, more than any other African country, had made the greatest headway in forging partnerships between the modern medical establishment and traditional healers, in directing efforts to enhance communication between them, in training traditional healers and in successfully encouraging traditional healers to organize themselves.

Cohen (1997), Stanley (2004), UNAIDS (2000), and WHO (2004) underlined the fact that the enhanced collaboration between modern and traditional medicine in Uganda was due to the advent of AIDS, the prevalence of malaria and preventable illnesses, as well as the mass poverty in the communities. UNAIDS (2002) described Uganda as one of the few countries that had "narrowed the gap between the traditional and biomedical health systems" (p. 8). Uganda, which was severely ravaged by HIV/AIDS in the 1980s, was among the first African countries to experience and recognize how the modern medical system was overwhelmed, in cities as well as rural areas. With the spike in the number of people experiencing various HIV/AIDS symptoms, it was noted (e.g., by Cohen, 1997; Stanley, 2004; UNAIDS, 2000; WHO, 2004) that, due to the unaffordable pharmaceutical products used to treat these symptoms, most community members turned to the more affordable products from traditional healers who were also more accessible to the communities.

Supported by international agencies such as the WHO and the World Bank, the Uganda government partnered with traditional healers for the dissemination of information and for public education relating to the prevention of HIV/AIDS and other STDs. The need to affect the subsequent partnership had led to the need for capacity building through training and the need to establish collaborative mechanisms to sustain the relationship. This necessarily involved acknowledging and recognizing the role of traditional healing. This acknowledgement of the potential role of traditional healing and assigning of significance to this role in different African countries has taken various forms. Green (1999), who carried out a World Bank study to assess the impact of education and communication programs on HIV decline in Uganda, asserted:

> Involvement of local opinion leaders such as traditional healers and clergy in government-sponsored HIV/AIDS prevention on a scale such as we find in Uganda is uncommon in Africa and the world; Uganda appears to lead at least the developing world in magnitude of HIV decline. (p. 2)

Green (1999) credited Uganda's education efforts, including efforts to engage community stakeholders and traditional healers, for the HIV decline. Umerah-Udezulu (2001) quoted the United Nations (UN), who reported that in Uganda, a ten-year public education campaign aimed at young individuals from 1987 to 1997, had succeeded in curtailing new HIV infections from 239,000 cases down to 57,000.

What the Changed Status and Role of Traditional Healers Has Entailed

In view of the incurable nature of HIV/AIDS, with respect to STD prevention in particular, and in light of the significant change in the role of traditional healers, some literature, including Monekosso (1990), King (2000), and Green (1999), has pointed to the numerous interactions and collaborations between traditional healers, modern medicine practitioners, and government health departments. In more concrete terms, traditional healers' new role is to promote aspects of primary health care. This has included providing prevention information about

STD/AIDS to as many community members as possible—for example, encouraging community members who seek their services to practice safe sex and promoting sanitation and aspects of child care, including immunization. King (2000) referred to the WHO, which in 1994 had suggested that upgrading the skills of traditional healers "made more sense than training new groups of health workers, such as village health workers" (King, 2000, p. 10).

Referring to collaborative programs in several African countries, including South Africa, Zambia, Mozambique, Swaziland, and Uganda, and pointing out that it was traditional healers "who see and treat (or attempt to treat) most cases of STDs," Green (2004) reported that, in these countries, the major objectives of the programs were "to develop healers as promoters of condoms and fidelity to one sexual partner," to prevent the spread of infections including HIV, hepatitis and tetanus "through sterilization of healers' instruments," "to modify healer's practices that may put them at risk themselves for HIV infection, and to encourage referrals of healers' STD patients to hospitals" (p. 1). Richter (2003) and Green (2004) also reported on the potential role of traditional healers with respect to care and counselling of patients who were already HIV positive. Green referred to healers in Dar es Salaam, Tanzania, who were counselling patients "about diet and exercise, avoiding alcohol and tobacco, and avoiding despair and depression" (2004, p. 1).

Acknowledgement and Recognition of Traditional Healers through Capacity Building Initiatives

Having recognized the need to involve traditional healers in formal health services, and in HIV programs in particular, it had become important for governments and their associates to examine the role that the traditional healers were playing with respect to HIV/AIDS treatment, to review their level of knowledge of the subject, and to determine what kind of education and training would enable them to successfully play any subscribed role. It was also important to establish how the traditional healers' role would be evaluated and how it would be overseen to protect the community (Monekosso, 1990, p. 21).

Indeed, some documents (e.g., Cohen, 1997; Devenish, 2005; Stanley, 2004) have focused on the interest shown by different African governments and by traditional healers themselves with regard to the modernization of traditional healing roles. Helwig (2001) noted the increased integration of traditional and modern medical practices through collaborative efforts and joint training. Rogerson (2002) stated how training and education for traditional healers had become a necessity, as the healers were consulting with many STD and HIV patients, often without adequate knowledge concerning HIV.

Hoff (1992) referred to a review of 18 projects in different countries, including Ghana, Nigeria, Sudan, Swaziland, Sierra Leone, and Zambia, in which traditional healers were successfully trained to work in primary care projects (p. 182). Hoff (1992) reported that, in the projects reviewed, topics covered during training included promotion of safe water, maternal health, childcare and immunization, promotion of prevention of local pandemics, procedures such as first aid, and provision of basic first aid medication such as aspirin (pp. 182-183).

Acknowledgement and Recognition of Traditional Healers through Partnerships and Collaborations

Many African governments' desire to engage traditional healers had also led to the creation and strengthening of partnerships with the traditional healing sector. Mohlala (2001) described some partnerships between traditional healers and the Department of Health in Uganda, as well as partnerships with local clinics. He also reported the involvement of traditional healers in the AIDS Council in South Africa.

Providing an example of a very successful collaboration between traditional healers and the modern medical sector in Uganda, Engle (1998) reported how the formation in Uganda of THETA (Traditional and Modern Health Practitioners Together against AIDS) had brought together traditional healers and modern medical practitioners. Engle (1998) reported how, in a two-year pilot project, the group had met frequently to share knowledge, experience, and resources on HIV/AIDS and other STDs, and to discuss counselling skills and educational strategies.

According to Engle (1998), the training that the traditional healers received had included demonstrations of proper condom use and information on how to educate and counsel their patients. At the end of the pilot project, the healers had received formal certification as AIDS educators and counsellors. According to Engle (1998), through the project the healers had found more effective methods to engage the broader community, going beyond their normal one-on-one practice, and one healer who was a graduate of the program had constructed a clinic and convinced partners from the modern health sector to work with him under the same roof.

Green (1999) estimated that between 1995 and 1998 alone, over 1,800 traditional healers in Uganda had been trained every year in, among others, referral and promotion of behaviour change with respect to HIV/AIDS. According to him, that amounted to "a greater number of Indigenous healers officially involved in HIV/AIDS prevention than most—perhaps any—other country in Africa that I am aware of" (Green, 1999). Engle (1998) wrote that following the success of the model, THETA had set up similar collaborative efforts in rural areas across Uganda and that this had set the stage for collaboration in other African countries, particularly as THETA was also a collaborative effort of Doctors Without Borders.

Wreford (2005), who carried out a review of scholarly literature on possible ways and means of improving and enhancing relationships between biomedicine and traditional healing, especially in HIV/AIDS interventions in South Africa, has provided an abstract as well as extensive bibliographical references on the relationship between African traditional healers and modern medicine practitioners in the area of HIV/AIDS in South Africa. Referring to Green, Zokwe, and Dupree (1995) and to King (2000), Wreford (2005) reported that, "despite the impetus that HIV/AIDS ostensibly offers to programmes of collaboration, actual examples are few and far between and have been 'seldom evaluated'" (p. 91).

In his literature review, Wreford (2005) referred to Anderson and Kaleeba (2002, pp. 31-46), who pointed out that compared to healers' organizations in the other countries reviewed, Uganda's THETA organization was the most innovative because it had an additional component involving the integration of biomedical health workers into a four-year training programme (Wreford, 2005, p. 104).

In terms of collaborative practice in Africa, Helwig (2001) also provided an example of a 48-bed hospital in Kwa-Mhlanga, South Africa, in which traditional African medicine was combined with Western healing methods. King (2000) provided a table which summarizes documented examples of collaboration in 18 sub-Saharan African countries (pp. 37-42). According to King, the literature she reviewed indicated that collaborations would increase traditional healers' knowledge and experience, create openness, and facilitate early referral to hospital (King, 2000, p. 9).

Governments' Subsequent Need to Formalize and Regulate Traditional Healing Practice

The decision to formally involve traditional healers in the health system, and in national AIDS programs in particular, necessitated the development of pertinent collaborative agreements, policy, and legislation. By 1990, the report from the WHO consultation on AIDS and traditional medicine was recommending the implementation of training as well as policy development (WHO, 1990, pp. 14-15). Others, including Richter

(2003), were also arguing for the regulation of traditional healers and traditional medicine in their respective countries (p. 27).

While the advent of HIV/AIDS presented a threat to the community health care system that had formed the major impetus for acknowledgement, collaboration, capacity building and, subsequently, formalization and regulation initiatives, some have recently drawn attention to an additional threat, mainly external, posed by Western multinational pharmaceutical companies claiming intellectual property rights on healing products from the region. This has added urgency to the need to speed up formalization and regulation of the traditional healing sector.

In an online article entitled "Uganda, Nigeria to Regulate Traditional Healers," published in *Afrol News* on September 14, 2009, for example, the *Afrol News* staff writer reported that Nigeria and Uganda had just announced plans to regulate traditional healers, joining South Africa as countries that had "decided to formally recognize the trade of traditional healers" the week earlier. The article not only quoted Nigeria's Minister of Health, Professor Eyitayo Lambo, who stated that the Ministry of Health gave traditional medicine "top priority" due to its popularity among Nigerians; it also referred to the need for regulation in both Uganda and Nigeria as a response to the increasing claims of intellectual property rights from Western multinational pharmaceutical companies on products that had been known to African traditional healers for many generations. It was reported in the same article that both the Nigerian and Ugandan Health Ministries had stated that they were going to focus on research, and that herbal research and treatments were "to become major studies at Uganda's medical school at Makerere University" (Afrol staff reporter, 2009).

Acknowledgement and Recognition of Traditional Healers

The modern medical community's acknowledgement, as well as recognition by international organizations—including the UN, WHO, IDRC, Doctors without Borders and World Bank—of the potential role of African traditional healers (particularly herbalists) in the provision of primary health care has played a major part in enhancing their role as partners in disease management and prevention.

As early as 1977, the WHO formally acknowledged the potential role of, and need to recognize and collaborate with, traditional healers (Richter, 2003, p. 10). Indeed, working through its Traditional Medicine Program, the many conferences and consultations organized by the WHO on this subject bear out its commitment. In the area of traditional healers and the AIDS/HIV epidemic, the WHO has supported various member countries that strive to develop national policies on traditional healing practice. The World Bank's interest in traditional healers can be affirmed by reading the World Bank website, where they also provide extensive bibliographic references to works written on the topic.

Ndhlalambi (2009) reported how, in 2003, the 56th World Health Assembly of the WHO had resolved "that its member states must ensure that their health care systems promote and support provision of training and, if necessary, retraining of traditional health practitioners, and a system for the qualification and/or accreditation or licensing of the practitioners" (p. 9). Ndhlalambi (2009) also gave the example of how the African Medical and Research Foundation (AMREF) had engaged in developing an inventory of successful HIV/AIDS collaboration between a traditional healers' forum and a primary health care program in Standerton, Mpumalanga province, in South Africa (p. 13).

Stanley (2004) reported that the Canadian IDRC had funded the computerization of inventory of Madagascar's medicinal and aromatic plants (p. 150). The IDRC also supports the Network on Medicinal Plants and Traditional Medicine in Eastern Africa, which brings together traditional healers, researchers, communities, entrepreneurs, development partners, and governments (Stanley, 2004, p. 150).

Taking Advantage: Self-Organizing and Advocating

In many African countries, but particularly in Uganda, traditional healers have organized themselves to advocate for recognition and for resources. As seen in Richter (2003) and Mohlala (2001), various forms of organization have been reported. As the National Council of Traditional Healers and Herbalists Associations (NACOTHA) website shows, self-organizing has enabled the National Council of Traditional Healers and Herbalists Associations of Uganda, for example, to liaise and to coordinate with the government. According to NACOTHA, advocacy has taken the form, not only of demanding more recognition and more resources, but also of demanding good practice from fellow practitioners (NACOTHA website, n. d.).

Reading the NACOTHA website, it is apparent that, even in a country such as Uganda, which is said to be ahead in terms of engaging with traditional healers, there are gaps. According to NACOTHA, these include gaps in policy development, difficulty evaluating traditional medicine due to gaps in defining standards, the need for greater collaboration and training with the modern medical establishment, and further government commitment in terms of budget allocation for research and awareness activities (NACOTHA website, n. d.).

Striving to Overcome Challenges

Several articles, including those by Devenish (2005); Ndhlalambi (2009); Colvin, Gumede, Grimwade, and Wilkinson (2001); Chipfakacha (1997); NACOTHA (n.d.); and WHO (1990), have also referred to challenges that hinder the recognition and improvement of the status of traditional healing practices. These include lack of full commitment by some governments, traditional healers' lack of knowledge of the HIV/AIDS disease, and the widespread abuses made by illicit healers, such that the traditional healers find themselves striving to separate good from bad practice.

Mohlala (2001) and Colvin et al. (2001) also highlighted challenges in the form of misunderstandings and tensions between Western and traditional medicine practitioners as well as tensions with the international community, particularly in the area of properties and patents. Ritcher (2003) elaborated on some of the reasons for tension between traditional and Western medicine (p. 12). WHO (1990) pointed to the distrust and the mystification of traditional medicine as one of the challenges particularly relating to research. It was also reported that, despite efforts in Ethiopia to draw up contracts with traditional healers that would stand up in court, the mistrust still remained a challenge (WHO, 1990).

Conclusion

From the discussion in this paper, the following assertions can be made: Even though organizations such as the WHO were advocating for recognition and inclusion of traditional healers in the modern health care system well before the advent of the HIV/AIDS epidemic, the latter lay bare the conspicuous failings of the modern medicine sector, exposing even further the inadequate functional infrastructure and lack of resources, including human resources, to adequately respond to new and old illnesses. The emergence of HIV/AIDS underlined, more than ever, most community members' long held confidence in, and respect for, traditional healers. Appreciating the importance of health education and of appropriate preventative information dissemination in stemming and managing not only the HIV/AIDS epidemic but also other STDs and illnesses, stakeholders in the African modern medicine establishment have conceded that the obvious route to accessing the majority of communities is to work collaboratively with the traditional healing sector. In efforts to succeed, they have had to develop and to make use of the tools, processes, and conditions necessary to facilitate partnerships and to accomplish health goals.

Drawing from the successes in Uganda, which the literature declares was among the most affected by the HIV/AIDS epidemic on the continent, it can be concluded that the accomplishment of health goals is more likely when there are impelling factors that create the desire by governments, health-related departments, modern medicine practitioners, and international agencies to take advantage of traditional healers' popularity and to form collaborations with them in disease prevention and care. Also drawing from Uganda, it can be concluded that, to succeed, there has to be formal acceptance of the practice and role of traditional healers by the government and by the modern medicine sector, underlined by the formal ascribing of roles and by the availing of resources for research and for capacity building, including training.

There have to be efforts to regulate and to formalize the traditional healing process to ensure protection of the public and to safeguard traditional healers' rights, including intellectual property rights. There also has to be support for efforts by the traditional medicine sector to organize themselves and to be accountable. As can be evidenced by Uganda in their desire to take advantage of the collaborations and partnerships with the modern medicine sector, traditional healers are, with some encouragement, likely to organize themselves and to take ownership. They are also likely to advocate for stronger links with the modern medicine sector, for more resources, and for more streamlined policy likely to protect their interests.

Despite the gaps and challenges still to be overcome, the spike in diseases such as diabetes and blood pressure—which are largely better managed with health education and behavioural change—as well as the persistence of mass poverty in the communities, is ensuring the growing role of traditional healers in a country like Uganda, where there is already respect for their work, and where the modern medical institution is unlikely to see great development in the very near future.

References

Afrol staff news reporter. (2009, September 14). Uganda, Nigeria to regulate traditional healers. *Afrol News.* Retrieved from http://www.afrol.com/articles/13950

Akosah-Sarpong, K. (2007, May 9-16). Traditional medicine should not be demonized. *The African Executive.* Retrieved from http://www.africanexecutive.com/modules/magazine/articles.php?article=2261

Anderson, S., & Kaleeba, N. (2002). Ancient remedies, new disease: Involving traditional healers in increasing access to AIDS care and prevention in East Africa. *UNAIDS Best Practice Collection.* Retrieved from http://data.unaids.org/Publications/IRC-pub02/jc761-ancientremedies_en.pdf

Chipfakacha, V. (1997). STD/HIV/AIDS knowledge, beliefs and practices of traditional healers in Botswana. *AIDS Care*, *9*(4), 417-425

Cohen, T. (1997, October 18). As Africa changes, so does traditional healing. In *PARKINSN Archives*, University of Toronto List Serve 15.5. Retrieved from https://listserv.utoronto.ca/cgibin/wa?A2=ind9710c&L=parkinsn&D=0&F=P&T=0&P=133571

Colvin, M., Gumede, L., Grimwade, K., & Wilkinson, D. (2001). Integrating traditional healers into a tuberculosis control programme in Hlabisa, South Africa. *Medical Research Council Policy Brief No. 4. December*. Retrieved from http://www.mrc.ac.za/policybriefs/tbtraditional.pdf

Devenish, A. (2005). Negotiating healing: Understanding the dynamics amongst traditional healers in Kwazulu-Natal as they engage with professionalisation. *Social Dynamics, 31*(2), 243-284. Retrieved from http://www.africanstudies.uct.ac.za/downloads/SD%20 31_2__%20Devenish_Revised-as.pdf

Engle, L. (1998). Traditional healing in a modern epidemic. *The Body Positive Magazine*. Retrieved from http://www.thebody.com/content/art30491.html

Green, E. C. (1999). Traditional healers and AIDS in Uganda. *Journal of Alternative and Complementary Medicine, 6*(1), 1-2. Retrieved from

http://www.stwr.org/africa/traditional-healers-and-aids-in-uganda.html

Green, E. C. (2004). The participation of African traditional healers in AIDS/STD prevention programs. Retrieved from http://www.stwr.org/africa/the-participation-of-african-traditional-healers-in-aids/std-prevention-programs.html

Green, E. C., Zokwe, B., & Dupree, J. (1995). The experience of an AIDS prevention program focused on South African traditional healers. *Social Science and Medicine, 40*(4), 503-515. Retrieved from http://www.stwr.org/health-education-shelter/the-experience-of-an-aids-prevention-program-focused-on-south-african-traditional-healers.html

Helwig, D. (2001, April 6). Traditional African medicine. *Encyclopedia of Alternative Medicine*. Retrieved from http://findarticles.com/p/articles/mi_g2603/is_0007/ai_2603000708/

Hoff, W. (1992). Traditional healers and community health. *World Health Forum*, 13. Retrieved fromhttp://centerfortraditionalmedicine.

org/pdf/web_articles/Traditional%20Healers%20and%20Community%20Health.pdf

Homsy, J., King, R., Balaba, D., & Kabatesi, D. (2004). Traditional health practitioners are key to scaling up comprehensive care for HIV/AIDS in sub-Saharan Africa. *AIDS, 18*(12), 1723-1725. Retrieved from http://journals.lww.com/aidsonline/Fulltext/2004/08200/Traditional_health_practitioners_are_key_to.14.aspx

King, R. (2000). Collaboration with traditional healers in HIV/AIDS prevention and care in Sub-Saharan Africa. *Best practice collection: A literature review.* Geneva, Switzerland. Retrieved from http://data.unaids.org/Publications/IRC-pub01/JC299-TradHeal_en.pdf

Mohlala, T. (2001, November 16). Turning to traditional healers: Natural herbs have no side effects and are less expensive than Western-based medication. *Daily Mail & Guardian.* Johannesburg, South Africa. Retrieved from http://www.aegis.com/news/DMG/2001/MG011113.html

Monekosso, G. L. (1990). Inaugural address at the WHO consultation on AIDS and traditional medicine: Prospects for involving traditional health practitioners, Francistown, Botswana, 23-27 July 1990. Retrieved from http://apps.who.int/medicinedocs/pdf/h2955e/h2955e.pdf

NACOTHA. (n.d.). National Council of Traditional Healers and Herbalists Associations of Uganda. Retrieved from http://www.blackherbals.com/nacotha1.htm

Ndhlalambi, M. (2009). Strengthening the capacity of traditional health practitioners to respond to HIV/AIDS and TB in KwaZulu, Natal, South Africa. *AMREF Case Studies.* Retrieved from. http://www.amref.org/silo/files/strengthening-the-capacity-of-traditional-health-practitioners.pdf

Richter, M. (2003). Traditional medicines and traditional healers in South Africa. (Unpublished discussion paper) Treatment Action Campaign and AIDS Law Project. Retrieved from http://www.tac.org.za/Documents/ResearchPapers/Traditional_Medicine_briefing.pdf

Rogerson, R. G. (2002). Traditional African healers: Their role in the fight against STDs, HIV and AIDS in South Africa. (Abstract No. E11522). *International Conference on AIDS, July 7-12.* Retrieved from http://gateway.nlm.nih.gov/MeetingAbstracts/ma?f=102249631.html

Stanley, B. (2004). Recognition and respect for African traditional medicine. *International Development Research Centre: Science for*

Humanity. Retrieved from http://www.idrc.ca/en/ev-55582-201-1-DO_TOPIC.html

Umerah-Udezulu, I. (2001). Resensitizing African health care and policy practitioners: The gendered nature of AIDS epidemics in Africa. *Jenda Journal of Culture and African Women Studies,* 1, 2. Retrieved from http://www.jendajournal.com/vol1.2/udezulu.html

UNAIDS. (2000). Ancient remedies, new diseases: Involving traditional healers to increase access to AIDS care and prevention in East Africa. *UNAIDS Best Practice Collection.* Geneva, Switzerland. Retrieved from http://data.unaids.org/Publications/IRC-pub02/jc761-ancientremedies_en.pdf

_____. (2000). Collaboration with traditional healers in HIV/AIDS prevention and care in Sub-Saharan Africa: A literature review. *UNAIDS/00.29E Geneva.* Retrieved from http://data.unaids.org/Publications/IRC-pub01/JC299-TradHeal_en.pdf

World Health Organization. (1990). Traditional medicine programme and global programme on AIDS. *Report of the consultation on AIDS and traditional medicine: Prospects for involving traditional health practitioners. Francistown, Botswana. July 23-27. WHO/TRM/GPA/90.1.* Retrieved from http://apps.who.int/medicinedocs/pdf/h2955e/h2955e.pdf

_____. (2000). WHO medicines strategy 2000–2003: Framework for action in essential drugs and medicines policy. WHO/EDM/2000.1. Geneva, Switzerland. Retrieved from http://apps.who.int/medicinedocs/pdf/whozip16e/whozip16e.pdf

_____. (2004, March 30). WHO welcomes South Africa's commitment to traditional medicine. (WHO/South Africa Press Release). Retrieved from http://www.afro.who.int/country_offices_press/2004/pr20040330.html

World Bank. (2009). Health system and financing: Traditional healer services. Retrieved from http://web.worldbank.org/WBSITE/EXTERNAL/TOPICS/EXTHEALTHNUTRITIONANDPOPULATION/EXTHSD/0,,contentMDK:20190826~menuPK:438812~pagePK:148956~piPK:216618~theSitePK:376793,00.html

Wreford, J. (2005). Sincedisa – We can help! A literature review of current practice involving traditional African healers in biomedical HIV/AIDS interventions in South Africa. *Social Dynamics, 31*(2) 90-117. Retrieved from http://www.africanstudies.uct.ac.za/downloads/SD%2031_2__%20Wreford%20_we%20can%20help_-as.pdf

Part B
Practical Examples of Indigenous Healing

Chapter Eight

CONCEPTS OF TRADITIONAL HEALING PRACTICES AMONG THE ACHOLI AND MADI IN NORTHERN UGANDA

Emilio Ovuga, MBChB, M.Med Psych, PhD
Dean, Faculty of Medicine, Gulu University

Abstract

Emerging economies in Eastern Central and Southern Africa have decentralized health services to districts aimed at promoting access to essential services in remote rural communities. However, owing to logistical problems, manpower shortages, and financial constraints, more than 80% of individuals with any form of ill health do not freely receive the care they need. Under the prevailing circumstances, traditional health care practitioners occupy a central role in the provision of health services in their communities and claim a sweeping ability to cure a variety of medical conditions including malaria, syphilis, epilepsy, infertility, hypertension, diabetes, and severe mental illness. Despite these claims, traditional healers in parts of the region have received negative publicity due to harmful practices such as human sacrifice.

In spite of the negative publicity, traditional health care providers are respected and protected by their communities and draw their clientele from all sectors of society. Accordingly, some governments in the region are under pressure to recognize traditional health care providers and give them equal status with conventional health care providers. In this chapter the author provides an overview of the concepts and practices of traditional healing systems among the Acholi and Madi ethnic groups of Northern Uganda. The chapter will discuss existing and future areas of collaboration between traditional health care providers and conventional medical practitioners, and suggest how collaboration might be achieved.

Background

Health care coverage in Uganda's rural areas is inadequate despite the decentralization of health services to the district level under the country's minimum health care package. Under the circumstances, traditional healers play a crucial role in providing health care to communities (Ovuga, Boardman, & Oluka, 1999). Research in Uganda revealed that 4 in 5 adults with mental illness receive treatment from traditional healers. Individuals who seek treatment from traditional healers and formal health care providers concurrently do better at three months follow-up (Abbo, 2009).

Mental health problems are a major public health issue worldwide (Weismann et al., 1996). The corresponding treatment gap for mental health problems is wide (Kohn, Saxena, Levav, & Saraceno, 2004; Thornicroft, 2004). Kasoro et al. (2002) have cited the involvement of traditional healers in the treatment and prevention of severe mental illness in Western Uganda. Okello et al (2006) and other Ugandan researchers have reported the preference by the Baganda for traditional healers to Western-trained doctors in the treatment of depressive illness that the Baganda attribute to cultural factors. For instance, Abbo and associates (2009) provide evidence from Busoga in Eastern Uganda suggesting that 60% of patients receiving care at traditional healers' shrines met DSM-IV diagnostic criteria for schizophrenia, affective disorders, anxiety disorders, and schizophreniform disorder. Work by Ovuga, Boardman, and Oluka (1999) revealed that 80% of traditional healers in Pallisa District, Uganda, were willing to collaborate with government doctors in the care of persons with severe mental illness.

Traditional healers in Uganda claim the ability to provide cures for a wide variety of ailments ranging from infertility, diabetes, hypertension, various forms of headache and body aches, through the casting out of evil spirits, as well as the ability to create wealth. The medium within which traditional healers claim these abilities in rural areas stems from the fact that the rural communities are inclined to attribute any "strange" disease that they cannot readily understand to witchcraft, the influence of supernatural forces, or personal faults of individuals or their families. Despite the lack of scientific evidence to support the claims of traditional healers, traditional healing is extremely popular in Uganda. Traditional healers are guaranteed the support and protection of their communities and pose a considerable challenge to modern health care systems that must tackle the problems of HIV/AIDS, tuberculosis, hepatitis E, malaria, diarrheal diseases, high maternal and infant mortality rates, and malnutrition. The tragedy with these health problems lies in the considerable amount of mortality, morbidity, and chronic disability associated with the health problems, with negative implications for social development, food security, human security, and the attainment of the Millennium Development Goals. Though the Ugandan government has, in principle, recognized traditional healers within the wider health care system, the process of enacting the necessary policy, regulations, and guidelines for the integration of traditional medicine into the official health care system appears to have been put on hold.

Available evidence, though limited in scope, suggests that it might not help to condemn or glorify traditional healers wholesale. While traditional healers might be seen to provide essential health care, the literature also seems to highlight the use of human sacrifice not only in the treatment and prevention of mental illness (Kasoro et al., 2002), but also for other purposes, including wealth creation and the protection of personal businesses and property. Despite the inevitable controversies that surround the practice of traditional healers, however, there are ample reasons supporting the need to integrate traditional healers into the formal health care system.

In this chapter, I describe prevailing concepts of common health problems, including mental illness among the Acholi and Madi ethnic groups in Northern Uganda. As there are several categories of alternate health care practitioners (including faith-based health practitioners, traditional surgeons, and bone-setters) in Uganda (Abbo, 2009), I limit my discussion throughout this chapter to traditional (native) health care providers who practice their trade either by providing herbs or animal products or by interceding with the spirit world on behalf of the living. I then describe the approaches to traditional health care provision, comparing these to modern health care practice. I conclude the chapter by highlighting the potential roles of traditional healers for health care provision, and propose a way forward to integrate these healers into the formal health care system.

Traditional Concepts of Mental and Neurological Disorders

Advances in the practice of psychiatry have developed through the formulation of scientific theories to explain the causation of mental illness, development of models for treatment and major mental health revolutions, and international legal reforms to protect and improve the welfare of individuals who suffer from mental health issues. Orley (1979),

Schulsinger and Jablensky (1991), Whyte (1995), Ovuga and Buga (1996), have provided cultural concepts of the aetiology of epilepsy in Uganda and Tanzania. In traditional thinking, common mental health problems (depressive illness, anxiety disorders, and alcohol use disorders) as recognized in modern medicine do not exist. In contrast, mental illness is equated with chronic deteriorating psychotic illness, which in modern medical terms refers to schizophrenia and severe affective disorders (Abbo et al., 2008). Ovuga and Boardman (2009a) have provided a model of mental illness from central Buganda in which various levels of mental health problems exist along a continuum of existential problems that culminate in death. In this formulation, transient forms of psychotic illness are all lumped together as the manifestation of spirit possession or cultural issues in human existence.

Concepts of Disease Causation

Common Taboos

The Acholi and Madi ethnic communities observe various accepted ways of leading their individual and collective lives (Ovuga & Boardman, 2009b). A major function of various taboos is to enforce uprightness in personal life in relation to the spirit world and the world of the living. For example, various taboos related to sexuality in Uganda aim to ensure fidelity and faithfulness within and outside of marriage. Among the Baganda, for instance, men are not supposed to see the used pad, a woman is not supposed to have sex when in menstruation, and a woman is not supposed to take any painkillers when in menstruation because then a woman, like in childbirth, has to withstand the pain. The Baganda also believe that a woman who is in her menstrual period is not supposed to go near the hut of the King of Buganda, as doing so would prevent her from giving birth. A female journalist had this to say about her experience on an assignment when she was in her menstrual period:

> I remember I went to do a story some time in Buddo, Nagalabi, where the kings of Buganda are enthroned and I entered one of the huts which is near the kings' chair (roots carved out as a chair) and when I walked out, the guide told me that women who are in their menstrual period are not supposed to go in there because they would never give birth. When I said I was in my period, he said it only because I did not know; otherwise, what I had done was terrible.

Menstruation is clearly shameful for most African women. It feels like walking naked. In Buganda, being naked in public is very bad and is equated to being a night dancer (sleep walker) or a witch. For Acholi warriors, abstinence from sex before going to war assures their purity from sin and contamination that aims to ensure victory in battle against the enemy.

Health taboos and related practices are many, and vary from one region of Uganda to another. In Buganda, when one is sick with *entunuka* (infection of the nail bed) the individual points the finger in the toilet/latrine as a way of treatment that is expected to magically cure the infection. When a child has measles in a home, the household does not eat meat. When someone is sick with chickenpox he/she would not be allowed leave the home till when the rashes have cleared. Among the Madi, to keep children from contracting conjunctivitis, they are not allowed to stare at strangers.

Illness Causation

Genetics and Clan History

Mental illness is believed to run in families or be related to clan history. The spirit of a mentally ill person who dies from causes related to neglect from family members becomes extremely annoyed and attacks other members of the family to draw their attention to the social responsibilities and obligations toward his/her welfare that the family ought to have provided. Thus, historically, In the past families and neighbours who lived with individuals suffering from severe mental illness never neglected their mentally ill. The mentally ill received food and drinking water wherever they went. Affected persons were left free to move about if they were not violent; those that were disturbed, violent, and destructive and posed a threat to social security and safety were tied in their huts for their own safety and that of their families and communities. If the mentally ill went missing from their homes and neighbourhoods, the communities readily searched for them, and always brought them back home.

Curse (kiir – Acholi*; ba aluka* – Madi*)*

Mental illness may be the result of a curse for wrongs committed by a member of an extended family, intended to avenge the wrong that this family member might have committed. If the offspring of an elderly individual do not respect the person concerned, the aggrieved might place a curse on the alleged ill-disciplined youths, the result of which is severe mental illness or other maladies that might even result in death unless the offender repents publicly. Curses may the take the form of an elderly woman showing her naked buttocks to a youthful offender, or a parent slapping the sole of his/her own foot in full view of everyone while chanting words of disapproval. Another example is the case of a family member who develops mental illness or epilepsy following the alleged killing of someone from another community. To avert this sort of misfortune, members of an alleged offender's family typically compensated the aggrieved community with the surrender of one of their own of the same sex and age, and performed a reconciliatory ritual.

Bad Omen

Typical rural communities scan their environments for signs of individual and collective calamity and act in time to prevent the occurrence of ills within their communities. For example, the hooting of the owl near a homestead at any time in the night was dreaded, as this was feared to bring to the community or individual families bad news of death, severe ill health among relatives, or some other catastrophe. The crowing of a cock inside a house, which is a very rare event during daytime, is an ominous sign of personal or collective calamity. The breaking off of a dry twig from an ageing tree in clear view of a passerby might signify death within the person's family network, and this might prompt the individual to seek the intervention of someone with special powers (traditional healer) to prevent the calamity from occurring.

Nyaru (In Madi; meaning a married person eating what is forbidden; read as sexual relation outside marriage)

Rural communities prescribed moral principles to guide how individual members led their daily lives. Deviation from prescribed moral principles is believed to bring a special form of illness referred to as *nyaru* that presents as physical ill health. An example of nyaru is the unexpected onset of severe illness in a family or an episode of difficult childbirth as a result of unfaithfulness by a married woman. Among the Baganda and Nyankore ethnic groups in central and western Uganda, respectively, the equivalent of nyaru is *amakiro.* Timely confession of nyaru by a woman was considered essential to the rapid resolution of illness or the successful end of labour.

Witchcraft

Mental illness or other forms of ill health may be the result of witchcraft instigated by an enemy or an envious person. The practice of witchcraft is believed to run in families and may take the form of a sleepwalking disorder or of sending evil spirits to inflict suffering on a victim. Elderly women who do not have children of their own, members of the community whose farm yield is lower than their neighbours', or those who do not have property may also face allegations of being witches. According to common belief, witches can send powerful evil spirits to cause considerable suffering in victims or lead victims to die from a variety of causes such as suicide, thunderstorms and lightning, HIV/ AIDS related causes, road traffic accidents, or any unfamiliar illness.

Spirit of the Dead

The spirit of a murder victim may attack someone from another family to avenge his or her death. Recent examples of murder victims are those who died during the recent conflict in northern Uganda. The psychotic-like behaviours seen in survivors of the recent war in northern Uganda are generally known as *cen* (spirit possession). Clinical evidence indicates that cases of cen may be diagnosed with severe anxiety states, major depressive disorder or brief reactive psychosis. The spirits of the dead may, however, possess the living from other communities in an effort to find a home among the living to seek solace from the harsh environment in which they live (Ovuga, 2005).

Satan

Mental illness may be interpreted as the God of the Land having sent Satan to punish the victim for alleged sins that he/she might have committed. Unlike in a curse, God's action in this case might also be interpreted as a message for the victim or their family to reconcile with God, or to repent and abandon their sinful ways.

Worrying

Too much worrying or too many negative thoughts may lead to chronic headache, which culminates in mental illness, referred to as the "disease of thoughts". (Okello et al, 2006)

Types of Mental Illness

Common types of mental disorder that traditional healers treat successfully include milder forms of depressive illness and milder forms of anxiety disorders. Among the Madi, at least four different forms of mental illness exist, namely mental sub-normality, anxiety disorders (*ori*), mild to moderate forms of depressive illness (*asi laza anzi rii*) and severe mental illness (*Ababa*—confused, does not know right from wrong; *Ta madi icadi ra rii*—a condition that is like mental illness, read as severe mental illness) (Ovuga, 2005). In this context, Ababa may be considered the same as Ta madi icadi ra rii and the difference between the two may be the level of severity, with the latter being more severe than the former. Abbo et al. (2009) have described two different forms of severe mental illness among the Basoga in eastern Uganda, namely schizophrenia (*Edalu*) and manic illness (*Akazoole*).

Recognition and Societal Response

The recognition of severe mental illness is based on an individual talking to, with, or under the influence of spirits. The first interpretation of spirit possession is that such a person may have found favour among the spirits and is meant to be a traditional healer. The first response is for clan elders to invite a traditional healer (*Ajwaka; Ojo*) to provide treatment and perform rituals in hopes of:

a) Reconciling the family with angry ancestral spirits or with the spirit of a departed family member;
b) Chasing away an offending and unwelcome evil spirit;
c) Restoring the health of the individual; and
d) Training the person to become a traditional healer.

Training and Diagnosis

The exact proportion of traditional healers who receive training through apprenticeship from senior traditional healers is unknown; however, 80% of traditional healers acquire their trade through personal experience of spirit possession (Ovuga, Boardman, & Oluka, 1999). A similar proportion of traditional healers claim a family history of spirit possession. Traditional healers in northern Uganda claim that they receive information about the health and personal problems of their clients and the type of treatment of their clients' problems through dreams prior to the visit of individual clients to their clinics.

Models of Traditional Health Practices

Figure 1, below, presents proposed models of traditional healing practices in northern Uganda in relation to how rural communities in northern Uganda perceive and explain poor health among them. Essentially, the models indicate that traditional healers provide interventions at four different levels, namely: biomedical models (herbs and or animal parts); traditional psychotherapy or counselling; intercession with the spirit world; and healing human relationships (akin to social casework).

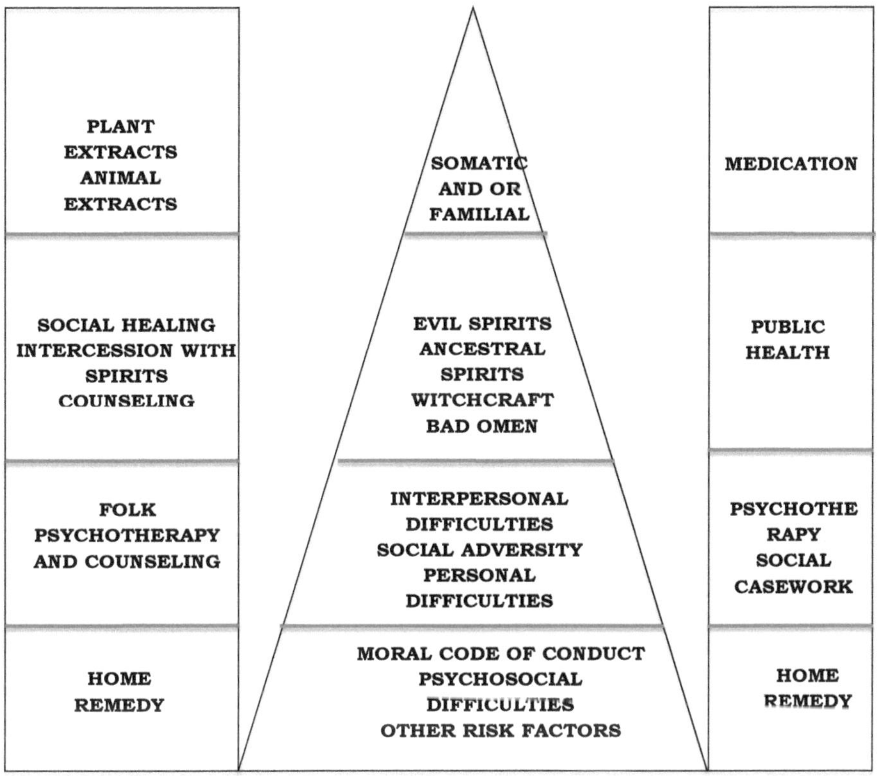

Figure 1 above.

Biomedical Model

Traditional healers may provide herbs and/or animal parts through scarification, sniffing, in suspensions or as solutions for the patient to drink and/or bathe in, or through fumigations to control fever or expel evil spirits. Plant pieces or animal parts may be worn as bracelets, bangles, or necklaces; sometimes these plants and animal products are planted in the doorway to protect young infants and other family members from various forms of disease and from the influence of evil spirits.

Traditional Psychotherapy/Counseling

The first source of help in rural communities is the world of family, relatives, and close friends. In rural communities, individuals share personal experiences, fears, hopes, successes, failures, and problems (Ovuga & Boardman, 2009a). In this context, family, elders, and/or friends provide emotional support and morale in confronting personal problems, giving advice and encouragement in the face of personal adversity.

Intercession with the Spirit World

If family and clan elders interpret the nature of someone's ill health as being the result of the supernatural forces, they may seek explanations from traditional healers. Traditional healers invariably invoke poor human relations between ill persons and the rest of their family members, or with the rest of their community. Spirits almost always feature as vehicles of ill health, as they would like to see that members of the living lead morally upright lives on earth, in harmony with each other. Traditional healers play the role of interceding with social foes or the spirit world on behalf of the sick to restore and maintain health, and prevent ill health.

Healing Social Wounds

As traditional healers usually live in the same communities as their prospective clients, they have inside knowledge of the social problems in the homes of their clients. A personal history of transient psychosis in a traditional healer places the healer in a special position of authority that enhances their interpretation of the sources of ill health. This special authority bestows upon traditional healers the ability to point out the possible interpersonal difficulties between their clients and the rest of their family as likely causes of illness.

Treatment

Traditional healers treat mental illness using:

a. Herbs, which may be applied through scarifications, orally, or by using steam that the individual inhales for a period of three days if the patient is male or four days if female, aimed to cast out evil spirits.
b. Performance of rituals, which involves the slaughter of animals aimed to appease ancestral spirits, to give a home to homeless spirits, or to cast out evil spirits.

Animal Sacrifice

The mode of action for rituals as a form of treatment in the alleviation of illness or the prevention of misfortunes is not known. It is possible that clients gain relief from their distress through complex psychological and physiological processes involving the hypothalamic-pituitary-adrenal-axis. Relief through placebo effects is also likely. Explanations provided by traditional healers for the efficacy of rituals involving animal sacrifice appear to point to the spirits' desire for human blood to satisfy their thirst and hunger. Traditional healers sacrifice animals to reconcile aggrieved spirits with their living kin or to substitute for human blood, and smear the blood and offal of the sacrificed animal on the body of the ill person to enable the possessing spirit to leave the victim. An Acholi traditional healer described the process of animal sacrifice as follows:

> Under the influence of the spirit the sick person runs round his/her village carrying the animal on the head. When exhausted from running around, the sick person falls to the ground in his/her home if he/she likes the possessing spirit. The traditional healer immediately slaughters the animal on the spot, where the animal is prepared and then consumed by the patient, his/her family, and community; the traditional healer then invites the possessing spirit to the home of the patient where a hut is constructed for him/her. However, if the possessing spirit is evil and the patient does not like it, the patient will run out of and far away from the village. Where the patient falls to the ground is where the traditional healer slaughters the animal. After the traditional healer casts out the evil spirit, the animal is left for vultures and wild animals to consume; no one in the family or community is allowed to consume that animal, as doing so might invite the evil spirit to the victim's home.

Duration

In most cases of mental illness that traditional healers treat, the problem resolves more or less permanently, permitting the person to carry on with their lives like anyone else in their community. In the case of fevers, body pains and aches, herbs or animal extracts in accurate doses for the correct malady may bring about immediate relief for reasonable periods of time. The following example illustrates a success story of how village elders successfully treated intractable and life-threatening diarrhoea that complicated an episode of measles in a 10-year-old boy.

> A 10-year-old boy suffered from severe measles that debilitated him severely when diarrhoea developed. As the illness progressed, village elders and herbalists reviewed the boy's health daily and consulted among themselves. Various forms of plant and grass roots failed to improve the boy's health. However, when the elders considered that it was time to control the boy's debilitating diarrhoea following the 'appearance of the (external) signs' of measles, they ordered red-hot charcoal and steaming water in a large calabash at about 4 p.m. The leader of the elders threw the

charcoal into the steaming water, and then he removed the large particle from the water, and gave the hot water to the ailing boy to drink as it was, with the ashes and small particles from the charcoal. The theory behind this was for the hot water to wash out the poison of measles from the stomach. Immediately thereafter, the eldest woman in the village bathed the boy with the rest of the water. The result was dramatic; the diarrhoea ceased and the boy was up playing the following day. *[Note: This treatment of diarrhoea by the rural elders was akin to using charcoal tablets in the symptomatic control of non-bacterial diarrhoea.]*

If treatment by an Ajwaka (Acholi) or Ojo (Madi) fails, this is usually interpreted to mean that the spirits that have taken hold of the person are just too powerful to manage, and he/she is left to deal with the sickness or possession (Ovuga & Boardman, 2009a), as we often see on the streets or on our roads.

Limitations of Traditional Healing Practices

The main criticism of traditional healing is the lack of theories and empirical evidence to back their practice—theories and evidence that would otherwise be subjected to scientific verification. However, traditional healers may further be criticized for being unable to control the purity of their plant and animal extracts and for being too secretive over the sharing of their knowledge and experience with modern health care providers. A more serious criticism of traditional healers, particularly those in the central region of Uganda, concerns the unending problem of human sacrifice. Despite these problems, Abbo et al. (2009) have produced evidence of the success of traditional healers in effecting relief from emotional distress due to certain forms of severe mental health problems within only three months.

Conclusion: Collaboration with Traditional Healers

Under the circumstances, it might be prudent to take a middle course and encourage good practices, discourage harmful practices, and tolerate traditional healers practices that are neither beneficial nor harmful. Beneficial collaboration with traditional healers based on this principle might require: a) cultivating trusting relationships with traditional healers; b) teaching traditional healers safe health care practices; c) expanding research with traditional healers on traditional healing practices; d) implementing public mental health education and awareness of treatments and preventive strategies against preventable illnesses; and, e) enacting policy, regulations, and guidelines to support collaboration with traditional healers.

In this spirit, the author of this chapter has established initial contact with traditional healers in the Acholi sub-region of northern Uganda, aiming to create a trusting relationship between the traditional healers and the Faculty of Medicine. The goal of this initiative is to eventually involve traditional healers in joint research ventures with researchers from Gulu University. It is our hope at the faculty that traditional healers will participate in joint efforts with the faculty in the control of infectious diseases, the prevention of common ailments that communities can take responsibility for, and the promotion of population health.

References

Abbo, C. (2009). *Profiles and outcomes of traditional healing practices in two districts in Uganda.* Unpublished doctoral dissertation. Karolinska Institute, Stockholm.

Abbo, C., Ekblad, S., Waako, P., Okello, E., & Musisi, S. (2009). The prevalence and severity of mental illnesses handled by traditional healers in two districts of Uganda. *African Health Sciences, 9*(S2), 16-22.

Abbo, C., Okello, E., Ekblad, S., Waako, P., & Musisi, S. (2008). Lay concepts of psychosis in Busoga, Eastern Uganda: A pilot study. *World Cultural Psychiatry Research Review, 3*(3), 132-145.

Kasoro, S., Sebudde, S., Kabagame-Rugamba, E., Ovuga E., & Boardman, J. (2002). Mental illness in one district in Uganda. *International Journal of Social Psychiatry, 48*(1), 29-37.

Kohn, R., Saxena, S., Levav, I., & Saraceno, B. (2004). The treatment gap in mental health care. *Bulletin of the World Health Organization, 82,* 858-866.

Okello, S. E., & Musisi, S. (2006). Depression as a clan illness (eByekika): An Indigenous model of psychotic depression among the Baganda of Uganda. *World Cultural Psychiatry Research Review, 1*(2), 60-73.

Orley J. (1970). Culture and mental illness: A study from Uganda, Nairobi, East African Publishing House, 1970.

Ovuga, E. (2005). Depression and Suicidal Behaviour in Uganda. PhD Thesis, Karolinska Institute and Makerere University, 2005

Ovuga, E., & Buga, J.W. (1996). *Epilepsy.* Makerere University Press

Ovuga, E., Boardman, J., & Oluka, G. A. O. (1999). Traditional healers and mental illness in Uganda. *Psychiatric Bulletin, 23,* 276-279.

_____. (2009a). The role of religion and different traditions in Uganda. In D. Wasserman & C. Wasserman (Eds.), *Oxford textbook of suicidology and suicide prevention: A global perspective (part 1, section 11).* London: Oxford University Press.

_____. (2009b). Prevention of suicide from the public health strategy: How to build suicide prevention in countries without such a tradition. In D. Wasserman & C. Wasserman (Eds.), *Oxford Textbook of Suicidology and Suicide Prevention: A global perspective* (part viii). London: Oxford University Press.

Schulsinger, F., & Jablensky, A. (Eds.). (1991). The national mental health programme in the United Republic of Tanzania: A report from the WHO and DANIDA, *Acta Psychiatrica Scandinavica (Supplementum), No. 364*, 83, 7-132.

Thornicroft, G. (2004, September 8). Most people with mental illness are not treated. *The Lancet, 370,* 807. Retrieved from http://www.thelancet.com.

Weissman, M.M.; Roger C. Bland,R.,; Canino,G.J; Faravelli, C.,; Greenwald, S; Hai-Gwo Hwu, H.G; Peter R. Joyce, P.R; Eile G. Karam., E.G; Lee, C.K; Lellouch, J; Lépine, J.P;. Newman, S.C; Rubio-Stipec, M; Wells, J.E,; Wickramaratne, P.J.; Hans-Ulrich Wittchen, H.U; Yeh, E.K. Cross-National Epidemiology of Major Depression and Bipolar Disorder, JAMA. 1996;276(4):293-299. doi:10.1001/jama.1996.03540040037030.

Whyte, R. S. (1995). Constructing epilepsy: Images and contexts in East Africa. In B. Ingstad & R. S. Whyte (Eds.), *Disability and culture* (pp. 226-245). Berkeley: University of California Press.

Chapter Nine

HEALING PSYCHOSOCIAL TRAUMA IN SOCIETIES RECOVERING FROM MASSIVE VIOLENCE: THE CASE OF RWANDA

Regine King and Izumi Sakamoto

Abstract

Wars and genocides have devastating consequences on individual and community psychosocial well-being (Lumsden, 1997). In 1994, an estimated 800,000 Tutsi were murdered in Rwanda by their Hutu neighbours. Rwandans were subject to physical and emotional cruelty such as rape and coerced participation in the murder of loved ones. The victims, often known to the killers, were murdered in public spaces (Des Forges, 1999). Different aspects of life die alongside people in a genocide. In addition to the experienced traumatic events, norms, morals and social networks that supported Rwandans were also severely damaged (Almedom, 2004). Psychosocial programs initiated by international organizations in Rwanda often focused on individual trauma-based models. These models are often criticized for lacking cultural sensitivity, being too individualistic, narrow, and inappropriate to post-conflict non-Western conditions, and more importantly, for overlooking local coping mechanisms (Pedersen, 2002). Trauma-based models contrast with traditional African cultures, which encourage shared observance of rituals to counter suffering and generate a sense of certainty and familiarity in community (Healey & Sybertz, 1996). Although the affected people always seek to restore their psychosocial well-being (Draguns, Gielen, & Fish, 2004), their efforts are often hindered not only by political and economic struggles, but also by ruling governments and humanitarian organizations that impose and legitimate certain intervention models and disregard others. Locally-initiated approaches often remain undocumented and understudied. In this paper, I suggest a framework of healing psychosocial trauma resulting from massive violence based on the existing literature and on my personal experience of living and working in post-genocide Rwanda.

Introduction

Over the last two decades, psychosocial interventions in post-conflict situations have been scarce and the little literature that exists has been dominated by models that were conceived and assessed in relatively peaceful Western societies. This chapter examines ways in which psychosocial models can be integrated into the existing local coping mechanisms of non-Western societies. Over the years, it has been argued that Western approaches to mental illness have failed to address issues of Africans on their home continent and among immigrant communities in the West. This is in part due to different conceptualizations of mental illness and to the neglect of studying preventive and curative approaches embedded in the local cultures across the continent. In many African societies, psychosocial well-being has been maintained through group rituals and healing processes that involve family, friends, and community, with the support of traditional healers. These Indigenous methods were weakened by colonialism and by the perception that Western theories and therapies were superior to local coping mechanisms. In more recent years, the traditional healing rituals and practices that survived colonialism have been further damaged by the HIV/AIDS pandemic, interethnic conflicts, and genocides that continue today. African approaches to mental and social distress have been challenged not only by the complexity of the issues at hand but also by the destruction of the socio-cultural structures that were used to solve conflict, heal emotional wounds, and re-establish stability. The present psychosocial issues encountered in many African post-conflict situations exceed the capacity of Indigenous approaches. However, this does not mean that the preferred solution is to replace them with individualistic and trauma-based models imported from the west. We submit that there is an urgent need to integrate effective practices of Western psychosocial models into traditional approaches in order to effectively address mental health issues in Africa. An appreciation of the socio-cultural and political context of the society in which programs are implemented is crucial to the conceptualization of successful psychosocial interventions. This chapter focuses on the case of post-genocide Rwanda to critically analyze the challenges and possibilities of psychosocial programs in post-conflict situations and to emphasize the need for contextualized models. After the introduction, the chapter will be composed of three main sections: (1) challenges and possibilities of healing psychosocial trauma in non-Western post-conflict societies, (2) psychological and psychosocial trauma, and (3) promoting healing.

Challenges and Possibilities of Healing Psychosocial Trauma in Non-Western Post-Conflict Societies: The Case of Post-Genocide Rwanda

The main part of this chapter is based on the first author's (King) ongoing doctoral dissertation research. Her supervisor (Sakamoto) is the second author for the edition and contributes commentary to the chapter to bring King's research into the broader context of social work research. Psychosocial healing programs in post-conflict situations are relatively rare. A few existing programs utilize models imported from Western societies, which were conceived of and assessed in relatively peaceful and fundamentally dissimilar places. These programs are often criticized for disregarding local approaches and lacking systematic monitoring and evaluation. On the other hand, local models, often known as 'traditional coping mechanisms,' frequently lack documentation, are understudied and undervalued. It is generally agreed that people of all cultures have the ability to overcome adversity. It is, however, questionable whether or not local existing coping practices in relatively peaceful non-Western societies can address psychosocial trauma that results from massive violence and genocide.

In this chapter, we argue that neither Western models nor local coping approaches alone are sufficient to restore the psychosocial well-being of individuals and communities in contemporary post-conflict societies. There is need to identify, document and systematically assess more contextualized models which integrate best practices in mental health programs in order to address the staggering levels of psychosocial trauma resulting from massive violence. From a structural violence framework, we utilize the case of the Tutsi genocide in Rwanda to demonstrate the complexity surrounding psychosocial trauma and the limitations of existing Western and non-Western models. We conclude the chapter with a description and preliminary observations of a study on a community-based mental health model initiated in post-genocide Rwanda, the Healing of Individual Emotional Wounds and Community Reconstruction (HIEWCR). The model combines traditional Rwandan practices and Western therapeutic techniques.

Healing Psychosocial Trauma in Post-Conflict Situations

Wars and genocides have a devastating impact on the psychosocial well-being of individuals and entire communities (Lumsden, 1997). Investigations done in post-conflict areas have shown that war and violence cause serious psychological and social damage to individuals and their communities (Métraux, 2004). War survivors in places as diverse as Sierra Leone, Bosnia, and El Salvador reveal feelings of hopelessness, low self-esteem, and the normalization of dehumanized social relationships (Carballo et al., 2004). High levels of depression and trauma-related symptoms have been observed among civilian survivors of violence (Abramowitz, 2005; Bolton et al., 2002). When not carefully assessed and addressed, these issues lead to the continued mental health deterioration of individuals and communities (Pupavac, 2004).

In stark contrast to the massive financial investment in the reconstruction of infrastructure and social institutions, there are scarce resources for programs designated to address psychosocial trauma in post-conflict non-Western countries. The existing psychosocial interventions are often implemented by international Non-Governmental Organizations (NGOs) with access to Western funding. These organizations tend to apply individual trauma-based models that were conceived and assessed in relatively peaceful Western societies. Although these programs may be implemented with good intentions, they are often criticized for being inappropriate and for undermining local coping mechanisms and practices (Kleinman & Kleinman, 1997). Such models usually focus on the needs of the individual without paying broader attention to collective needs, and tend to have time-limited mandates.

Imposing individual psychological models as a panacea in non-Western settings (Pedersen, Tremblay, Errázuriz, & Gamarra, 2008) prevents local people from transforming personal stories of suffering into healing narratives within affected communities (Papadopolous, 1998). It is often argued that, in situations of adversity, people of all backgrounds seek avenues to restore physical health, promote psychological and social well-being, and achieve spiritual serenity (Draguns, Gielen, & Fish, 2004). In societies destroyed by massive violence and ongoing economic struggles, these local capacities are weakened by policies of ruling governments and humanitarian interventions that place a priority on restoring material infrastructure and legitimatize certain forms of psychosocial intervention at the expense of others (Alexander, Eyerman, Giesen, Smelser, & Sztompka, 2004). Local people have little say in the conceptualization and implementation of such programs. More importantly, the implemented models lack systematic evaluation in terms of health outcomes and their overall impact on the quality of life and well-being of people (Pedersen et al., 2008).

On the other hand, it is questionable whether local coping mechanisms adopted in stable and normal conditions are sufficient to deal with psychosocial trauma after massive violence. In this chapter, local coping mechanisms or practices mean healing processes that ordinary people of non-Western societies, and of Africa in particular, put in place to overcome adversity through a mutually caring network of family, friends, and community. Such practices bind community members together and ensure their protection during difficult times of loss. In times of death for instance, neighbours and friends participate in mourning rituals in order to fully reintegrate the grieved people back into daily functioning. In this context, healing means the restoration of the mental well-being of individuals with the support of community through a shared experience of performed practices and symbolized rituals.

However, this sense of belonging and mutual caring is often absent in times of massive violence. This is particularly significant when members of the same communities inflict suffering. Those targeted by violence are usually running for their lives. After violence has stopped, survivors are frequently overwhelmed—not only by the traumatic event of violence but also by the loss of loved ones. Their grief is intensified by isolation and a lack of support from other community members. Situations like these require the creation of new strategies that may be rooted in the past, but are restructured to adapt to the new realities of post-conflict situations. The imposition of imported models and the failure to recognize these more contextualized approaches may complicate the healing of individual emotional wounds and the rebuilding of shattered communities.

The inability to overcome adversity and restore psychosocial well-being is well represented in Edkins' (2003) definition of trauma. This author postulates that people become traumatized when the powers that are supposed to protect and provide them with security become their tormentors, when their community turns against them, or when their family dwelling is no longer a place of refuge. This definition helps us to understand the complexity of such trauma, both at the individual and social levels. The term "psychosocial trauma," commonly utilized by scholars, who examine the impact of massive violence from a structural violence framework, is more appropriate in this context.

The structural violence framework enables the reader to understand the issues at stake when violence erupts within a collective social setting. It points toward a multiple dimensional perspective of psychosocial trauma and the need to restore the well-being of individuals and communities at different levels. In the following section, we provide a brief explanation of psychosocial trauma from a structural violence framework.

Structural Violence and Psychosocial Trauma

The term "structural violence" was originally used by Johan Galtung (1969) to denote "a form of violence which corresponds with the systematic ways in which a given social structure or social institution kills people slowly by preventing them from meeting their basic needs" (p. 169) and maintaining their psychosocial well-being. Structural violence exists in social structures characterized by extreme poverty, inequality, exploitation, and other forms of social marginalization (Farmer, 2004; Galtung, 2001; Uvin, 1998). Structural violence, embedded in systems of dominance and observed in socio-cultural, economic, legal, and political institutions (Christie, Wagner, & Winter, 2001), ranges in a continuum from indirect to direct violence. The internalization and normalization of violence in society often leads to the eruption of acute violence such as interpersonal, group, and state-sponsored violence.

Structural violence is contextualized to each historical and social setting. Recent forms of massive violence in different parts of Africa and elsewhere have their roots in the legacy of colonialism (Ganguly & Taras, 2006). Colonial rule destroyed local social structures through military power, economic exploitation, and cultural subordination. European culture and forms of government were regarded as superior while the culture and government of the colonies were classified as primitive and backward (Anghie, 2002). Thus, the experience of colonial oppression had severe psychosocial impacts on many African communities and societies.

Historical trauma is a theme that requires ongoing research in the former colonies. Attempts have been made to explore the psychological impact of colonialism among Aboriginal people in North America and Australia. The system of removing children from their families and communities and the resulting loss of cultural heritage have been at the base of the social and psychological destruction of colonialism. The impact of the social, economic, and political abuses of colonialism, or the accentuation of the patterns of inequality and exclusion characterizing many post-colonial states, remains largely unknown. However, we concur with Farmer (2005) that people who struggle to survive under a perpetual state of anxiety or terror experience psychological and social distress that may negatively affect their mental well-being. Indirect violence results in emotions of pain, grief, and fear that are often mixed with feelings of anger, betrayal of trust, frustration, and desires for revenge (Edkins, 2003; Fierke, 2004; Hutchison & Bleiker, 2008). These feelings often motivate actions of acute violence against other people. In the following section, we utilize a structural violence framework to examine the case of Rwanda, providing the highlights of factors that led to the 1994 Tutsi Rwandan genocide as well as its subsequent psychosocial consequences.

Geopolitical and Historical Description of Rwanda

Rwanda is a small, mountainous, landlocked country located in central-east Africa. It spans 26,336 square kilometres and is bordered by Uganda in the north, Tanzania in the east, Burundi in the south, and the Democratic Republic of Congo, formerly known as Zaire, in the west. The country's economic livelihood largely depends on agricultural production and its main foreign currency is generated from the exportation of coffee and tea, and gorilla tourism. Rwanda's population is comprised of three ethnic groups: the Hutu, the Tutsi, and the Twa, whose representation in the 1930s was estimated to be 84%, 15%, and 1%, respectively (Des Forges & Longman, 2004). To this day, these groups continue to live intermingled in the same communities where they speak the same language and share the same cultural rituals and practices.

The history of Rwanda can be divided into four main political periods: (1) pre-colonial (before 1900), a period during which Rwanda was governed by a hereditary monarchy from the Nyiginya and Abega clans of the Tutsi group; (2) colonial (1900-1961), a period during which Rwanda remained a Tutsi-governed monarchy, but was under the colonial rule of Germans at the beginning of the 20th century and of the Belgians after World War I; (3) post-independence (1961-1994), an era during which the country became a republic and was governed by two successive Hutu presidents until the eruption of the 1994 Tutsi genocide; and (4) post-genocide, a period of many challenges, including psychosocial trauma, resulting from the genocide.

There are two main schools of thought about the historical evolution of Rwandan society, and they stand in contradiction to one another. The first perspective asserts that the Tutsi and Hutu were socio-economic groups that co-habited Rwanda in relative symbiosis and harmony for centuries (Newbury, 1998). The boundary between the Hutu and Tutsi was economic and fluid. Overdulve (1997) attributes the tensions in social relations to the expansion of the territorial rule of the Nyinginya (Tutsi) kingdom, which consolidated its power by accumulating wealth during the 19th century through the exploitation of the lower classes.

The second perspective proposes that ethnic groups in Rwanda were never cohesive and peaceful (Logiest, 1988; Lugan, 1997). This explanation purports that the Twa first occupied Rwanda as hunters. They were later followed by Hutus, a segment of the Bantu people who settled in communities and cultivated the soil. This perspective maintains that the Tutsi were the last group that entered Rwanda from regions of the Nile, and used military power and cattle to disrupt the peaceful communities they found in Rwanda. This version of history is based on the European colonial theory that the Tutsi were a Hamitic group superior to other Bantu ethnic groups. The colonial administration used this narrative to favour the Tutsi elite. However, it was turned against all Tutsi when the Hutu independence movement categorized them as foreign invaders and not legitimate Rwandan citizens. This ideology became the basis for the 1959 revolution and the violent outbreaks against the Tutsi that culminated in Tutsi genocide in 1994.

Mamdani (2001), a Ugandan researcher and scholar, defines the 1959 revolution as the turning point in the geopolitics and history of Rwanda because it nationalized discriminatory policies by building on "bipolar racial identities" (p. 35). These racial identities had been established by the Belgian colonial administration in the 1930s when they introduced a discriminatory system of identity cards for the three groups living in Rwanda based on body features and number of cows owned by a family unit. As Mamdani (2001) comments, the identities of the Tutsi and Hutu were permanently frozen (p. 101), and the narratives of communal solidarity were silenced.

These divisions were hardened by the proclamation of independence on July 1st, 1962, and the subsequent policies of the two Hutu-led republics. For the first Hutu government, more than formally ending Belgian colonization, independence meant abolishing the memory of the Tutsi kingdom. Their ideological orientation resulted in violence against the Tutsi. Houses were burned and Tutsi were killed or forced into exile. Between 1959 and 1963, an estimated 200,000 Rwandan Tutsi fled to the neighbouring countries of Burundi, Uganda, Tanzania, and the former Zaire, now known as the Democratic Republic of Congo. They became the first UNHCR refugee group linked with the decolonization process in the Great Lakes Region of Africa (Kuperman, 2001). The Tutsi who remained in the country were defined as aliens and unwanted invaders. Their presence was tolerated on the condition that they remain outside of the country's political life (Mamdani, 2001). However, national politics consistently pushed them to the center of discriminatory policies.

During the second republic (1973-1994), the basic identity of the Tutsi shifted from that of unwanted foreigners to expendable Rwandan citizens. Tutsi people could participate in civil and political life under new conditions that restricted their representation through a control system of quotas. Publicly, the quota system was explained as a means "to redress the grievances of a hitherto oppressed majority"—the Hutu (Mamdani, 1996, p. 17). The legalization of the Tutsi as a national ethnic group actually helped the government exercise tighter control of the Tutsi in all sectors of life. Passports were restricted, university education was limited, Hutu males in higher bureaucratic and military positions were banned from marrying Tutsi women, and Tutsi refugees were denied return on the basis that the country was full and there was no space for them. Post-colonial Rwanda was characterized by normalized discriminatory policies, both written and unwritten. These policies and practices often silenced the voices of Hutu and Tutsi people who lived side by side in the same communities.

Although one could argue that people in communities continued to express solidarity in times of major events such as death, birth, and weddings, the underlying ethnic tensions were never discussed or addressed as important social issues in civil society or in the political life of the country. During colonialism, the Tutsi elite received privileges from the colonial state on the condition that they help impose forced labour, using physical abuse as discipline, to support colonial projects. During and after independence, the homes of the Tutsi were burned and families were forced to leave the country or relocate to inhospitable areas. The Hutu members of the same communities watched passively or actively participated in such violent actions without remorse. In 1973, a number of Tutsi intellectuals were fired from their jobs and students expelled from schools. While Hutu families rose in groups to defend some Hutu students who were mistaken as Tutsi, they were silent regarding the violence inflicted against their Tutsi neighbours. After such occasional outbreaks of violence, however, the Hutu and Tutsi went on with their lives as if nothing had ever happened. Ethnic-based violence became a normalized way of life. Rwandan communities failed to create constructive ways to overcome state sponsored enmity. Many people were intimidated into silence and passivity. The Hutu-Tutsi categories and the structural violence that characterized their relationships became the foundation of a dangerous ideology that eventually erupted into war and genocide.

Over the course of only 100 days in 1994, an estimated 800,000 Tutsi people were murdered by their Hutu neighbours in a government-sponsored genocide (Melvern, 2004). The Tutsi genocide is infamous for its efficiency and intimacy in the killing of neighbours and even family members who had intermarried. Rwandans were subject to acts of physical and emotional cruelty such as rape, coerced participation in the murder of loved ones, and forced displacement from their communities. HIV was utilized as a secondary weapon to slowly kill those who might survive.

The 1994 Tutsi genocide was possible because of the history of systemic oppression and dehumanization that normalized different patterns of abuse and granted impunity. The genocide resulted in the deterioration and deep disruption of the remaining social systems that had previously helped to alleviate suffering. Murders took place in public spaces such as churches and government buildings. Two-thirds of the Tutsi population and some moderate Hutus were killed. In many instances, the victims were known to the killers.

During the genocide, an estimated 250,000 to 500,000 women were raped (de Brouwer, Ka Hon Chu, & Muscati, 2009) and a large number of them were infected with HIV/AIDS (Kayitesi-Blewitt, 2006). After the genocide, more than 13% of Rwandan households were headed by orphans as young as 10 years of age (Human Rights Watch, 2003). A wave of approximately one million Tutsi refugees from different continents returned to Rwanda without any support of the UNHCR after more than three decades of life in refugee camps in foreign countries. Over two million Hutus fled the country after the former government's propaganda instilled fear about the potential reprisal of the Rwandan Patriotic Front (RPF) troops, the army that stopped the genocide. The vast majority of these Hutu refugees returned to Rwanda after two years in refugee camps, where many people were subjected to internal violence. By 1996, Rwanda had more than 120,000 prisoners accused of genocide crimes. The Tutsi survivors, many of whom were the sole living members of their families, lived in isolation and extreme poverty with the haunting memories of the experiences of the genocide (Hatzfeld, 2005). However, both groups continued to live side by side in the same communities.

The psychosocial issues surrounding the Tutsi genocide profoundly damaged the mental well-being of individuals and communities. People who survive extreme forms of violence live in a state of mental chaos (Gasibirege, 2009) and lack sufficient words to describe the abyss between the time before and after the traumatic event (Gobodo-Madikizela & Van der Merwe, 2007). Violent experiences destroy both internal and external feelings of continuity and order which cannot be re-established without consideration of the different dimensions affected by violence.

Psychosocial trauma is a social problem that needs to be treated within the social world or contexts in which the violence occurred (Martín-Baró, 1994; Summerfield, 1999). This requires approaches that give voice to those who are silenced and that address the needs of individuals and communities simultaneously. Thus far, existing models in stable and peaceful societies, such as individual trauma-based models from the West and pre-existing local coping mechanisms, are of limited value. Priority must be given to programs that consider contributory factors to violence and combine therapeutic models and practices that pay attention to the emotional needs of individuals and the rebuilding of healthy communities. Such programs require contextual conceptualization and implementation, and systematic monitoring and evaluation. In the following section, we offer a brief description of such a model of intervention.

The Healing of Individual and Emotional Wounds and Community Reconstruction (HIEWCR) Model

Historical Evolution of the Model

The Healing of Individual and Emotional Wounds and Community Reconstruction (HIEWCR) Model was introduced in Rwanda in 1995 under the name of "Personal Development Workshops" (PDWs) by a Rwandan, Dr. Simon Gasibirege. His initial goal was to heal the emotional and psychological wounds of individual survivors of the Tutsi genocide. Soon, he realized that many Rwandans, both Tutsi and Hutu, had experienced traumatic events that required urgent intervention. He started facilitating the PDWs for professionals who interacted with groups of people (e.g., teachers, social workers, and nurses) with the aim that they would in turn help others in their respective communities. The model included staff and/or beneficiaries of different international and local NGOs such as World Vision Rwanda, Avega (genocide widows' association), members of various religious groups, and some government institutions such as universities and prisons. From the list of graduating participants, a selected group received training as instructors with the objective of multiplying the number of facilitators who could later utilize the model.

Over the last decade, Dr. Gasibirege and the trained facilitators from different organizations have adapted a model that suits the needs of different groups such as widows, prisoners, orphans, ex-prisoners, and survivors. Many participants anecdotally reported benefiting from these healing workshops and recommended extending the model to other Rwandan communities. Based on his observations and evaluations, Dr. Gasibirege introduced a second phase to the healing workshops. The focus moved to therapeutic actions at the grassroots levels of community in order to help people who live in close proximity to become agents of change in their villages through mutual healing and support.

The second phase included the creation of healing spaces in two pilot areas. The first location, called the Center for Healing Life Wounds, is found in a rural community in the southern province. The other centre, known as the Promotion of Community Mental Health, is on the outskirts of the capital city of Kigali. Participants invited to the healing process are expected to address their own psychological and emotional wounds and to potentially act as agents in repairing the damaged social fabric of their communities.

Healing workshops organized in different categories are conducted by a trained community facilitator with the voluntary participation of community members. Those who need further follow-up are accompanied by a psychosocial animator appointed to do outreach and home visits. The implementation of the model combines Western therapeutic techniques and skills and Rwandan coping mechanisms to address the individual and collective wounds of participants, an approach reflected in the name of the model, the Healing of Individual Emotional Wounds and Community Reconstruction (HIEWCR).

The HIEWCR model is still evolving. In its early stages, the founder of the model and the trained facilitators implemented the HIEWCR workshops. As the program expanded, it integrated the work of trained volunteers who cared for those most vulnerable in their respective communities, such as orphaned children and widows. Following recommendations from the graduates of the second phase and in keeping with the national goal to fight against domestic violence, a recent innovation has been the integration of couples into the program. The family unit, represented by each couple, is considered to be the foundation of mutual support and agency for improved mental health in communities.

Key Components of the HIEWCR Model

The HIEWCR consists of sensitization sessions and in-depth healing workshops for groups of individuals and couple participants.

a. *Sensitization Session*

The HIEWCR sensitization session consists of raising awareness about psychosocial wounds among Rwandan individuals, families, and communities. Initially, Gasibirege employed a single day for an information session. In the second phase, this was expanded to a three-day session organized to discuss psychosocial issues through a projective method that utilizes drawings. Participants are invited to observe and reflect on these drawings and assess related issues in their own lives. Individuals who express the desire to further explore their issues are encouraged to participate in an in-depth healing process. Further, participants who express the need to address domestic-related issues are encouraged to participate in the model designed for couples.

b. *The HIEWCR: An In-depth Healing Process*

The actual workshops comprise three modules: (a) living and sharing the bereavement process; (b) dealing with emotions; and (c) forgiveness and reconciliation. Each module includes plenary psycho-education presentations and a series of small group activities during which participants share their experiences. These modules were initially conducted in three-day sessions. However, they were expanded to five days in the second phase of implementation. Time for the workshops was increased based on observations that as the years passed, psychosocial trauma has evolved into a very complex phenomenon characterized by increased domestic abuse, uncontrollable traumatic crises, and heightened ethnic tensions associated with the *gacaca* community courts.

Gacaca, which literally means "grass" in the Kinyarwanda language, is a modification of a traditional Rwandan justice mechanism for dispute resolution. This model was renewed and introduced in 2002 as a form of truth commission to judge cases of thousands of genocide suspects. Gacaca increased psychosocial distress and traumatic breakdowns as genocide perpetrators who had confessed their wrongdoings were returned into their communities. The traumatizing testimonies during gacaca hearings were made without sufficient psychological preparation or follow-up for members of different communities.

The first session of the HIEWCR on bereavement helps people to mourn the multiple losses experienced before, during, and after the 1994 genocide. The second session deals with the deep and varied emotions that come out during the bereavement session. The third session on forgiveness and reconciliation helps people to discover ways to live at peace with themselves, others in the community, and their social environment, and to initiate reconciliatory actions.

c. *Couples' Healing Workshops*

Couples' workshops consist of a five-day session that examines the problems faced by couples and helps them to manage their own emotional wounds as well as those found in their families and communities. The participants, with the support of a facilitator, explore issues related to gender-based violence rooted in the socio-cultural structures of the Rwandan communities. People who complete the couples' healing workshops are invited to identify at least three other couples in their respective communities who may benefit from the same workshops and find ways to invite them to the next sessions.

Group Composition and Process of the HIEWCR Model

All modules are conducted in a group setting using both large and small group activities. The groups are formed to deliberately create heterogeneity in ethnicity, gender, and age. Participants are required to set up guidelines constituting a safe space for them to share their stories in a more authentic manner. This exercise allows them to think about and share their individual expectations, concerns, and ways to reach their objectives.

Individual participants are allowed to express their opinions verbally or artistically, and they are often supported when group participation is requested. Members of small groups first do the exercise individually, and then share their answers with others orally through storytelling and listening. The process encourages participants to move at their own pace and share their stories according to their own perspectives. In order to benefit from the workshops, participants are urged to pay attention to their own needs and those of others, and share as much as they can. With the exception of the sensitization sessions, other modules are conducted in a residential setting, which offers time and space for participants to bond and interact outside of the group.

Some General Observations about the HIEWCR Model and Concluding Remarks

This section provides a few remarks from an ongoing data analysis of a qualitative case study the first author (King) of this chapter collected in Rwanda from January to April, 2010, under the supervision of the second author (Sakamoto). The data consists of pre- and post-intervention in-depth interviews, notes from participant observation, audio-recordings from the HIEWCR workshops, documents including HIEWCR workshop materials, internal evaluation reports about the model, and data obtained from concept mapping techniques with facilitators who have used the HIEWCR model. Far from a complete analysis of the collected data, the following lines offer a few general observations from notes taken during the HIEWCR intervention.

Participants who are initially hesitant to interact with a person from a different ethnic background report a breakthrough in realizing that they are not the only ones who suffered loss. Anecdotal stories from Rwandans and research findings with survivors and perpetrators show that many Rwandans chose silence or superficial accounts in regard to private life stories (Hatzfeld, 2009). The realization of shared suffering may be the beginning of compassion between persons who would not otherwise choose to interact at a social level.

The sharing of personal experiences takes place in small groups. Aspects of confidentiality, respect, and self-esteem are discussed and contextualized by each participant before stories can be shared. By contributing to these guidelines as a group, participants may develop some level of mutual accountability and ownership of the healing process, and an opportunity to confront feelings of fear and intergroup prejudice identified as an obstacle to individual well-being and social relationships. One participant reported feeling comfortable telling others how she contracted HIV/AIDS through rape she experienced during the genocide. She had never shared this story with her family, not even her husband before he passed away. After sharing this experience with others in the small group, she reported feeling great relief. Her telling such a painful story seemed to invite others to console her and share their own experiences.

Based on the preliminary results, we can say that the HIEWCR model has managed to integrate Western knowledge of psychology and mental health with Rwandan cultural practices and skills. Participants are invited to use their own knowledge and abilities within the intervention. This researcher (King) noticed that participants at times suggested games during breaks, or songs to lift up the spirit of the group. The plenary sessions offered Western theoretical explanations of certain phenomena, such as grief and emotions. This new understanding seemed to motivate participants' reflection and interpretation from the cultural context, and urge them to support those who experienced traumatic crises during the intervention through evening visits. These visits continued between sessions, according to their reports.

The conceptualization and implementation of the HIEWCR at the grassroots levels of community in post-genocide Rwanda demonstrates the importance of building on local resources in more sustainable ways. The beneficiaries of the model are challenged to not only heal themselves, but also to contribute to the rebuilding of the social fabric disrupted by massive violence. Models like the one under study require systematic monitoring and evaluation in order to assess their effectiveness in promoting mental well-being in post-conflict situations.

In this chapter, we demonstrated the challenges encountered by programs that fail to conceptualize and implement psychosocial programs without giving importance to realities of non-Western post-conflict societies. Utilizing a structural violence framework, we demonstrated how both indirect and direct forms of violence weakened the social structures of Rwanda over the last century, resulting in genocide and related psychosocial issues. We provided an example of a community-based mental health model that combines Western and non-Western theories, techniques, and skills that take into account the needs of both individuals and communities. We suggest systematic monitoring and evaluations of such models in order to determine the most effective approaches to address psychosocial trauma that results from massive violence.

References

Abramowitz, S. A. (2005). The poor have become rich, and the rich have become poor: Collective trauma in the Guinean Languete. *Social Science & Medicine, 61*(10), 2106-2118.

Alexander, J. C., Eyerman, R., Giesen, B., Smelser, N. J., & Sztompka, P. (2004). *Cultural trauma and collective identity.* Berkeley, CA: University of California Press.

Anghie, A. (2002). Colonialism and the birth of international institutions: Sovereignty, economy, and the mandate system of the League of Nations. *International Law and Politics, 34*, 513-633.

Bolton, P. et al. (2002). Prevalence of depression in rural Rwanda based on symptom and functional criteria. *The Journal of Nervous & Mental Disease, 190* (9), 631-637.

Carballo, M., Smajkic, A., Zeric, D., Dzidowska, M., Gebre-Medhin, J., & Van Halem, J. (2004). Mental health and coping in a war situation: The case of Bosnia and Hersegovina. *Journal of Biosocial Science, 36*(4), 463-477.

Christie, D., Wagner, R. V., & Winter, D. D. (Eds.) (2001). *Peace, conflict and violence. Peace psychology for the 21st century.* New Jersey: Prentice Hall.

de Brouwer, A-M., Ka Hon Chu, S., & Muscati, S. (2009). *The men who killed me: Rwandan survivors of sexual violence.* Vancouver: Douglas & McIntyre.

Des Forges, A., & Longman, T. (2004). Legal responses to genocide in Rwanda. In E. Stover & H. M. Weinstein (Eds.), *My neighbour my enemy. Justice and community in the aftermath of mass atrocity* (pp. 49-66). London: Cambridge University Press.

Draguns, J. G., Gielen, U. P., & Fish, J. M. (2004). Approaches to culture, healing, and psychotherapy. In U. P. Gielen, J. M. Fish, & J. G. Draguns (Eds.), *Handbook of culture, therapy, and healing* (pp. 1-11). Mahwah, NJ, US: Lawrence Erlbaum Associates Publishers.

Edkins, J. (2003). *Trauma and the memory of politics.* Cambridge: Cambridge University Press.

Farmer, P. (2004). An anthropology of structural violence. *Current Anthropology, 45*(3), 305-325.

_____. (2005). *Pathologies of power: Health, human rights and the new war on the poor.* Berkeley: University of California Press.

Fierke, K. M. (2004). Whereof we can speak, thereof we must not be silent: Trauma, political solipsism and war. *Review of International Studies, 30*, 471-491.

Galtung, J. (2001). After violence, reconstruction, reconciliation, and resolution. In M. Abu-Nimer (Ed.), *Reconciliation, justice, and coexistence* (pp. 3-23). Lanham, MD: Lexington Books.

Galtung, J. (1969). Violence, peace and peace research. *Journal of Peace Research, 6*(3), 167-191.

Ganguly, R., & Taras, R. (2006). *Understanding ethnic conflict: The international dimension.* New York: Longman.

Gasibirege, S. (2009). *Lien entre guérison du traumatisme, réconciliation et développement. Casdu Rwandan: Deux expériences qui tentent de retisser ce lien et de le consolider au niveau des communautés locales.* Unpublished document.

Gobodo-Madikizela, P., & Van der Merwe, C. N. (2007). *Narrating our healing: Perspectives on working through trauma.* Newcastle, UK: Cambridge Scholars Publishing.

Hatzfeld, J. (2005). *Into the quick of life, the Rwandan genocide: The survivors speak: A report.* London: Serpent's Tail.

_____. (2009). *The antelope's strategy. Living in Rwanda after the genocide.* New York: Farrar, Strauss and Giroux.

Hutchison, E., & Beleiker, R. (2008). Emotional reconciliation. Reconstructing identity and community after trauma. *European Journal of Social Theory, 11*(3), 385-403.

Kayitesi-Blewitt, M. (2006). Funding development in Rwanda: The survivors' perspective. *Development in Practice, 16*(3-4), 316-321.

Kleinman, A. & Kleinman, J. (1997). The appeal of experiences; The dismay of images: Cultural appropriation of suffering in our times. In A. Kleinman, V. Das, & M. M. Lock (Eds.), *Social suffering* (pp. 1-24). Berkeley: University of California Press.

Kuperman, A. J. (2001). *The limits of humanitarian intervention: Genocide in Rwanda.* Washington, DC: Brookings Institution Press.

Logiest, G. (1988). *Mission au Rwanda: Un Blanc dans la bagarre Hutu-Tutsi.* Bruxelles: Didier Hatier.

Lugan, B. (1997). *Histoire du Rwanda: De la préhistoire à nos jours.* Etrepilly: Bartillat.

Lumsden, M. (1997). Breaking the cycle of violence. *Journal of Peace Research, 34*(4), 377-383.

Mamdani, M. (1996). From conquest to consent as the basis of state formation: Reflections on Rwanda. *New Left Review, 216*, 3-36.

Mamdani, M. (2001). *When victims become killers. Colonialism, nativism, and the genocide in Rwanda.* New Jersey: Princeton University Press.

Martín-Baró, I. (1994). *Writings for a liberation psychology.* Cambridge, Mass.: Harvard University Press.

Melvern, L. (2004). *Conspiracy to murder: The Rwandan genocide.* London: Verso.

Métraux, J. C. (2004). *Deuils collectifs et création sociale.* Paris: La Dispute.

Newbury, C. (1998). Ethnicity and the politics of history in Rwanda. *Africa Today, 45*(1), 7-24.

Overdulve, C. M. (1997). *Rwanda: Un people avec une histoire.* Paris: L'Harmattan.

Papadopoulos, R. K. (1998). Destructiveness, atrocities and healing: Epistemological and clinical reflections. *Journal of Analytical Psychology, 43*, 455-477.

Pedersen, D., Tremblay, J., Errázuriz, C., & Gamarra, J. (2008). The sequelae of political violence: Assessing trauma, suffering and dislocation in the Peruvian highlands. *Social Science & Medicine, 67*(2), 205-217.

Pupavac, V. (2004). *International therapeutic peace and justice in Bosnia. Social & Legal Studies.* London, Thousand Oaks, CA and New Delhi: Sage Publications.

Sarkar, S. (2008). Nationalism and poverty: Discourses of development and culture in 20th century India. *Third World Quarterly, 29*(3) 429-445.

Summerfield, D. (1999). A critique of seven assumptions behind psychological trauma programmes in war-affected areas. *Social Science & Medicine, 48*(10), 1449-1462.

Uvin, P. (1998). *Aiding violence: The development enterprise in Rwanda.* West Hartford, Conn: Kumaria Press.

Chapter Ten

CHEWING KOLANUTS IN CANADA: AN ANALOGUE OF AFRICAN TRADITIONAL HEALING PRACTICES AND MODERN PSYCHOTHERAPEUTIC METHODS

Edna Aryee (PhD Candidate)[i] & Roy Moodley[ii] (PhD and Associate Professor)

Department of Applied Psychology and Human Development , University of Toronto

Abstract

The authenticity of African traditional healing has been garbled by the various intrinsic opinions of many people despite the crucial role played by traditional healers in building the health systems of African-Canadian communities. The Indigenous healing practice is alive in the diasporic African-Canadian community, where a large number use the system secretly on a daily basis. Two African traditional healers[iii] in the Greater Toronto Area were interviewed. This chapter reports on: (1) how they received their calling and training in traditional healing; (2) how they diagnose illnesses and heal the people they work with; and, (3) how they work with mainstream psychological services and professionals in the Greater Toronto Area. The thematic analysis revealed that in spite of the prevalence of Western medicine, individuals and families in North America continue to consult African traditional healers for mental health treatment and life solutions. Typically, God, ancestors, and spirits are viewed as the main source or relief in all presenting situations. On the whole, the chapter identifies the urgent need for close collaboration between Western psychological programs and services and African traditional healers in Canada. In addition to advocating for the regulation of the African traditional healing profession in Canada, the study also acknowledges the recognition and integration of African traditional healing practices in mainstream psychotherapy.

---

i The first author of the chapter and worked as an associate researcher on the project.

ii The second author of the chapter and the prinicipal investigator of the research which was funded by SSHRC

iii We would like to express our gratitude to the healers who participated in the study, particularly, the Sangoma and Ifa healers. The writing of this chapter and the completion of the project wouldn't have been successful without their support and insightful information.

Introduction

In working with the African traditional healing system in psychotherapy, it is important to understand the practices, the role of African traditional healers, and how African traditional healing complements Eurocentric forms of medicinal intervention. In this chapter, we have emphasized the importance of engaging African traditional healers in diagnosis and how traditional healing processes can be incorporated into mainstream psychological practice. Before we discuss the themes in this chapter, we would like to introduce you to some of the misconceptions about the African traditional healing practice. First, for centuries the practice of African traditional healing has been portrayed negatively by the Western world and, to a large extent, the Western world has managed to devalue the richness and quintessence of our cultural and traditional healing practices. As a result, most individuals of African descent on the continent and in the diaspora have resorted to Western ways of understanding and treating mental and physiological illnesses. Second, some have misunderstood the role of our ancestors and traditional healing practices to mean ancestral and satanic worship. However, having said this, like with any other human group, there are always the extremists (including traditional healers) who may misuse their roles and spiritual abilities to the disservice of the entire community. This study therefore aims to bring to light the prodigious role played by African traditional healers. The overarching aim of the study are as follows: (a) describe and critically examine the processes within which traditional healers consult, assess, diagnose, and treat clients; (b) record the various kinds of herbal medicines and other medical substances they use; (c) analyze the types of training and skills development of traditional healers; and finally, (d) compare the roles of traditional healers to those of the Western counsellors.

One of the striking features of modern advanced societies is the significant representation of government-sanctioned cultural diversity. Statistics Canada (2003) has reported that between 1991 and 2000, 2.2 million immigrants (representing 18.4% of the Canadian population) were admitted to Canada. Immigrants to Canada include cohorts from Africa, whose population in Ontario alone has increased from 0.4% in 1961 to 6.8% in 2001 (Statistics Canada). Whereas diversity and multiculturalism in Canada has some obvious political, social, and economic benefits, it also poses challenges, especially in the area of mental health. African immigrants have been reported to be one of the visible minority groups that under-utilizes mental health facilities (Jackson, Neighbors & Torres, 2007; Nasir et al., 2006). Studies attribute this apparent lack of interest in mental health care to stigma (Adewuya & Makanjuola, 2005; Edge et al., 2004; Nadeem et al. 2007; Schreiber, Stern, & Wilson, 1998) and general dissatisfaction with or mistrust of the health system (Secker & Harding, 2002). As convincing as these reasons may be, it is important not to ignore the significant role culture plays in influencing the health-seeking attitudes and behaviours of African immigrants. As a cultural group, African immigrants have their own conceptualizations of abnormality and well-being, as well as ways of coping with mental health problems (Lee & Armstrong, 1995; Myers, 1999).

The hallmark of African traditional healing is Africans' understanding that mental illnesses have both physical and spiritual dimensions (Ndege, 2001). That is, it is grounded on the core belief that there is unity in creation and that "interconnections between the dimensions of natural and supernatural are far more important than the differences between them" (Nelms & Gorski, 2006, p. 186). Vontress, Johnson & Epps (1999) provides support for this claim by describing traditional healers' methods for diagnosing mental problems as "religiously-based" (p. 327). Good (1980) further suggests that a mental disease is symptomatic of a "rupture of life's harmony" (p. 25). Fosu (1981) also suggests that to most Africans even "natural" illnesses have metaphysical etiology and meanings. The cultural beliefs about health issues are so central that African immigrants still hold onto their beliefs as they go through processes of acculturation. As Wahrisch-Oblau (2001) rightly states, African immigrants bring with them a "consciousness that life is always influenced by numinous powers in both positive and negative ways" (p. 92). Consequently, their views about the healing process are in many ways different from those of the dominant culture and the philosophies from which mental health services have developed. It is in this sense that many African immigrants address their mental health issues by substituting or complementing what is provided within the dominant culture with alternative healing options. African immigrants seek this alternative or traditional healing through the herbalist/diviner medium (Green, 1999) on the one hand, and pastors of Charismatic/ (neo) Pentecostal Churches on the other (Wahrisch-Oblau, 2001).

Considering the largely secular nature of current psychotherapies and the tendency for the West to summarize African religious beliefs as superstitious, it is easy to infer that the mental health needs of most African immigrants are not being fully met. Richter (2003) highlighted the fact that traditional healers are generally divided into two categories: those who serve the role of diviner-diagnostician (or diviner-mediums) and those who are healers (or herbalists). He argued that the herbalist chooses and applies relevant herbal remedies, while the spiritualist heals through prayer and rituals. Beck (1985) and Nelms and Goski (2006) explained that, unlike their Western counterpart, traditional healers do not receive formal training in medical procedures or medicinal dispensation, but rather acquire their healing methods and skills from the spirit of a deceased family healer or are chosen by an unknown spirit, namely a *mudzimu*, meaning ancestral spirit. Chavunduka (1986) noted that of 195 healers, 145 claimed to have been possessed by a spirit and 25 claimed to have learned the profession through an apprenticeship with other healers. Thus, the traditional healing practice is a well-guarded family possession and is handed down through the generations from one family member to the next. In support of this, Nelms and Goski (2006) show that herbalists are frequently taught in this manner as well. They also argued that diviners would often look for "signs" in their children to distinguish those to whom they might eventually pass on the traditional healing art.

The African community (including those in the diaspora) recognizes traditional healers as experts in the provision of health services. According to Ulin (1980), traditional healers make use of the customary knowledge and beliefs in the community about the causes of illnesses and make remedies using plant, animal, and mineral substances. To formulate the traditional practice successfully, traditional healers develop a holistic approach that considers the whole individual—mind and body—and works with the individual, not in isolation but as a member of the family and the community. According to Mzimkulu and Simbayi (2006), African traditional healers generally locate the cause and treatment of psychological distress within the community and describe psychosis in mystical terms by relating to the archetypes of the collective unconscious of individuals (Mabunda, 2001). Mogale (1999) Kale, 1995) identified and described the symptomology of a psychiatric illness called *moriti wa le tswele* ("the shadow of the breast") from accounts given by traditional healers and patients. Mogale (1999) concluded that the symptoms of *moriti wa le tswele* are similar to the symptoms of somatoform pain disorder of the *Diagnostic and Statistical Manual of Mental Disorders* (DSM-IV-TR) of the American Psychiatric Association) but have some cultural features that include mental confusion and psychosis. Mzimkulu and Simbayi (2006) noted similar traditional conceptualizations and beliefs about the causes of psychosis in cultures found in other African countries such as Zimbabwe and Ethiopia. For example, Patel, Musara, Maramba, and Fuyane (1995) suggested that spirits in Zimbabwe cause mental illness and the most common types of spirits thought to cause psychosis are known as "*ngozi*." Mutebirwa (1989) also specified that ngozi are the spirits of persons killed either by the patient or by one of his or her ancestors. He further cited the potential reason for psychosis as the violation of a taboo by either the patient or his/her family. The spirits would be angered, which in turn would cause the illness. Mutambirwa (1989) noted that a cycle of family psychosis could be broken if sufficient or adequate compensation ("*Kuripa*" in Shona) was given to the aggrieved family.

The Sangoma Traditional Practice[i]

As mentioned earlier, we interviewed two healers, the Sangoma of South African origin and the Ifa healer of Nigerian origin. The Sangoma is normally a female healer who is called by the ancestors, and a refusal of the calling leads to an ongoing physical or mental illness. The Sangoma is described as a practitioner of herbal medicine, divination, and counselling. She performs a holistic and symbolic form of healing, embedded in the beliefs of her culture that the ancestors in the afterlife guide and protect the living. She is formally trained under another Sangoma for a period of years, performing humbling service in the community. The trainee Sangoma undergoes purification through steaming, washing in the blood of sacrificed animals, and the use of herbal medicine. They work in a sacred healing hut or *Ndumba*, where their ancestors reside. They have to wear specific coloured clothes to please each ancestor, and in their hair they often wear the gallbladder of a goat sacrificed at their graduation ceremony. They summon the ancestors by burning a plant called *Imphepho*, dancing, chanting, and, most importantly, playing drums.

The most common indicator of diagnosis and healing is the Sangoma's ability to access advice and guidance from the ancestors for their patients, which is often accompanied by the possession or channelling of an ancestor, throwing bones, and interpreting dreams. In the possession states, the Sangoma works herself into a trance through drumming, dancing, and chanting, and allows her ego to step aside so an ancestor can possess her body and communicate directly with the patient, providing specific information about his or her problems. It can be very dramatic, with the Sangoma speaking in tongues or foreign languages according to the specific ancestor, or dancing fervently beyond her normal ability. The

i The Sangoma who participated in this study was born and raised in South Africa. Currently, she practices and lives in the GTA. She has also provided consultation around the globe including Africa and Europe. She has extensive experience in diagnosing, healing, and supporting clients. She is a fully licenced Sangoma, well trained and educated.

Sangoma possesses a collection of small bones and other small objects like seeds and shells, each with a specific significance to human life. Accessing the ancestors' advice through the bones is an alternative to the exhausting possession states.

As an earthly being, this fragile connection to the spiritual world offers the Sangoma a limitless stream of information and the ability to tap into the ethereal source. Once the Sangoma has linked with her particular ancestor, she is then able to communicate with the deceased, angels, guides, and spirits. The spiritual exchange is often directly related to past life experiences, soul-connected incidences, and psychic phenomena. As a healer, the Sangoma is known to use a variety of roots, bark, herbs, flowers, and a wide range of land and animal products when making medicine, or "*muti*" as it is called in Zulu. Most of the treatments are focused on the balance of ethereal energies and the human body. It is the source of the ailment that is the primary concern; therefore, before centering on the physical effects of the ailment, the Sangoma will investigate if indeed there is a spiritual or metaphysical reason behind the symptoms. According to Milingo, the connection between the two worlds is important because these divine beings possess the ancestral keys—that is, they are able to unlock the universal information and share it with those who seek answers or require help and assistance (Callaway, in Struik, 1970).

The Sangoma healer has many different social and political roles in the community, such as healing, protecting the society, and narrating the history and myths of that society. In southern Africa, for example, the Sangomas far outnumber Western-style doctors and are consulted first (or exclusively) by approximately 80% of the Black population. The Sangomas are highly revered and respected because they know the local dynamics and can counsel appropriately. It is important to note that the formal health sector has shown continued interest in the role of Sangomas and the efficacy of their herbal remedies. To a large extent, some Western-style scientists have continued to study the ingredients of traditional medicines used by Sangomas. In addition, Public Health specialists are now enlisting Sangomas in the fight against the spread of HIV/AIDS.

Traditional Practice of the Ifa[i]

Drawing on the Ifa practice in Nigeria, it is important to highlight that, of all the methods of divination employed by the Yoruba, Ifa divination is considered the most reliable and popular means of divination (Awolalu, 1979; Bascom, 1969). Ifa divination is described as a body of knowledge and a system of social, emotional, and pathological control. Awolalu (1979) acknowledges that it is the most complex system of divination both in its repertoire of verses and in its range of applications. The divination process involves employing relevant historical and mythological precedents contained in the special divinatory verses to be recited, chanted, or sung by the *Babalawo*—the trained, dedicated Ifa priests and diviners. The divination or consultation by the Babalawo with the supreme divinity *Orunmila* is of crucial spiritual importance because emphasis is placed on the part played by Orunmila in guiding the destiny of man and the divinities (Ajayi,1996).

Ifa divination processes have been divided into three broad structural parts: prologue, narrative,and epilogue (Akinnaso, 1983). This is a process that starts from the moment the client enters the Babalawo's house until he or she departs. The internal structure of the divination is as follows:

The Prologue

a) The preliminary exchange of greetings
b) The client's intention expressed
c) The Babalawo paying homage
d) The Babalawo divines for an *Odu (spirit)* to emerge

The Narrative

e) The interpretation of the Odu sign
f) The narration of related stones
g) The explication of the message contained in *ese Ifa*

The Epilogue

h) The client's view of the revelation
i) The detailed findings with the use of *Ibo*
j) The prescription of sacrifice
k) The performance of sacrifice

---

i The Ifa healer in this study was born and raised in Canada; however, she identifies herself as African. She describes herself as a level ii healer and was trained by a Babalawo in Nigerian. She has extensive experience in diagnoses and healing.

The Ifa healer or the Babalawo in traditional Yoruba society is called a doctor, pharmacist, or herbalist, and is the most popular resource for people to consult for advice, guidance, and medical treatment. A Babalawo is generous, faithful, knowledgeable, and is a good traditional counsellor to the members of his community. He is highly respected for his wisdom and intelligence. Also, Bascom (1969) describes the Babalawo as the most organised and most knowledgeable, magic-religious sect among the Yorubas. Unlike the Sangoma, the Babalawo's role is not attained through lineage or honour. However, common to some aspects of the Sangoma training, an individual is called to the office of a Babalawo or Ifa after many years of rigorous training and experience (Bascom, 1969).

It is highly essential that one who aspires to be an Ifa priest (Babalawo) receive adequate training from an experienced Babalawo. While in training, the trainee is taught the Odu signs and commits to memory a great number of *Ese Ifa* (stories) associated with the *Odu,* starting with *Ejiogbe* (the first Odu in the corpus). After the mastery of the required stories in each of the 16 principles of Odu, they then proceed with the stories in the minor *Odu.* In the work of Abimbola (1976 & 2006), it is noted that before a trainee Babalawo lays his hand on anything, divination has to be performed in order for him to know the Odu that is destined for him. Following this, the trainee continues his/her education with the identification of the signature of each of the 16 principal Odu and the Opele as the major instructional materials. After a trainee has mastered the signs of the 16 Odu, he is then examined by his master, perhaps in the company of a few fellow Babalawos. The performance of the trainee determines whether or not he will proceed to the minor Odu. No Babalawo makes any diagnosis without using either the *opele* (the divining chain) or the *ikin* (the sacred palm nut). The use of these instruments will enable the Babalawo to know the nature of his client's problem. In addition to knowledge of Ifa and the process of divination, an aspiring Ifa healer or Babalawo learns the appropriate sacrifice for each Odu and also receives an enormous amount of herbal and pharmaceutical lore with its accompanying repertoire of charms and incantation (Idowu, 1962).

Methodology

The in-depth interview method, qualitative research method, and grounded theory were employed in this study. The in-depth interview was chosen because it is open-ended and is conducted in an informal setting.

We interviewed two African traditional healers (a Sangoma[i] and an Ifa Priestess[ii]) practicing in the Greater Toronto Area. The Sangoma is an extensively experienced female South African traditional healer who practices in Toronto and other parts of the world, while the Ifa Priestess is a Yoruba female healer who is still in training. They both identified themselves as African. They have been in practice for approximately 7-15 years. Their ages ranged from 32-48 years. Both were registered or affiliated with a recognized Traditional Healer's Institution in Africa. The recruitment of the sample was based entirely on contacts made through various acquaintances. They were not registered with any official institution in Canada because Canada does not recognize the practices of African Traditional Healing; hence, there is no such group available to register with. Thus, a purposeful sampling method was used in the selection of participants and, most importantly, we included participants who provided rich and vivid accounts of traditional forms of healing. This approach was chosen because it was suitable for the study and the healers. To aid in selection of participants, we used the following criteria: adult healers who identify with an African ethnicity, actively practicing in one of the following forms of healing in Toronto—Voodoo, Shango, Spiritual Baptist (Orisha), Ifa, Pastoral healing, Ayurveda, homeopathy, and astrology.

This strategy ensured that the participants and their expertise are related to the study's focus of inquiry.

Grounded Theory

Grounded theory is a research method most often used in qualitative research. It focuses on generating a theory using certain steps that include reading and re-reading data from a corpus of data, labelling emerging themes/variables/concepts and assessing interrelationships between these themes. In the final step, the task is to formulate a theory that is central to all the themes and relates most or all of the concepts prevalent in those themes (Dick, 2005).

---

i *The Sangoma is referred to as participant 1*

ii *The Ifa priestess/healer is referred to as participant 2*

For our study, we first interviewed the healers and recorded their transcripts. Second, we used their transcripts as the data corpus for the application of grounded theory analysis. We later identified and labelled the themes or concepts that emerged from the data and categorized them. Although grounded theory is considered to be complete upon formulation of a theory, for this study, the analysis ended at identification of themes. Third, we compared the methods of these healers with common counselling methodology used by Western counsellors under categories such as: education and training of counsellors, assessment and diagnostic tools used, treatment process, client profiles, illnesses treated, and relationship between counsellors and clients. Overall, the documentation of various researchers on the commonalities between Western forms of counselling helped in our comparison with the traditional forms of healing (Abudabbeh & Nydell 1993; Bojuwoye, 2001; Fukuyama, 1990; Lee & Armstrong, 1995; Semela, 2001).

Since constructivism theory states that the values, perceptions, and experiences of researchers can influence the research, we found it imperative to conduct a relatively non-biased approach during the study. We maintained self-reflexive journals to document our thought processes pertaining to the research. These emerging self-understandings were examined and incorporated into the research and analysis (Morrow, 2005; Patton, 2002). In addition, we used triangulations of analysis strategy (Patton, 2002) whereby two independent people (i.e., the research coordinator and the research supervisor, who is the second author) were used as judges. In this case, multiple analysts reviewed the findings obtained from the research to help reduce bias that may have resulted due to the data collection and interpretation, since we share the same background as the healers (Pannon, 2002). We believe that by doing this, the same data can then be compared to assess any biases. In addition to the self-reflexive journal and triangulation of analysts, we went through an expert audit review. According to Pannon (2002), this method allows experts related to the field to evaluate the research findings and thus increases the credibility of the research.

Although using self-reflexive journals, triangulation of analysts, and expert audits can significantly raise the credibility of the research, we will also emphasize that the findings are highly contextual and that it may not be possible to generalize or extrapolate them to other situations, time periods, or people (Pannon, 2002).

Research Procedure

1. *First stage: Preparation.* This stage involved the identification of participants through community contacts and the negotiation of participation in the study. Once the healers were identified, we had a preliminary phone discussion on their practices; an explanation of the research process was also provided. It has been observed that qualitative studies typically focus on relatively small samples, usually selected purposefully (Pannon, 2002).

2. *Second stage: Data collection and ongoing analysis.* Prior to each interview, the participants read and signed a consent form that explained the nature of the study, confidentiality, risks, benefits, and uses of information. The interview lasted for about 60 minutes and was tape-recorded. For the Sangoma, the interview took place at a Sangoma shrine and for the Ifa priestess, we met in a private office at the University of Toronto. All the interviews were conducted in English by the first author. The interviews covered the five topics mentioned below. The interviews were transcribed verbatim and then prepared for team review. After confirmation of authenticity of the interviews, we continued with the qualitative analysis.

3. *Third Stage: Data analysis and synthesis.* At this stage, the transcripts were analyzed using the grounded theory analysis procedure. The following steps adapted from McLeod (2001) were followed: Each interview will be analyzed following its collection, this concurrent analysis serves to sensitize the researcher to themes or concepts that may be addressed in the next interview, and data collection will end when the category system or theory gets saturated.

Instruments

The aim of the study is to examine the importance or role of African Traditional practice in psychotherapy. It was important for us to remain as accurate and close to the listed questions as possible without influencing the healers' pre-conceived ideas about psychology and psychiatry. The interviews were structured in two main groups and they are as follows:

1. *Demographic information*. A brief form was created to collect demographic information. The form consisted of five questions inquiring about each participant's name (pseudonym), gender, religion, and ethnicity.

2. *Semi-structured interview.* We used a semi-structured interview (60 minutes) to gather data from the participants. The questions were fully worded before the interview, although certain questions were

followed by probes. The benefits of using a semi-structured interview is that the instrument can be replicated by different researchers and the variation can be minimized. In addition, analysis is facilitated as the participant responses are categorized under the interview questions (Pannon, 2002). Previous research on interviewing traditional healers (Moodley, 2005; Vontress, 1991; Vontress Johnson, & Epps 1999) was cross-referenced for the development of the interview questions and probes.

The interview questions were organised into five themes:

1. Reasons for being a healer
2. Healer's practice
3. Healer's client group
4. Process of healing
5. Relationship to Western methods of healing

To delve more deeply into the interviewee's responses, we asked for clarification but we made sure that leading questions were avoided. The aim of an in-depth interview is to obtain rich and detailed descriptions of the respondent's own concerns, opinions, and actions in their own words rather than eliciting stimuli.

Data Analysis and Synthesis

In this stage, the transcripts will be analyzed using the grounded theory analysis procedure. The following steps adapted from McLeod (2001) were followed: Each interview was analyzed following its collection, and this concurrent analysis served to sensitize the researcher to themes or concepts that may be addressed in the next interview. As mentioned earlier, data collection ended when the category system or theory was saturated.

1. Process of open coding. We repeatedly read the transcripts to generate as many alternative categories or units of meaning as possible within the text. We wanted to grasp the wholeness of the data and avoid any personal preconceptions and judgements.

2. Labelling and filling categories. In this case, we broke the interview into naturally occurring units that conveyed a particular meaning, using each participant's own vocabulary as related to the list categories. Upon identification of categories, themes were organized by labelling the categories. The categories were then examined as a whole to identify higher order categories that included clusters of the categories found earlier. The transformed labels were then expressed as central themes and each central theme expressed more than one meaning.

3. *Axial coding.* This process refers to the identification and assessment of connection between the categories. In this step, the various categories were assessed to find any connections that may have existed between them.

4. *Constant comparison.* This method allowed for constant refinement of categories by continual contrast and comparison of the categories within and across cases.

Findings

Findings from the Sangoma healer and the Ifa healer are presented first, and identified themes and extended descriptions are provided under the listed interview questions.

How did you become a traditional healer?

According to the Sangoma healer, one can only become a Sangoma healer if they are called and initiated by a Sangoma, who is typically an elder, traditional priest, healer, or the spirit of an ancestor.

In plain words, the Sangoma in the study stated: "One becomes a traditional healer by being discovered by a Sangoma, a discovering and diagnosing process known as the 'Sangoma illness.'"

According to this participant (participant 1), "Sangomas are primarily psychologists; and they deal with the consciousness, subconsciousness, the DNA, and so on through divination and different processes of assessment and diagnosis." She emphasized that they are not "medicine people" nor do they use charms in any of their practices.

- *Feeling inner uneasiness and spiritual search for answers*

She revealed that prior to visiting her ancestral home, she was diagnosed with a psychotic disorder and prescribed antipsychotic medications. She also added that in experiencing the Sangoma illness, she felt an inner uneasiness and a spiritual search for answers for her discomfort (which were spiritual, psychological, and physiological). She relayed that she was spiritually lead to her ancestral home in South Africa, which led to the spiritual diagnosis of her inner "struggles or uneasiness" and the release of a "total and permanent" peace in her spirit. In describing the discovering and diagnosis process (Sangoma illness), she mentioned that after careful inner reflection and a discussion with her sister, she visited a Sangoma in her village. Upon arrival at the Sangoma shrine, the Sangoma began to prophesy about her entire life and lineage, revealing that her mother was supposed to be a Sangoma but it was suppressed. The same was reported about her paternal family. Following this, she began speaking and praying in a particular way along with mentioning her ancestral names. She relayed that it was a call to the ancestors and she was provided with a stream of events, people, and experiences in her life and family.

According to her, the sickness she experienced was an indication of her ancestors rising in her DNA and basically purging anything that was stopping her spiritual purpose from coming to life. She concluded that toward the end of the process, the Sangoma picked up a bottle of water, shook it from side to side and prayed for more specific information about her calling and any areas that were blocked in her spirit.

Initiation Process and Training

The initiation process comes in several levels, such as looking at the talents of the spirits, talents that you are born with, talents through childhood, youth, and adulthood, and on through to full maturity. There is a specific way that the psyche of the person must be acknowledged, which means that there are distinct passages that the soul goes through and each passage must be marked and engineered in a specific way. If it is not engineered in this way, the psyche of the spirit will become corroded. This is emphasized in the following quotes:

"The initiation process in a sense is the training because for us the talent and the calling, the channels and the power that is within you individually come from your genes that we call the ancestors. So genetically, if you inherited the power of being a great speaker, a great artist, a great writer, whatever it is, first of all you have to address whether that being and trait has been given the permission so that your ability to fulfill or to express what is genetically in your heritage is not cut off."

"The primary priority of this training is teaching you how to mix medicine. You learn orally because you have a mentor who takes you to the plants and trees so you are taught mechanically—what this tree is good for... cleansing of the body of trauma or subconscious influences that have affected the physical flesh of the body.... so that becomes a mechanical process of learning that we can learn anywhere, anyhow, through a particular process."

Clients

Participant 1: She reported that often people who come to her are "people who are gifted and need to go through the initiation process or want their psyche cleaned up a bit." She mentioned that most of her clients are women, and her client base has shifted from primarily Caucasian to African-Canadians "but I don't know why, Caribbean, African women population. I would say I have about 95% women and 5% men, 1% Caucasians and the rest [of the] people of African descent. I don't have Asians. I don't have oriental people. I feel [most of my clients are] African because of the cultural relevance. I am from the continent [so they can] relate to my practices and feel they can discuss and openly talk about their issues, [as] I can understand. The majority of my clients are in their late 20s to their mid-40s but on average their cut off is 50. The range is 20-50 years. My clients are from Toronto and outside of Toronto in the Brampton area, Markham, Mississauga, and Scarborough. I [also] have patients in Greece, South Africa and North America."

"I have a balance of people who can say they are spiritual but not religious and people who come from very Christian religious backgrounds."

"There are many things that are curable without a physical element. I believe [strongly] in energy medicine and I believe that the mind is a very powerful place. And I believe that the conscious mind in collaboration with the subconscious mind [will] stimulate the body itself to generate healing."

"My first inspiration comes with anything that can be used with thoughts, using the spoken word, the mind, and the consciousness versus sub-consciousness; and changing energy and thought forms. My practice is trying to empower the patients and this is what I give them, the empowerment to first of all understand what illness is because when they understand what illness is from my perspective, training, and knowledge, [then] do they have tools within their own reach that they can use on a daily basis to heal and to change."

"The roots of illnesses is the lack of awareness of what is wrong and often times when I meet patients for the first time, I read their energy and give them the root causes of their problems."

Participant 2: According to the Ifa healer, the term client, in this study, refers to the person who consults a healer for advice and guidance by means of divination. She indicated that before a client consults an Ifa, he or she must share the belief in the institution of traditional divination because of the role of faith in the healing process. She emphasized that in spite of the client's status, religious inclination, age or educational attainment, a client must submit himself to the authority and direction of the Ifa healer. The client is required to remain passive and attentive to the divine message from the Ifa healer. She relayed that the divine message to the client is contained in Ifa stories and such mediums are used when the divining chain is employed.

- *Presenting Problems*

"I have seen all types of illnesses that patients bring in—everything from childhood brain damage from birth [for a patient] who is now 26 years old, a mentally ill patient, a patient who is in a psychiatric ward. I have had an immigrant patient from the Congo who is suddenly ill and has gone through peculiar symptoms of what would be called delusional in psychotherapy, that is, seeing things, feeling and having weird conditions of scratching himself."

"Also, I have had mental patients that have come to me for solutions; those with knee operations, uterus operations and seeking a change that necessarily won't be going to surgery, so they are looking for options; and I have patients who have had surgeries in the past but the conditions haven't changed and they still feel sick; people with relationships and looking to find direction in counselling, be it spousal or mother and daughter [relationships]; people who want to set proper goals; or those who want to manage their money because they are making a lot of money but can't see it at the end of the month—I give them more kind of life coaching skills."

- *Diagnosis*

Participant 1: "I use divination tools and I have various divination tools. Most sangomas have used objects to divine like bones and we use water to divine. I use bones, water, and divination cards that I constructed myself. I will use physical objects to pick up energy."

Participant 2: According to the Ifa healer, the prominent Ifa instruments used for divination include the Ikin (the 16 sacred palm nuts of divination), the Opele (the divining chain), and the various objects which form the *ibo* (instruments for casting lots). Others are the Iyerosun (divination powder), Opon Ifa (the divining tray), Osun (ornamental Ifa metal staff), Iroke (the carved ivory rattle) and *apo Ifa* (bags for keeping Ifa divination instruments). She added that the *ikin* and the *ibo* are very crucial for a better understanding of the Ifa divination process.

- *Can you talk about the process, time, and techniques involved in the treatment?*

"The first is the diagnosis and this is from conception to adulthood, so this becomes my template of all that the person needs to address. The person has the choice to address all the issues or not, and there are rituals involved, so most of the time I have a counselling package so that people can better understand the issues."

"Usually, I have a package of three months and this includes the atonement, the blood cleansing, medicine taking, and some form of plan for them to do things that they can do on their own or to research something that they didn't know. Some [plans] might involve exercises that would help them change their psyche in conjunction with doing a ritual, having a bath, or taking medicine. Sometimes, when I do a workshop with a patient, I bring in the element of education and sometimes all my patients are involved in group work like healing circles where we ask questions related to the system of healing themselves and being healed in this particular way."

"In the trans-state I was able to travel to a state where [the patient] was in her mother's womb, and hear and see the dialogue that was spoken between her parents and grandparents. In this situation, her paternal grandparents were against the reunion of her parents and this was causing her mother to wonder if she should have the child. Through the umbilical cord, the condition that the mother was in was transmitted to the child so the condition of the child for five months involved the state of the mother, wanting to terminate the pregnancy [and] communicating [this] to a very intelligent embryo that was aware of all of this. [When] the woman was in the flesh and older, she was unaware of all of this, other than in the physical. Other than in the physical, when they are flesh and older." Thus this situation was this women's subconscious reality. Through clairvoyance I was able to go through a scene and tell her what it was and she said to me exactly, my mother was ... and she knew her history so she was able to give me her feedback and we collectively understood that her issue came from something that existed before she was born, something that is a strong driving force in her subconscious. So the psychologists were right—it is a self-manifesting thing but it is coming from a place where she won't necessarily know how or why she was doing it but she was playing out the drama that she absorbed in her mother's womb...for the first time, she told me she feels she has been healed and putting all the pieces together has made her feel better already."

Treatment

- *What do you give to your clients when they come?*

"I tend not to give anything to my clients when they come unless it is required specifically because there is a culture among our society that when you go to a Sangoma you must leave with something, something you can lick on your tongue or a magic pill."

- *Atonement*

"If I have to do an initiation for a person I need to pray over the goats and speak over the animal or offering, and then once it is slaughtered there is the bile that has to be put in the medicine. The herbal medicine of that initiation needs to have a few drops of the bile added to it."

"What is vital in the treatment is the atonement, and this is the controversial part of our discussion that I have been avoiding till now. The thing that has anchored me as a Sangoma is the use of blood atonement [...] I mean the offering of a cow, goat, and chicken on behalf of the person to release a particular ailment or cleanse the person. My interest in that came very late in my practice because I practiced and live here and it's not the easiest place for that kind of work...in the last years I have been exploring what would work best for my patients and until the last three years I discovered blood atonement was the most effective. I don't know how it works, and the ancestors don't know, but it works. I don't have any scientific theory to prove why it works. Until three years ago, I decided that in order to give my best to my patients I would have to bring in that element of atonement, and with that I was able to cure serious ailments."

"[We use] medicines, rituals, and sometimes we have to do rituals with candles. I have worked different candle colors crafted in different elements. We use candles, water to break cycles, break patterns to bring people together or to set goals, create visions, and in some cases to lift up spirits. So if I have a patient diagnosed with depression or bipolar, I will do a different ritual to redirect their thinking. We believe in cleansing through the mouth, cleansing by voicing, by speaking...I also teach them how to prepare the medicine and how to take it."

- *Psychological*

"One example is a male patient who came to me in his 60s. He came to me because he had gone through divorce seven years prior; he had two grown children and had gone through series of failed relationships. He was on medication for depression and was diagnosed possibly with bipolar disorder. In diagnosing him the first thing that was really prominent was that he had lost his mother at the age of 10, the mother figure that came into his life later on was his stepmother, and most of the issue that came up was anger management. The prominent thing in his diagnosis was that he was the last person his mother spoke to before going to the hospital to say that he had to take care of his brothers and the house. That was the first thing, and the second thing that I could find with clairvoyance was that he didn't know that his father had him [in a relationship] before his mother. He was the first born and he never knew he was from a different mother so when we were discussing what I had found, he was shocked, but not surprised, because he had always looked at himself and his brothers, and he looked different."

- *Health education for clients*

"Apart from the one-on-one sessions with the patients, the workshops and healing circles are places where education and healing take place. We talk about a broad range of issues and not just specific issues; we talk about spiritual health, how spiritual health to me is critical to physical health, emotional health, and mental health. Thus, the health of the psyche reflects the health of the body."

- *Referrals to Western practitioners*

"It's harder for that to happen the other way around. I have spoken to Western practitioners regarding immigrant women, children, and their families, and they have told me that there is a need for a form of culturally supportive service that their own patients are familiar with, considering their home background. This doctor said her patients have mental and psychological issues but they would not feel confident going to a Western psychologist for treatment for fear that they would be admitted into a psychiatric ward. And she feels the health of these individuals would be enhanced if they were looked after by a traditional practitioner. The Congolese patient I spoke about before, for instance, was referred to me by a lawyer who works with refugees."

- *Collaborating with psychologists, counsellors, therapists, medical doctors*

Participant 1 "Well I'm part of a group of psychologists called the spirituality network of psychologists and they look into emerging alternative healing into therapy. I think naturally that what is going to be made available to patients is a holistic service to address health."

Both participants stated, "Unfortunately, we have reached a time in the world where Western medicine says we have to prove everything. Until I prove it, it cannot be accepted, so people will keep dying of strange diseases and illnesses and be psychologically and mentally unstable. We are not able to cure AIDS, cancer—all of which we cannot cure through scientific conventional medicine methods. I think there is an understanding now that we do not know everything, and there is a slight humility that is coming into play. This humility is making that particular sector of health (i.e. Western medicine) look elsewhere and they will find that there is room to collaborate and to do better. And on the other hand, I think my traditional practices and all forms of traditional practices can learn from what has happened to Western science's thorough processes to prove and to theorize. There is a need to report and to challenge, to systematize and to operate in a system that makes it possible to transport an individual perspective of practices globally. The Chinese practice has not taken that long—I would say about three decades—to make its presence known in the Western tradition...it has benefited the profession and the Asian and Chinese traditions..., until we as Africans let the world know about our practices, their benefits will be for only a small group of people."

Conclusion

It is evident that the healers focused on various aspects of traditional practice and treated illness mainly with plants, animal products, prayers, and incantations. They also used spiritual resources to augment their healing process. Even though the number of participants in the present study is limited, the findings suggest that both participants work with varied issues, including mental health. Their processes of training, diagnosis, and treatment are similar to those of Western psychotherapy. In sum, there is an urgent request for recognition and incorporation of Africa traditional healing into Western psychotherapy.

References

Abimbola, W. (1976 & 2006 reprint). Ijinle Ohun Enu If, Apa Keji. University Press, Ibadan Nigeria.

Abudabbeh, N., & Nydell, M. (1993). Transcultural counseling and Arab Americans. In J. McFadden, (Ed.), Transcultural Counseling: Bilateral and International Perspectives, (pp. 261-284). Alexandria, VA: American Counseling Association

Adewuya, A. O., & Makanjuola, R. O. (2005). Social distance towards people with mental illness amongst Nigerian university students. Social

Psychiatry and Psychiatric Epidemiology, 40, 865-868.

Ajayi, B. (1996), Ifa Divinision, Its practice among the Yoruba of Nigeria, Ilorin, Nigeria; Unilorin Press

Akinnaso, F. N. (1983). The Structure of Divinatory Speech: A Soc to linguistic Analysis of Yoniba " Sixteen Cowry " Divination. Ph.D., Thesis, Univ. of California, Berkerly

Awolalu, J. O. (1979). Yoruba Beliefs and Sacrificial Rites. London: Longman Group Limited.

Bojuwoye, O. (2001). Crossing cultural boundaries in counselling. *International Journal for the Advancement of Counseling, 23*, 31–50.

Bascom, W (1969), *lfa Divination; Communication between gods and Men in Went Africa.* Indiana: Indiana University Press.

Callaway, H. The Religious System of the Amazulu ((Springdale: Springdale Mission Press, 1868-70; rpt Cape Town: C. Struik, 1970), 74-75, 104

Chavunduka, G. L. (1986). *'Development of African Traditional Medicine: The Case of Zimbabwe' in African Medicine in the Modern World*: Proceeds of a Seminar, Edinburgh: Centre of African Studies

Dick, B. (2005). Grounded theory: A thumbnail sketch. [On line] Retrieved from http://www.aral.com.au/resources/grounded.html

Edge, D., Baker, D., & Rogers, A. (2004). Perinatal depression among black Caribbean women. *Health and Social Care in the Community, 12*, 430-438.

Fosu, G.B. (1981). Disease classification in rural Ghana: Framework and implications for health behaviour. *Social Science Medical Journal. 15B*, 471.

Fukuyama, M. A. (1990). Taking a universal approach to multicultural counseling. Counselor Education and Supervision, 30, 6-17.

Good, C. M. (1980). A comparison of rural and urban ethnomedicine among the Kamba in Kenya. In P. R. Ulin & M. H. Segall (Eds.), *Traditional healthcare delivery in contemporary Africa.* New York: Syracuse University.

Green, J.A. (1999). *Cultural Awareness in the Human Services: A Multi-ethnic Approach.* Needham Heights, MA: Allyn & Bacon.

Jackson, J. S., Neighbors, H. W., & Torres, M. (2007). Use of mental health services and subjective satisfaction with treatment among Black Caribbean immigrants: Results from national survey of American life. *American Journal of Public Health, 97*(1), 60-67.

Kale, R. (1995). Traditional healers in South Africa: A parallel health care system: South Africa's health. *British Medical Journal, 310* (6988), 1182-1186.

Lee, C. C., & Armstrong, K. L. (1995). *Indigenous models of mental health intervention: Lessons from traditional healers.* Thousand Oaks, CA: Sage Publications, Inc.

Mabunda, M.M. (2001). Perceptions of Disease, Illness and Healing among Selected Black

Communities in the Northern Province, South Africa. *South African Journal of Ethnology, 24* (1), 11-16.

McLeod, J. (2001). Qualitative research in counselling and psychotherapy. London: Sage.

Mogale, C.C. (1999). "Moriti wa letswele" (The Shadow of Beast), A Stress-related Somatoform Pain Disorder. *South Africa Journal of Psychology, 29,* 72-75

Moodley, R. (2005). Shamanic performances: Healing through magic and the supernatural.

In R. Moodley, & W. West (Eds.), Integrating traditional healing practices into counseling and psychotherapy (pp. 2–14). Thousand Oaks, CA: Sage

Morrow, S.L., (2005). Quality and trustworthiness in qualitative research in counselling psychology. *Journal of Counselling Psychology, 52,* 250-260.

Mutambirwa, J. (1989). Health problems in rural communities. Zimbabwe. Social Science & Medicine, 29(8), 927–932

Myers, L. J. (1999). Transforming psychology: An African American perspective. In R. L. Jones (Ed.), *Advances in African American psychology* (pp. 9-26). Hampton, VA: Cobb & Henry.

Mzimkulu, K.G., and Simbayi, L.C. (2006). An investigation of perspectives and practices of Xhosa-speaking African traditional healers when managing psychoses. *International Journal of Disability, Development and Education, 53*(4), 417–431

Nadeem, E., Lange, J. M., Edge, M. S., Fongwa, M., Belin, T., & Miranda, J. (2007). *Psychiatric Service, 58,* 1547-1554.

Nasir W., Kamaldeep, B., Tom, C., Sarah, C., Salaad, M., Stephen, S., Paul, M., & Graham, T. (2006). Post-migration geographical mobility, mental health and health service utilisation among Somali refugees in the UK: A qualitative study. *Health and Place, 12*(4), 503-515

Ndege, G. O. (2001). *Health state and society in Kenya.* Rochester, NY: University of Rochester Press.

Nelms, L. W., & Gorski, J. (2006). The role of the African traditional healer in women's health. *Journal of Transcultural Nursing, 17*(2), 184-189.

Patel, V., Musara, T., Butau, T., Maramba, P., & Fuyane, S. (1995). Concepts of mental illness and medical pluralism in Harare. *Psychological Medicine,* **25**, 485–593.

Patton, M.Q. (2002). Qualitative research and evaluation methods (3rd ed.). Thousand Oaks, CA: Sage

Richter, M. (2003). Traditional Medicines and Traditional Healers in South Africa. Discussion paper prepared for the Treatment Action Campaign and AIDS Law Project.

Schreiber, R., Stern, P. N., & Wilson, C. (1998). The contexts for managing depression and its stigma among Black West Indian Canadian women. *Journal of Advanced Nursing, 27*, 510–517.

Semela, J.J.M., (2001). Significance of cultural variables in assessment and therapy. *Folia Phoniatr Logop;53*:128–134

Ulin, P. (1980). Introduction: Traditional healers and primary health care in Africa. In P. R. Ulin & M. H. Segall (Eds.), *Traditional healthcare delivery in contemporary Africa.* New York: Syracuse University.

Vontress, C.E. (1991). Traditional healing in Africa: Implications for cross-cultural counseling. Journal of Counseling and Development, 70(1), 242–249

Vontress, C., Johnson, J., & Epps, L. (Eds.). (1999). Cross-cultural counseling: A casebook. Alexandria, VA: American Counseling Association.

Wahrisch-Oblau, C. (2001). God can make us healthy through and through. *International Review of Mission, 90*, 87-100.

Chapter Eleven

AN ACT GOVERNING TRADITIONAL MEDICINE PRACTICES: AN EXPERIENCE IN TANZANIA

Edmund J. Kayombo, Muhimbili University of Health and Allied Sciences—Dar-es-salaam

Abstract

Traditional medicine has been in place for health care in Africa since time immemorial. There has emerged a contradiction in the practice of traditional and conventional medicine in the provision of healthcare to the community in recent years. The legal systems in Africa are expected to serve as an arbiter that determines the acceptable policy in the provision of health care. Incidentally, traditional and conventional medicines draw on different legal jurisprudence to anchor them. The rules and regulations of the practice of traditional medicine are coined in the socio-cultural system of the community and were passed from one generation to another. Common laws often contradict traditions with regard to the use of traditional medicine. For example, common laws and regulations define punishment for those who breach the governing laws and regulations on the use of traditional medicine. These can be very punitive at times, recommending long jail terms or even the death penalty. The need to harmonize African traditional practices and current legal systems with regard to the use of traditional medicine is urgent, especially at this time when there is an HIV/AIDS crisis. Limited availability of conventional medicine in many resource-poor countries increases this need. The World Health Organization, for example, advises developing countries to utilize traditional medicine to provide primary health care to a vast majority of the population who are excluded from the formal health system. Contradictions in legal jurisprudence concerning traditional medicine suggest a need to develop appropriate institutional frameworks that may facilitate the integration of traditional medicine in resource-poor countries. This paper presents the experience of developing such a framework in the case of Tanzania. Tanzania is an ideal focus because of its steward position in doing this work since 2002, when it adopted an Act of Parliament, The Traditional and Alternative Medicine Act, 2002.

Introduction

Tanzania is one of the countries in sub-Saharan Africa that has a plurality of health systems, providing a wide range of options to clients who might not respond to one health system. Since the area of medicine is one of the major keys to the overall health of human beings, it needs regulatory machinery for the betterment of healthy communities. Not only should the regulatory machinery be in place, it should also be known to the people and stakeholders who use it, stakeholders such as the traditional healing practitioners (THPs), policy makers, and conventional health workers. By creating awareness, the regulatory system will operate to ensure that the management process within medical pluralism is offering services that are efficacious and safe for the health and well-being of people.

Before the arrival of missionaries and colonial governments, like other African countries south of the Sahara, Tanzania had her Indigenous traditional health care systems, referred to as traditional medicine (TM). "TM is the sum of all the knowledge and practical skills, whether explicable or not, used in the diagnosis, prevention and elimination of physical, mental or social imbalance and relies exclusively on practical experience and observation handed down from generation to generation, whether verbally or in writing" (WHO/Afro, 1976, p. 8). TM is part of the socio-cultural systems that have developed the control mechanisms of the practitioners (Kayombo, 1996, 1997, 1998), which everybody in the given community knows and demands in the provision of healthcare. The practitioners of TM are called traditional health practitioners (THPs). These include traditional healers (*waganga*): Traditional Healers (THs) of all categories (witchdoctors, shamans, diviners, sorcerers, herbalists, circumcisers, bone setters, witchcraft eradicators, fortune-tellers, etc.) and traditional birth attendants (TBAs) (United Republic Tanzania, 2000).

THPs are defined as "persons who are recognised by the community in which they live as competent to provide health care by using vegetable, animal and mineral substances and certain other methods based on social, cultural and religious background" (WHO/Afro, 1976,

p. 9). Through experience, THPs have developed a variety of ways for maintaining health and dealing with health conditions, and have advised people on how to use available remedies to deal with diseases and their consequences—leading to what we now call popular medicine. In some communities, THPs enjoyed the privilege of advising the chiefs in administrative matters, including wars and environmental protection. In some communities, THPs were rainmakers and were used when there was a prolonged drought or to temporarily prevent rain when there were important events (Kimambo & Temu, 1969). Above all, THPs are the custodians of traditional cultural practices and thus deserve respect.

There is no written evidence of the rules and guidelines that show how THPs should practice; it is based purely on memory. Some of the known rules and regulations governing the practice of TM are: "i) to be honest to their respective clients; ii) patients should be seen as their children and practitioners should work in collaboration with family; iii) when the woman was in her monthly period she should not touch *mkoba wa uganga* (bag that contain remedies and divination tools); if she does, the remedies lose their potency in healing the health condition; iv) THPs are strictly forbidden to have love affairs with their clients during the process of treatment; and v) THPs should offer *tambiko* (sacrifice) of thanksgiving at least once a year or when it is needed, and also tambiko of forgiveness if they have transgressed the norms of the ancestors or elders" (Kayombo, 1996, 1998, 1999, 2000). To be allowed to practice TM, one has to be selected by *mzimu wa mkoba wa uganga* (the spirit of the bag of medicine), an adult of at least 30 years old, and married. With this age, he/she is expected to make a sound decision in the process of treatment. Failure to observe rules sets forth deserved immediate punishment. It has to be stressed here that not just anybody can practice TM. He/she must be "called" by ancestors to practice (Kayombo, 1998; Peek, 1982). The poor practitioners of TM that we see today in our communities are very likely not called to practice TM.

The THP should be able to tell who initiated him/her, connecting them to a lineage of authentic practitioners, as well as explaining the comparison in practices of TM as they relate to the originator. In my village (Mlangali village, Ludewa District, Iringa region), I witnessed a case where the THP, who was treating a certain illness in a clan, died. A similar illness to the first appeared in another person in the community and the patient had to seek the THP who initiated the dead THP. The point that is being traced here is that people have strong confidence in information passed down through lineages and in the competence of certain THPs to manage certain health conditions, which is to say that there are specialists within the THPs.

During the colonial period, conventional Western medicine was introduced in Tanzania through the help of missionaries, first in urban areas and Christian mission centers. Western medicine was for elites, those working in government, and people living near missionary centers—typically new converts. Later, it spread to other parts of the country. The penetration of conventional medicine was associated with the demise of TM. During the German rule, healers were persecuted because they were taken as a threat to German sovereignty. During the British rule, the Witchcraft Ordinance Act of 1929 was introduced and THPs were persecuted and harassed once again as threats to sovereignty (Feierman, 1979, 1986). THPs are custodians of tribal secrets and are entrusted with the survival of their society; hence, they were regarded as a threat to foreign religions, cultures, and rules (Iwu, 2001; Kayombo, 1998; United Republic of Tanzania, 2000). The overall impact of labeling traditional remedies as *za kishenzi* and associating them with witchcraft created a mindset that discouraged the practice of TM, and those seeking traditional health services had to do so in great secrecy.

Notwithstanding, TM was entrenched in societies and, for many, it was the only means of health care; conventional medicine was for a select few. As argued earlier, TM is part and parcel of African culture and, therefore, the early missionaries' and colonizers' campaigns against TM demonstrated a typical means of imperialist power, introducing something new to kill the traditional culture of Tanzania and to create a dependency on conventional medicine. This move not only had an eye for the present, but also looked to the future, seeing Tanzania and other African countries as a profitable market for conventional medicine and pharmaceuticals. This is what most African countries are witnessing now—a greater dependency on conventional medicine that many cannot afford.

At some stage, the colonial government did accept the practice of TM in their respective areas because conventional medicine and its staff could not meet the demand of the growing population. Before the government could accept TM, it had to be assessed. For example, Germany in 1907 incorporated traditional medicine into the health care system of the then "German East Africa" (Kuelker, 2001). THPs in Tanganyika were given certificates indicating their locations of practice and the illnesses they were allowed to manage. During the British colonial rule, despite the introduction of the Witchcraft Ordinance in 1929, THPs were still allowed to practice TM in communities where respective traditional elders allowed them to do so (Mbwambo, Mahunnah, & Kayombo, 2007).

Surprisingly, the practice of TM was neither addressed at independence nor during the first to third development plans (1964-1969). Further, even after the Arusha Declaration (1967) when a lot of emphasis was put on the development of appropriate rural health facilities and rural health personnel, the contributions of traditional healers and TBAs were not taken into consideration (United Republic of Tanzania, 2000). Gradual positive changes toward TM in Tanzania began to take place. In 1968, the Ministry of Health issued a new Medical Practitioners and Dentists Ordinance of 1968 (United Republic of Tanzania, 2000) that took into consideration practitioners of TM. In 1969, the government took a new initiative aimed at the integration of conventional and traditional medicine (United Republic of Tanzania, 2000). This was due to the following factors: There was an awareness of the value of TM; the realization of the shortage of the resources and manpower essential for continued expansion of all type of curative and preventive services; and the practice of TM was flourishing even in urban centers despite the otherwise rapid changes toward modernization (United Republic of Tanzania, 2000). In 1969, the Chief Medical Officer in the Ministry of Health directed the regional medical officer to collect information from THPs on TM practices, including which drugs were being used.

The outcome of the Chief Medical Officer's directive was that THPs were seen by the Ministry of Health as continuing to maintain the centuries old relationship between the THPs and the patient, whereby a diagnosis was carried out, followed by customary formulation and dispensation of the medication (United Republic of Tanzania, 2000). Further, it was argued that the current situation of Western medicine was impractical and uneconomical, although it was the best means of guaranteeing the quality, safety, and efficacy of the medicine prepared. It argued that THPs must have appropriate accreditation to be seen as competent THPs. Despite the gains, the key issue here is the maintained superiority of the conventional medicine over the Indigenous medicine as a necessity of cultural imperialism.

Despite forced acculturation through foreign influence, it is estimated that there are over 80,000 THPs in mainland Tanzania (ITM, 2005) and it is estimated that at least 60% of Tanzanians in urban areas and 80% of the rural population rely on TM for their primary health care needs (Mahunnah, 2002). The importance of traditional health practitioners has been given due respect with the emergence of HIV/AIDS, where many patients in rural areas use TM. A caution has to be made: people use TM not only because of the unavailability of health services and the inability to pay for them, but also because there are some specific illnesses/ diseases that respond better to TM/Complementary/alternative medicine

(CAM) than to conventional medicine. For example, some kinds of mental illness, infant illnesses, impotence and infertility, cancer, diabetes, blood pressure, and degenerative diseases, respond better to TM/CAM than to conventional medicine (Kamiah et al., 2008; Kayombo, 1997; Richard et al., 2006; Thomas et al., 2006).

In recent years in Tanzania, we have witnessed the increase in interactions within and outside of the country as a result of technology, development in transport, and improved communication systems. The health outcome of this has been the penetration of other health and healing systems into Tanzania, referred to as CAM because they are not part of traditional Tanzanian culture. With this pluralism, there is the possibility for better provision of healthcare to the community but also the need for regulatory mechanisms that can control provision of healthcare and, at the same time, prevent quacks and charlatans.

The Tanzanian government at the policy level has seen the importance of TM and CAM in healthcare and has developed policy and legal frameworks to govern their practice. The issues in the legal framework include the National Health Policy of 1990, the TM and TBAs guidelines of 2000, Traditional and Alternative Medicine Act no.23 of 2002, regulations on the registration of traditional and alternative health practitioners and facilities, regulations on the registration of traditional and alternative health practitioners and their facilities, regulation on ethics and codes of conduct, and practice and regulation on the registration of medical material in 2008. Other initiatives are the forming of standard guidelines for traditional and alternative health facilities in Tanzania and supportive supervision guidelines for traditional and alternative health care services.

The government has demonstrated its political commitment to promoting TM. At present, the Tanzanian Health Policy recognizes TM along with other CAM systems of health care (MoH, 1996). In 2000, the government established the National Traditional and TBAs Implementation Policy Guidelines. In 2002, legislation was passed by the Parliament to establish the Traditional and Alternative Medicine Act with its regulations by 2008. Among the other things the Act and regulations aim for are the following:

i. To ensure high standard of conduct and practices among THPs;
ii. To foster good relations among THPs, patients and other health practitioners; and
iii. To increase THPs awareness of the existing rules and regulations governing the practice of TM and CAM (United Republic of Tanzania, 2000; MoH, 2001).

The overall goal of the legal framework is the promotion of TM in Tanzania by focusing on the following areas: product quality improvement, services quality improvement, promotion of TM/CAM professionalism, sustainable conservation of natural resources of TM, and collaboration that intends to bridge the gap between the systems (WHO, 2004). The major output is the socio-cultural-economic growth and overall health and well-being of the nation. But how does this policy and legal framework work with THPs and CAM practitioners to achieve the above aims and the overall goal in the country and, in general, the improvement of healthcare in the underserved rural areas?

The Health Situation of Tanzania

Tanzanian health services are provided by the government, parastatal organizations, volunteer agencies, private institutions, and traditional healing systems (URT MOH, 1983, 1989). The volunteer sectors provide 30-40% of health services, both curative and preventive, and most of their health institutions are located in rural areas (URT MOH, 1983, 1989).

In all developing countries, poverty-linked diseases account for about three quarters of all deaths of total population. For example, the major cause of morbidity and mortality in most developing tropical countries is infectious and parasitic diseases associated with poor sanitation and water supply, poor nutrition, and inadequate health knowledge (Lorenz & Mpemba , 2005; Report from the Joint Swedish/Tanzanian Health Sector Review in Tanzania, 1982). All of these diseases could be handled with public health services, including THPs who are with the people in the communities. Again, about one-third of childhood deaths are due to some form of malnutrition as a contributing cause, and approximately 16% of reported deaths in children under five years old are attributable to diseases which could be prevented through immunization (Lorenz & Mpemba, 2005; Report from the Joint Swedish/Tanzanian Health Sector Review in Tanzania, 1982). In Tanzania, the major causes of deaths reported in hospital are pneumonia, diarrhoea, defective nutrition, measles, conditions of early infancy, tetanus, tuberculosis, malaria, anemia (severe), and meningitis (Lorenz & Mpemba, 2005; Report from the Joint Swedish/Tanzanian Health sector Review in Tanzania, 1982) (See Table 1). All these could be prevented if the government had the money and qualified health personnel in both rural and urban health facilities, as well as if they used the traditional health practitioners who employ available and safe remedies as first aid.

Table: 1 Type of illness or injury Reported by Age Group and Sex HBS (2007)

Age group and condition	Male		Female		Total	
	2000/01	2007	2000/01	2007	2000/01	2007
Children (under 15 years)						
Fever /malaria	68.7	76.7	77.5	77.5	69.3	77.1
of which fever	N/A	49.7	50.8	50.8	N/A	50.3
Malaria	N/A	39.7	39.2	39.2	N/A	39.5
Diarrhea	14.1	12.4	12.0	12.0	14.4	12.2
Accident	3.0	2.8	2.2	2.2	2.5	2.5
Dental	2.4	1.2	0.9	0.9	2.4	1.0
Skin condition	2.9	4.2	4.1	4.1	3.6	4.1
Eye	7.4	2.4	2.6	2.6	7.1	2.5
Ear, nose or throat	10.7	6.8	7.7	7.7	10.5	7.3
Chronic illnesses	N/A	2.8	2.1	2.1	N/A	2.4
Other	12.3	8.0	8.5	8.5	12.0	8.3
% who reported multiple complaints	17.8	16.4	16.5	16.5	18.5	16.5
Adult (15+ years)						
Fever /malaria	60.4	61.0	63.1	63.1	60.1	62.2
Of which fever	N/A	39.5	41.5	41.5	N/A	40.6
Malaria	N/A	30.2	31.5	31.5	N/A	31.0
Diarrhea	9.7	7.3	7.0	7.0	9.9	7.1
Accident	8.7	7.9	3.6	3.6	5.0	5.4
Dental	5.1	3.5	4.1	4.1	5.6	3.8
Skin condition	2.2	2.6	2.1	2.1	2.1	2.3
Eye	5.2	4.6	4.7	4.7	5.2	4.6
Ear, nose or throat	7.8	6.0	9.2	6.5	8.6	6.3
Chronic illnesses	N/A	13.2	N/A	13.5	N/A	13.4
Other	25.1	15.1	29.2	17.8	27.5	16.7
% who reported multiple complaints	19.9	17.9	19.6	19.6	19.6	18.9

Source: *Household Budget Survey and National Budget Survey,* 2007.

Through the effort to provide comprehensive health services to all citizens by 1980, 72% of the Tanzanian population is living within 5 km of a health unit—i.e., within one hour walking distance (URT MOH, 1989; 1983; Lorenz & Mpemba, 2005). The government put an emphasis on rural health development, on preventive medicine, and promotion of curative services. In addition, Tanzania adopted the public health care (PHC) approach following the Alma Ata Declaration of 1978 (URT MOH, 1983). Since PHC is commensurate with the National Health Policy, its adoption has provided added impetus to the ongoing effort of achieving the social goal of health for all (URT MOH, 1983). It has to be pointed out that PHC is not just about providing more resources at the level of the remedial health services that most people come into contact with, as it is far more proactive than that. It is about giving people the skills and knowledge they need in order to stay healthy in the first place (Report from the Joint Swedish/Tanzanian Health Sector Review in Tanzania, 1982). It is about helping people to understand the causes of ill health and enabling them to make changes that will not only improve their quality of life but will also reduce demand on the health services—enabling limited and valuable resources to be stretched further (The Report from the Joint Swedish/Tanzanian Health sector Review in Tanzania, 1982). It is not known to what extent Tanzania has achieved the stipulations in the PHC policy. However, despite being where most of the Tanzanian population seeks healthcare, and despite their vast knowledge of various useful plants and methods of first aid, THPs are rarely included in that program. There is no way that developing countries can provide health care to all without including THPs. For example, the estimated total population of the WHO Africa Region in 2001 was 655,477,000. Over 50% of this number, the poor and most disadvantaged, do not have access to existing essential medicines (DeJong, 1991) and, therefore, had to seek health care from THPs for their health care needs. This percentage varies from country to country and from one region to another (Sambo, 2003). Nonetheless, reports from Member States to the WHO show that there is an increasing number of people seeking healthcare from traditional healers in Uganda and Tanzania (60%), Benin and Rwanda (70%), and Ethiopia (90%) (Sambo, 2003); hence the need for regulatory machinery in TM so that people can get safe remedies and, at the same time, THPs can be recognized as providers of health care in line with conventional medical practitioners.

Process of Development and Regulations of Act no. 23 of 2002

A government Act has a special mission to fulfill and it requires experts who have the will, commitment, and knowledge of the issues. Implementing the Act, on the other hand, requires the resources for creating awareness so that people can understand the Act and how it is going to operate. In the creation of awareness, areas of ambiguity and biases are going to be identified. These would be areas for consideration during the time of revision.

In Tanzania, the main objective of Act no.23 is to provide a legal framework for the promotion, control, and regulation of TM and other alternative medicine practices. The process of developing the Act was, at first, difficult because of the conflict of interest between conventional health practitioners, on the one hand, and policy makers and THPs on the other hand. Many conventional health practitioners denied the important role played by THPs. As shown elsewhere in this chapter, 60-80% of the population of Tanzania visits THPs for various ill health conditions and more than 50% of child deliveries are done at home by THPs (Kayombo, 1996; Tanzania, 2005). The conventional health practitioners argued that most of these home deliveries are done with the help of grandmothers, aunts, older sisters, or mothers-in-law, and very few are attended by TBAs. Conventional health practitioners deny the important role that TBAs play in health provision and child delivery. In one study, my colleague and I requested to meet with the THPs of the Kisarawe District of the coastal region of Tanzania. We were told that we could be allowed to see the THPs but not the TBAs because they were killing their wives. We asked how many mothers were killed by TBAs in this district—there was no answer (ITM, 2005). This is the type of continuous conflict that is unjustly directed toward practitioners of TM.

I faced a similar problem when I presented a paper on the role of TBAs in child delivery in rural areas at the 1990 Scientific Conference of Gynecologists and Obstetricians of Tanzania at Muhimbili University College of Sciences. During the discussion of the paper, most obstetric and gynaecology doctors argued TBAs were killing women and this accounted for a lot of the present maternal mortality rate (570/100,000 live births). A senior specialist in obstetrics and gynaecology asked his fellow doctors if they had data to substantiate their claim that TBAs kill women at delivery because of poor services rendered. He even went further by pointing a finger at them: How many women die in their hands because of poor mishandling and are not reported? He rescued me on that day. However, this is indicative of how TBAs are perceived in Tanzania.

The denial from the conventional health practitioners on the important role played by the THPs/TBAs can be seen in the government documents regarding health in Tanzania. For example, in the National Act on Mental Illness, even though it is known that many patients with mental illness are treated by traditional healing systems, there was no mention of TM or of including THPs until the late 1990s, with the advent of HIV/AIDS (DeJong, 1991; Kayombo, 2010; Mhondwa et al., 2004; WHO, 2000). Above all, there are no government budgets for traditional medicine activities involved with the intervention on infectious diseases like cholera, TB and HIV/AIDS.

The three paragraphs above give a picture of how difficult it was to develop the Traditional and Alternative Medicine Act in Tanzania. Nevertheless, at the end of 1989, there was a series of meetings with different stakeholders such as the chairperson of the THP associations, alternative medicine practitioners like homeopaths, and the Institute of Traditional Medicine at the School of Public Health of Muhimbili University College. More meetings were held in the 1990s on the development of the National Traditional and Birth Attendants Implementation Policy Guidelines, led by Dr. Sabina Mnaliwa, who was heading the Traditional Medicine Unit in the Ministry of Health. The output from this series of meetings was the establishment of the National Traditional and Birth Attendants Implementation Policy Guidelines of 2000. After developing this policy, major concerns and constraints within the traditional health services sector were identified and these are:

i. In the existing ordinances there is no legislation to govern, control and co-ordinate traditional health services (e.g., registration of THPs and licensing);

ii. THPs and their clients continue to operate in secrecy and fear with ambiguous legal and medical status;

iii. There is no formalized system of collaboration between conventional practitioners and THPs;

iv. There has been no attempt to introduce or incorporate the science and discipline of traditional health services in the training curriculum of the allopathic medical cadres;

v. The biodiversity that has harboured the medicinal resources is declining in certain localities as no deliberate protection measures exist; and

vi. The number of THPs is declining through old age and lack of apprentices.

Based on the above constraints, the overall goal of the national traditional health services is to improve the health status of people through the utilization of effective and safe elements of traditional healthcare and other alternative systems of healing in organized health care systems. Thus the following policy guidelines were developed:

a. Promotion of safe, effective, and ethically and socially acceptable THP services and other alternative systems of healing;
b. The practices which demonstrate efficacy and acceptable safety be promoted and integrated into health care delivery systems;
c. Any practice proven fatal, deceptive or harmful to the health of people shall be banned;
d. Fatal traditional surgical practices such as tooth bud extractions and female circumcision shall be banned;
e. Any practice whose primary intention is not to promote health shall not be adopted as part of traditional health care practice (e.g., bewitching);
f. Traditional healthcare and other alternative systems of healing facilities shall be encouraged to open and will be promoted to the people for use; and
g. Research on TM (material medica) shall be conducted at grassroots and advanced levels, involving THPs where necessary.

Using these guidelines, the major stakeholders of TM and lawyers developed the Traditional and Alternative Medicine Act no.23 of 2002. The legislation had to take on board other alternative medicines because the practitioners of these medicines were already in the country and practicing. For example, Homeopathic medicine was introduced in 1991 and other alternative medicines continued to mushroom thereafter. These included radionics, chiropractic, Ayurvedic, massage, acupuncture, magnet therapy, reflexology, and many others. Alternative medicine diagnostic procedures involve modern medicine diagnostic facilities, radionic computer methods, acupressure methods, iridology, etc.

Components of this legislation include statements on: health policy, traditional birth attendants' policy guidelines and implementation, vision for traditional and alternative medicine, and organization and management structures. Other components include the role and responsibility of stakeholders as identified by the Ministry of Health: traditional and alternative health care practitioners, the community/ clients, universities and research institutions, the pharmacy board, and the chief government chemist.

The legislation also provides for regulation on the ethical conduct of traditional and alternative medicine practitioners, registration of entitled persons, and letters of authorization. More areas covered under this legislation are the regulation of material aspects of traditional and alternative medicine remedies and the rights, duties, and limits of traditional and alternative health practitioners. Provision is also made for information dissemination among the stakeholders and general public, training, titles and designations, associations, and research development. The legislation concludes with issues pertaining to offences and penalties, finances, and development.

The expected outcome from the legislation is provision for registration, regulation, and control of the practice of traditional health practitioners and matters either incidental or connected with the foregoing. Further, the Act would safeguard the interest, security, and rights of the practitioners and clients and provide appropriate control measures on traditional medicine resources, conservation, multiplication, harvesting, and import and export of foreign remedies and practices. We also worked toward removing the inbuilt bias against traditional health care practices as contained in the Pharmaceuticals and Poisons Act of 1978, section 68(1)(2) regarding research methodologies, formulation, and utilization of traditional medicines. The Act recognizes training institutions inside and outside of Tanzania (since the country has no such facilities for training for the time being, though efforts shall be made to establish relevant institutions within the country), categorizes the THPs and their titles, standardized procedures on licensing, remedies, case management, and research methodologies.

Implementation of the Act of Traditional and Alternative Medicine Act, 2002

The aim of the Act and regulations is to have a legal tool to guide and regulate the extensive and growing practices and practitioners of traditional and alternative medicine. While historically, practitioners of TM were old people (Kimambo & Temu, 1969; Swantz, 1990) we are now seeing the younger generation practicing TM, and not only in their home communities, but also in urban centers where no one can ascertain for sure how they became THPs and who initiated them (Kayombo et al., 2006). In addition, the Act and regulation are expected to fill some of the gaps existing in the fragmented legal framework for control of natural resources of medicinal value (United Republic of Tanzania, 2000; Ministry of Health, 2001).

The chairperson for the Traditional and Alternative Health Care Practitioner Council was appointed by the President. The Ministry of Health, on the other hand, has appointed the registrar of THPs, who is a medical personnel and member of the council. All these are now in place. The Traditional and Alternative Medicine council has held a series of meetings to review the Act and develop a code of ethics, conduct and practices for TM and CAM. Through these meetings and others, and in cooperation with other stakeholders who were invited to these series of review meetings, the regulations of Traditional and Alternative Medicine Regulations were published on the 26th of December, 2008.

In addition, the council, with the financial support of the WHO, has organized and implemented two sensitization workshops—one at the Iringa District and the other in the coastal region. Key issues addressed during these sensitization workshops were the creation of awareness about the Act of Traditional and Alternative Medicine and the process of grassroots registration. The local government will be key when THPs start registering themselves because local government leaders know them and even know how they became THPs. The participants of the workshops were local government leaders, ward executive officers, District Medical Office staff, and other administrative staff at the district level. The sensitization workshops were to be expanded into other districts before starting registration of THPs that need to be registered according to the regulations of 2008. Financial constraints became the major bottleneck for implementing the sensitization workshops in other districts of Tanzania and even registration of THPs has not yet started in any of the districts.

Besides the above constraints in the attempt to implement the Act, it has come to my attention that the working principle of practice and remedies involved in traditional and alternative medicine are not well understood by conventional medicine practitioners and the elite class of Tanzania, who were the main stakeholders in ensuring that the Act was implemented. Practices of TM still rank highly in providing healthcare for Tanzanian people but unfortunately, the existing regulatory framework lacks competent personnel well versed in traditional medicine regulations, remedies, and practices involved (MOH, 2001). The issue of helping the larger population understand traditional and alternative medicine is further complicated by the existing alternative healing systems in Tanzania that include disciplines already established internationally, such as homeopathic medicine, chiropractic, massage, back flower remedies, aromatherapy, acupuncture and pressure, Ayurvedic medicine, reflexology, magnet therapy, radionic medicine, sauna bath, fasting therapy, crystal therapy, polarity therapy, naturopathy, hydrotherapy, and other established systems. All these need experts who can help advise the council and the Ministry of Health on their effective control, lest they create more serious health problems and become a burden to the country.

Furthermore, with regard to the Witchcraft Ordinance Act of 1929, to date it is difficult to pinpoint the witchcraft practitioners because THPs could also have knowledge of witchcraft. As is it is with conventional medical practices, the medical doctor knows both the healing and killing methods. Similarly, the THPs might also know the healing and witchcraft mechanisms and can use either if their clients need it. In one of the training workshops, a lawyer from the attorney general's office warned THPs that they could be in trouble because objects used in the treatment/ healing of patients may be associated with witchcraft in the Witchcraft Ordinance Act of 1929. There needs to be a review of the Witchcraft Act of 1929 so as to allow THPs to practice TM without fear.

Above all, even though TM is now legally recognized, it is not yet fully institutionalized. Gaps exist, as mentioned earlier, in the understanding of health issues and management of cases between traditional and conventional health practitioners. As shown earlier, many THPs are not aware of policy and regulations governing traditional medicine in the country and the institutional arrangements that deal with TM's promotion and development.

Implication of the Act in the Practice of TM and CAM in Tanzania

It is a good start for Tanzania. In the two sensitization workshops the THPs were willing to participate in, researchers and conventional health practitioners came together to discuss research and treatment especially for diseases that do not have cures in conventional medicine. Because of the different philosophy of disease causation and treatment, the problem is getting researchers and conventional health practitioners to see THPs as partners in research and health care. With the growing population in Tanzania, it has to be known that THPs have the human resources and, in order to improve health and well-being, there is no way conventional health practitioners can work without them (Kayombo, 1996, 1999, 2005, 2006).

Besides the willingness to collaborate with researchers and conventional health workers, there were other issues from the THPs that were raised during the sensitization workshops and these were: security of their remedies, intellectual property rights, harvesting herbal remedies in restricted areas, bio-piracy, and THPs being marginalized by conventional health practitioners. Similar concerns were noted in workshops on Traditional Medicine and HIV/AIDS (2003-2007) and on Traditional Medicinal Plants and Traditional Medicine Network in Eastern Africa (2003-2007). Even though the issues raised are only from a segment of the country, they still suggest that THPs are suspicious of researchers and conventional health workers, and conventional health workers do not trust THPs.

This calls for the cultivation of trust, transparent dealings, confidence and appreciation in experts in the three healing systems of the country, that is, the traditional, conventional, and alternative medicine practitioners (Kayombo et al., 2006). This should start in the early stages of the process of implementing the Act, through seminars, workshops, visits, having lunch together, exhibitions, etc., as a way of sharing knowledge and understanding the competency of other practitioners in each heath provision arena. This process requires time, but researchers are interested in rapid results. The THPs, on the other hand, are interested in finding people they can trust to work with in research and treatment (Kayombo et al., 2006).

The issue of harvesting the herbal remedies in restricted areas should be discussed at the community level to see how it can be solved. One of the roles of the Institute of Traditional Medicine of Muhimbili University is to train THPs on conservation. Four training seminars on how to grow medicinal plants have been done in Dar es Salaam and in the Morogoro region for THPs and other stakeholders who are interested in cultivating medicinal plants. Some of the THPs and other stakeholders in Dar es Salaam and the coastal region now have small plots of herbal medicinal plants. If THPs and other stakeholders will start conserving herbal plants in home gardens or on farms, it will reduce the conflict with foresters who are restricting THPs from harvesting herbal remedies in certain areas. In any meeting with THPs, there is the loud cry of the bio-piracy of herbal plants, where Indigenous knowledge of nature, originating with Indigenous peoples, is used by others for profit without permission. With the help of the Traditional and Alternative Medicine Council, useful medical and aromatic plants should be listed and restricted.

Conclusion

Introducing an Act like this one requires human resources well versed with both the Act and the important content and reason for which the Act is being developed. The case presented in this text is a case in point. Tanzania has a political will to introduce the Traditional and Alternative

Medicine Act, and with the help of experts, has managed to come up with an Act. In the process of its implementation,, the Act has succumbed to financial constraints and the lack of culturally qualified personnel in TM and CAM in Tanzania. As shown in the chapter, there is a lot to be done in sensitizing the conventional health workers and researchers to TM, CAM, the Act, and how it can help THPs and practitioners of CAM to improve the provision of health care. There is the need for highly qualified and dynamic experts who know the practice and malpractice of TM to help in implementing the Act, ironing out ambiguous issues, and taking up key issues in an amicable manner based on trust, transparency, respect, and appreciation of one another's expertise.

We sum up by arguing that this is a good start for Tanzania because only a few countries in Africa have given traditional medicine an official place, and Tanzania is one of them. There is need to continue reviewing the Act through research, with the possibility that they might touch other areas which are not included in the Act but are useful and should be included. The government, through its channels, should source money for sensitization, awareness, and registration so we can wipe out charlatans and quacks in the practice of TM. We can then focus on genuine THPs who can help the government in provision of efficacious and safe healthcare, especially in areas where conventional health services are not available. In this way, TM and CAM can become a viable option.

Reference

DeJong, J. (1991). Non-governmental organizations and health delivery in Sub-Saharan Africa. *Policy, research and external affairs: Working Paper 708*. Washington, DC: World Bank.

Feierman, S. (1979). History of pluralistic medicine systems: Change in African therapeutic system. *Social Science Medicine, 13b*, 277-284.

Feierman, S. (1986). Popular control over the institutions of health: A history study. In M. Last & G. L. Chavunduka (Eds.), *The professionalisation of African medicine* (pp. 205-220). Manchester: Manchester University Press.

Institute of Traditional Medicine Profile. (2005). Dar es Salaam: Muhimbili University of Health and Allied Sciences.

Iwu, M. M. (2001). Forward. In S. Laird (Ed.), *Introduction from biodiversity and traditional knowledge* (pp. xx-xxii). London, UK: Equitable Partnership in Practice.

Kayombo, E. J. (1996). Tambiko as healing therapy. In S. N. Madu, P. K. Baguma, & A. Pritz (Eds.), *Psychotherapy in Africa*. Vienna: WCP.

_____. (1997). Traditional birth attendants (TBAs) and maternal health care in Tanzania. In E. Kalipen & P. Thiuri (Eds.), *Issues and perspectives on health care in contemporary Sub-Saharan Africa by studies in Africa health and medicine* (Vol. 8, pp. 288-305). Lewiston, NY: The Edwin Mellen Press.

_____. (1998). Initiation of healers: An example of Tanzania. In *Ethnotherapien Therapeutische Konzepte Im Kulturvergleich Ethnotherapies Herausgegeben von Christine E. Gottschalk-Batschkus und Christian Ratsch* (pp. 25-28), VWB-Verlag fur Wissenschaft und Bildung.

_____. (1999), "Kupinga Tego" in Southern highlands of Tanzania: A case of one African: Traditional methods of healing. In S. N. Madu, P. K. Baguma, & A. Pritz (Eds.), *In quest for psychotherapy for modern Africa, third issue* (pp. 20-34). Pietersburg: WCP.

_____. (1999). Traditional healers and treatment of HIV/AIDS patients in Tanzania: A case of Njombe rural areas district, Iringa region. Unpublished doctoral dissertation, Wien University.

_____. (2000). Can dreams be a source of knowledge in traditional healing therapies? A case of six traditional healers in Tanzania. In S. N. Madu, P. K. Baguma, & A. Pritz (Eds.), *Psychotherapy and African reality* (pp. 95-119). Pietersburg: WCP.

_____. (2003). Mzimu in traditional healing in Africa: A case of Tanzania. In N. S. Madu (Ed.), *Contributions to Psychotherapy in Africa* (p. 5). Polokwane, Pietersburg: World Council for Psychotherapy: African Chapter.

_____. (2010). Traditional knowledge for health project in Tanzania. *Literature review on traditional knowledge for mental health in Tanzania* (Consultancy report submitted to Swedish Development Cooperation).

Kimambo, I. N., & Temu, A. J. (1969). *A History of Tanzania.* Nairobi: East African Publishing House.

Kuelker, R. (2001). The history of health care in Tanzania: An exhibition on the development of the health sector in more than 100 years. National museum of Tanzania. Dar es Salaam: Tanzania Printers Ltd.

Lorenz, N., & Mpemba, C. (2005). *Review of the state of health in Tanzania 2004: Independent technical review on behalf of the Ministry of Health, the president's office regional and local government and the government of Tanzania.* Swiss Centre for International Health.

Mahunnah, R. L. A. (2002). Ethnobotany and conservation of medicinal plants in Africa: The way forward in the decade. In Adenji (Ed.), *Proceedings of 15th Meeting of Inter-African Experts Committee on African Traditional Medicine and Medicinal Plants.* Arusha, Tanzania: AU Lagos.

Ministry of Health. (1983). *Guidelines for the implementation of primary health care in Tanzania.* Dar es Salaam: Government Printers.

_____. (1989). *National family planning programme plan for operation 1989-1993.* Dar es Salaam: Government Printers.

_____. (1996.) National health care policy. *Ministry of Health, United Republic of Tanzania.* Dar es Salaam: Government Printers.

_____. (2001). Key features of the proposed national traditional and traditional and alternative medicine legislation. Dar es Salaam: Government Printers.

National Bureau of Statistics. (2005). *Tanzania HIV/AIDS indicator survey 2003-2004.* Tanzania Commission for HIV/AIDS.

Niemtzow, R. C., Pham, N., Burns, S. M., Alston, C., & Lundgren, J. B. (2006). Macular degenerative disease and acupuncture safety precautions. Retrieved from: http://www.medicalacupuncture.org/aama_marf/journal/vol17_3/case_1.html

Peek, M. P. (1992). Introduction: The study of divination, present and past. In P. M. Peek (Ed.), *African divination systems.* Bloomington and Indianapolis: Indiana University Press.

Report from the Joint Swedish/Tanzanian Health Sector Review In Tanzania. (1982).

United Republic Of Tanzania. (2002). The National Traditional and Birth Attendants Implementation Policy Guidelines. Dar es Salaam: Ministry of Health.

United Republic of Tanzania. (2008). Supplementary no. 43 Subsidiary Legislation, The Traditional Medicine and Alternative Medicine, Code of Ethics, Conduct and Practice, Regulations, Arrangement of Regulations. *The Gazette of United Republic of Tanzania*, No. 52, Vol.89. Dar es Salaam: Government Printers.

United Republic of Tanzania. (2007). Household Budget Survey. National Bureau of Statistics. Retrieved from www.scribd.com/.../Tanzania-Household-Budget-Survey-2007

World Health Organization. (2004). Tools for continuing education of traditional health practitioners in primary healthcare. *WHO/Afro tools for continuing education of traditional health practitioners in primary health care.*

World Health Organization/Afro. (1976). *African traditional medicine.* (Technical Report Series, no. 1). Tanzania: World Health Organization Regional Office.

Chapter Twelve

HEALING PRACTICES OF KENYAN TRADITIONAL HEALERS: A DIALOGUE/INTERVIEW

Erica Neeganagwedgin and Simon Murangiri

I was born on the island of Jamaica, or Xayamaca, as the Indigenous people there call it. I am a woman with African and Taino ancestry: my ancestors were brought to Taino territory by European slave masters. In Jamaica, I frequently witnessed people turn to traditional forms of medicine when western conventional ways of healing failed to work, in order to obtain spiritual, physical, and mental health and wellness.

Gina Robinson (2010) speaks to the significance of traditional healers, noting that many formally trained Jamaican physicians will refer patients to herbalists and other medicine people in cases where they have difficultly diagnosing a patient. My experiences confirmed this: as a mere three-year-old, I learned about traditional medicines. I knew their names and I could go into the bush and pick the one I needed if I had a stomach ache or some other type of ailment. I would simply say, "Mama, mi a go a bush go pick bush." Medicines such as rosemary, leaf and life, cirrosy or bitter bush, and aloe, to name a few, were used for everyday treatment of ailments. Children and adults alike knew when to pick them and how to prepare them in order for them to work effectively. Plants were multipurpose, and we knew all of their applications. For instance, not only did we use scotch bonnet pepper in various foods to provide flavour, but we also knew how to use the leaves to help our bodies heal. This was a medicine that grew naturally in the soil and required no chemicals—only rain and sunshine.

The notion of the bush for me is connected to the importance of the bush to us as a people. The people who lived in my small rural community called the bush Burnt Ground, or Bun Grung Bush in the Jamaican language. The name Bun Grung Bush is symbolic of the everyday interaction we have with the land and our environment, and provides us with the medicines that we use to physically and spiritually heal ourselves. Having a connection to the bush and an understanding of plants and medicines helped to ground me, and others from my community, in our everyday lives. Coming from a people deeply rooted in the land and plants is a significant part of my identity—and, as I have come to understand, these Caribbean traditions are themselves rooted in African contexts and traditional healing practices.

In 2008, I had an opportunity to engage in a conversation with an herbalist from Kenya, Dr. Simon Murangiri, at a conference organized by scholars from the Ontario Institute for Studies in Education at the University of Toronto. The conversation that follows is a dialogue driven by curiosity about comparing ways of Indigenous healing between those who left the African continent as a result of chattel slavery and those who remained. I wanted to compare notes with Dr. Murangiri based on what I knew or what I had learned growing up in Jamaica. I had often wondered whether the practices were similar to those still practiced in Africa. Do we use similar herbs to cure common colds? Are Indigenous ways of knowing perceived as *primitive* and *backward* in Africa as they so often are in the Western world? What are our similarities and commonalities when it comes to Indigenous ways of healing? Do we have similar stories about our Indigenous teachers?

The following is the dialogue I engaged in with Dr. Simon Murangiri, an herbalist from Kenya, at the University of Toronto in 2008. It has been edited for clarity.

Erica Neeganagwedgin (EN): Dr. Murangiri, I must say that I thoroughly enjoyed your keynote address. It was interesting to note how conversant you were with different herbs and plants. It was refreshing to learn how you became a practicing herbalist. Maybe you can share with us a little bit more about your experiences and what motivated you to pursue herbal healing as a full-time occupation.

Dr. Simon Murangiri (SM): Erica, I never thought I would have an opportunity to talk about Indigenous healing with one of my African daughters. You must be one of the few young people I have met so far who is interested in traditional healing. My observation is that, more and more, young people do not want to have anything to do with traditions, or anything to do with old people in the village. Yes, it is very rare to find a traditional healer who is your age.

EN: Let me make a correction. I am not a healer, but a person who carries my African blood in my veins. I want to know more about African ways of knowing and healing. Your keynote today triggered lots of memories of home remedies that my parents prepared for me if I was sick.

SM: What makes you interested in knowing what I know about herbs or how I administer them?

EN: I teach in the area of Indigenous studies and as a Jamaican who grew up in the bush surrounded by many different medicines, I think our conversation will be interesting.

SM: Let me explain about healing. We have healers in Kenya who will pray for you. Others will mix herbs to give to their patients.

I learned to identify the healing plants before I was 10 years old. I used to be fascinated watching my maternal grandfather pick out roots in the forest. I used to follow him and watch him prepare the roots. Sometimes I would stay with him when clients came to see him. My grandfather, without knowing, planted the first seed, and when I retired at 55 years old, I became a full-time herbal healer.

You see, from my grandfather's teaching on practical applications, such as collections of the plants from the forest and preparation and administration of the right dosage, I was confident that I would be a good healer. But once I decided to follow in my grandfather's footsteps, I thought I should collect more information on herbal medicine.

I joined an alternative healing college in Kenya and studied traditional medicine. In particular, I was interested in the chemistry aspect of the plants, as well as their efficacy. Despite all the knowledge I gained from books, in the initial years of my practice I would still talk to my grandfather, who would confirm what the books were saying. He was a living library. The informal education from my grandparents was actually rubberstamped, or confirmed, by the laboratory tests I have done.

EN: Earlier today, you mentioned to the audience that the plants that surround our school are medicinal and most of what you use in Kenya can be found here. It is one thing to know the names of plants, and it is another thing to know their efficacy. Can you talk about that?

SM: Let me explain about the process of becoming a healer. Remember, I was not an only child. For my grandfather to hand over his healing kit, he had to be convinced without a doubt that I could be trusted—trusted with the knowledge, trusted to keep other people's affairs out of the public. My grandfather had to be sure that I would not engage in money-making ventures, but that I would be a healer who had integrity and the community's needs at heart.

EN: Yes. You are a walking dictionary, a science dictionary; and yet, you are a very humble person.

I do not want to ask you how many diseases you can cure or what type of sicknesses you deal with. I will leave you to decide what you want to share with me. Also, if you wish, you can talk about ways of preparing your herbs.

SM: Currently, we have two major diseases in Kenya. We have malaria, which is parasitic, and we have amadiasis, which is also parasitic. On the bacterial side, we have typhoid, which is very common in many areas.

The way I treat any of these diseases is very complex. When a client comes to see me, I have a discussion with him or her about their well-being. If they have any waterborne diseases, I give them some basics on cleanliness and on the clearing of swampy areas, and explain the importance of ensuring that there are no containers with stagnant water [in their homes]. I check their tongue, check their eyes, nails–these physical aspects of a patient can reveal a lot about their illness.

I then ask them some questions. If they have been to see a doctor in a hospital, I ask them to bring their medical records and any drugs they might be taking. Any herbs that I give my clients have been laboratory tested to confirm the degree of efficacy. In some cases, one plant may not be able to clear specific bacteria. For example, you might find that one plant will cure one type of bacteria and another plant another kind of bacteria, so you have to mix the two to remove the bacteria from the body. On the other [hand], you might find one that will cure both bacteria and parasites at the same time. You can combine two plants to cure a bacterial disease and a parasitic disease. For example, if one is suffering from typhoid fever, which is bacterial, and at the same time malaria, which is parasitic, they both can be flushed out by salmamalria. So, you give one medicine to cure the two diseases by mixing a broader spectrum of herbal medicine.

EN: What are some names of common medicinal plants that you use?

SM: For the purpose of treating malaria, aloe has been very effective, but not in the last ten or so years. This is because aloe products are in our supermarkets in Nairobi, in soaps, oils, teas, shampoos. This is good, but also not good. When a medicinal plant is applied as an everyday commodity, the body becomes immune to the curative aspects of the plant. My advice to you is: use herbal plants when you need them and not as a household food or tea. That is, do not misuse herbs. By "misuse," I mean when our bodies resist the herb but the parasites are not reacting to it.

We also have other plants, like *Shkuhuria pinata*. We have *Ajuga remota*. We have *Calsepinia Volkensii*, which does very well on malaria, especially in places where aloe has been misused.

My grandfather emphasized to us while growing up that anything used in excess is not good. However, he did emphasize the importance of preventative medicine—like taking mint tea or boiling roots that he would give us to drink—to purge out anything foreign in our bodies. For instance, we all knew the value of the mint plant. (He introduced it to my village—I am not sure where he got it from.) If you come to my home today, I have a botanic garden with all types of bushes.

I also want to mention that sometimes, I randomly select samples of plants—their leaves or their roots—and bring them to the university to test whether they are toxic or curative or preventative. By preventative, I mean whether they have any nutritional value.

During my keynote, I did not get a chance to talk about how I prepare my herbs. I will give you a glimpse into the world of herbalists.

Herbs can be prepared in different ways. For instance, if it is an emergency and I have no time for laborious preparation, I use the simmering system. This means boiling the herbs for a few minutes, a maximum of five minutes, so that you can extract the medicine within a very short time. Then, I let it cool and give the medicine to the patient. Other times, if it's a routine treatment, I prepare powder from different herbs. This is the best method. When the client comes for their weekly or monthly check up, they take the powder home with instructions to infuse one teaspoon in a half-glass of boiling water. You cover it to cool, then take it accordingly.

EN: Do you plan to pass this knowledge on to anyone else?

SM: Right now, I have one of my grand-daughters, who is a professional in this field and has a clinic. Then I have my last-born son, who is also a professional in herbal medicine.

EN: I think you mentioned during your keynote that traditional healing is usually passed on to males. So, your grand-daughter, how did she get to do this?

SM: Currently, the male factor has been taken out of the line, because women are also included. Right now, I am a lecturer and I am teaching both men and women. These days, we can produce female herbal doctors in addition to male herbal doctors because we have to develop as the world is being developed.

EN: What are some of the tensions between traditional healing practices and contemporary medicine?

SM: The major challenge for these two practices is regulation. Contemporary medicine is the preferred medicine and is under the Ministry of Health, while traditional medicine is under the Ministry of Culture. One practice is viewed as an essential element for people's health, while the other one is regarded as an artifact.

Another issue is that of the pharmaceutical industry. They have a big say in the types of drugs that should be allowed onto the market. That's my personal view.

Also, managing perceptions is a big thing in this industry. I have contemporary doctors who come to me and ask my opinion of certain cases, and I give them herbs in capsule form or tablet form to give to their clients. The contemporary doctors' patients have no idea that they are taking herbs for their condition. I keep telling my doctor friends, we should have a way of working together, because one cannot exist without the other. Both practices complement each other. For example, I know that in case of an emergency, herbal medicine does not work in some situations. Take, for example, a fracture. The contemporary doctor or surgeon has to do a bone setting in the theatre, and it is necessary to operate. As a traditional healer, I will come with herbs, which will accelerate the restoration of the body parts. One is not supposed to be supreme [over] the other.

I have a clinic that has been in operation for the last four years, and the current number of the clients at the time I left Kenya one month ago was 12,000. The diseases that I treat and find success in treating are often ones that have been declared terminal, such as diabetes, cancer, hypertension, hypoglycaemia, and asthma. I have so many cases of asthmatics that I have treated and cured. People are very happy. This is because, when I do the treatment, I do not just deal with the symptoms and the cause. I have to deal with the cause, the symptoms, and the source because, unless you eliminate the source of the cause of the symptom, you are doing nothing in the treatment. I'll use an example of a diabetic. Lowering blood sugar in a diabetic is not a cure. That is just dealing with the symptom and the cause. The pancreas has to be revaporized because it is the source of the cause of the raising of the blood sugar. If the pancreas is brought back to normal, the diabetes goes away.

Discussion

My experiences with healing practices in my rural community and my dialogue with Dr. Murangiri are indicators that Indigenous traditions play an important role in health and wellness, whether in a rural Jamaican context or in the Kenyan context. These healing practices continue to be deeply rooted in who we are as people of African ancestry and in the ways we see the world in which we live. They are rooted in our ancestral ways of knowing, traditions that have maintained and sustained us for the more than 400 years.

Leonard Barrett (1976) notes that many of the herbs, barks and roots used as medicine in Jamaica originally had African names, such as Cudjoe weed and Kwaku bush (p. 68). This suggests the passing down of traditional medicines from one generation to the next by African descendants and the importance of plants in the healing process. Many medicine people continued to utilize herbs even while being chattel slaves (Barrett, p. 76). According to Payne-Jackson and Alleyne (2004), knowledge of African medicinal treatments and rituals was brought from Africa to Jamaica by healers who were already professionals in their own villages. The most powerful *obeah* (medicine) persons, especially in earlier years of the colonial era, were described as African.

Robinson (2010) points out that the ethno-medicinal practices in Jamaica are deeply rooted in spirituality. For example, she notes that "bush doctors," the term for herbal healers in the Caribbean, diagnosed symptoms and prescribed treatments using "divination." Whether by the use of tape measures, tea leaves or Book of Psalms, these healers had a remarkable accuracy rate. Even when Western medicine was introduced to Jamaica, many rural people would go to the Western-trained doctor for a diagnosis and still go to the bush doctor for treatment.

Despite the widespread trust and confidence in medicine people even today, I have still observed some resistance to Indigenous healing methods. On a recent trip to a rural community in Jamaica, at my request, my relatives and I drove into the hills to seek the help and expertise of a traditional healer. To this day, my relatives refuse to speak about the visit because they believe it clashes with their Christian worldviews and values. The legacy of the colonial mindset is still very pervasive throughout the island. For example, the practice of *obeah*, in which medicine people utilize herbs and bush to help provide wellness to people in the community, was made illegal by British colonizers, a prohibition that continues to this day. However, today this does not stop medicine people from practicing their science, nor does it prevent people in the community from seeking the assistance of such practitioners. Indeed, as a child and even into adulthood, my father made visits to medicine people in various communities.

As noted by many Indigenous scholars, Indigenous healing practices remain important to people of African ancestry, whether directly from the continent or those living in the diaspora. They are a vital part of African thought systems and health practices. Many Indigenous scholars who have researched Indigenous healing practices have found them to be dynamic and complex. Dr. Murangiri reminds us that practitioners of Indigenous medicine and conventional medicine can work collaboratively.

References

Barrett, E. L. (1976). *The sun and the drum.* London: Heinemann Educational Books.

Payne-Jackson, Mervyn C. Alleyne (2004). *Jamaican Folk Medicine: A source of ealing.* Kingston: The University of West Indies Press

Robinson, G. (2010). Ask Doctor Gina: Jamaica's ethnomedicine. Retrieved March 14 at http://www.askdoctorgina.com/Jamaica%27s-Ethnomedicine.php

Chapter Thirteen

SPIRITUALITY AND ETHICS IN SOUTH AFRICAN TRADITIONAL HEALING: IMPLICATIONS FOR THE HELPING PROFESSIONS

Eleanor Ross, PhD, University of the Witwatersrand, South Africa

Introduction

This chapter takes as its point of departure a statement by Martin Luther King: "If we are going to go forward, we must go back and rediscover those precious values - that all reality hinges on moral foundations and that all reality has spiritual control" (Carson, 1999, p. 33).

South African traditional healing appears to be derived from—and inextricably linked with—spirituality, morals, and ethics. There are important principles to be learned from traditional South African approaches to healing—even for those who do not share the specific South African cosmology or worldview (Manda, 2008). This chapter adopts an etic or outsider perspective in that the author is not a member of the South African culture. Efforts are made to discuss the main tenets underpinning South African religion and spirituality; the differences between Western allopathic healthcare and African traditional healing; and the South African conceptualization of health, illness, disease, and healing that is predicated on the ethical principle of *ubuntu*. Examples are provided of ethical dilemmas arising from the application of traditional healing approaches within a rights-based society. Finally, the implications of integrating the South African and Western landscapes of healing into a pluralistic approach to healthcare are discussed.

Commonalities in African Religion and Spirituality

Within sub-Saharan Africa, the term African Religion, or African Traditional Religions, accommodates a wide variety of concepts and practices that distinguish the religious systems of various language or cultural groups from one another (Mbiti, 1989). However, even though there are differences between Zulu, Xhosa, Ndebele, Tsonga and other groupings, there would appear to be commonalities across the various South African cultures. Below, a number of these commonalities are discussed in order to set up the context for a discussion on healthcare and their spiritual aspects.

In view of the fact that, historically, many schools and hospitals in rural Africa were run by church-related organizations, the process of cross-fertilization between the African ethos and Christianity in Southern Africa has resulted in the emergence of so-called African Indigenous Churches. Although it is impossible to estimate the number of adherents of African Religion in Southern Africa, next to Christianity, it is believed to have the largest number of adherents in the region (Lubbe, 2004). However, Thabede (2008, p. 241) cautions that some Africans have adopted the Christian faith by and large without forsaking their Indigenous notions of the Supreme Being and their beliefs in ancestors and the power of witchcraft.

One of the key features of this spiritual or religious orientation is the belief in a Supreme Being—a God that created the world. According to African traditions, one can only gain access to the Supreme Creator through intermediaries in the form of ancestral spirits. It is generally believed that only those who have married and produced children, who will remember them, become ancestors when they die. Hammond-Tooke (1974, p. 325) defines ancestors as the spirits of the dead members of the lineage or clan. However, only those who have lived honourable and exemplary lives are destined to become ancestors (Kruger, Lifshitz, & Baloyi, 2007, p. 333). It is the responsibility of each family to remember its own ancestors until they have faded into oblivion. While the ancestors are respected and honoured by the living, by being included and remembered in family functions and in decision-making processes, the living family members also rely on the ancestors for protection and prosperity. However, the ancestors can also mete out punishment to people who do not listen to their wisdom, obey their norms and customs, or who violate taboos. Moreover, people can restore their relationship with their ancestors through offerings and sacrifices. Belief in the influence of ancestors in daily life is particularly prevalent in times of sickness (Magubane, 1998). In African society, only certain persons are chosen by the ancestors for mediatory work. These chosen individuals are the diviners and traditional doctors.

There is also a widespread belief in the spirits of nature, which are found in certain mountains, or hills, in specific rivers or lakes, or in special stones. The African animistic worldview "sees the world as a community of living organisms, and espouses respectful and conscious relationships with, among others, humans, rivers, trees, rocks, plants, animals, birds and ancestral spirits who are also members of the wider community of life" (Kruger et al.., 2007, p.333).

From birth, many South Africans are socialized to be part of a family and community, both of which are regarded as indispensable for security and for the development of a sense of wholeness. The performance of rituals plays a major role in the lives of individuals and the community (Thabede, 2008). In order to help a person move successfully through the various stages of life, life-affirming rites of passage are maintained and center primarily on life cycle stages such as birth, puberty and initiation, marriage and death, when the ancestors are revered and their blessings and benevolence are requested. Death is not seen as the end of life but rather as a way of moving on to join the company of the departed in a state of collective immortality (Lubbe, 2004).

According to Thabede (2008, p. 240), African knowledge of God is expressed in proverbs, idioms, songs, prayers, stories, and religious ceremonies passed on to succeeding generations through a predominantly oral history. Oppong (1992); Elion and Strieman (2001); and Bar-On (1999) as cited in Smith (2005), provide the following examples of traditional African religious rituals and practices:

(1) When parents complain that a child is difficult, cries often, wets the bed or is often ill, enquiries are made as to whether [or not] the birth rituals were performed. These rituals involve the introduction of the baby to the ancestors and the ritual slaughtering of a goat whereby the goat's skin is used to carry the child on the mother's back. This particular ceremony is referred to as *imbeleko*. If these rituals have not been performed, the parents are encouraged to have them done.

(2) Initiation marks the end of boyhood and ushers in the beginning of manhood/adulthood. Culturally defined rites of passage are performed when initiates are circumcised and withdraw from other people to live in seclusion in the mountains or in specially prepared huts away from the villages (Thabede, 2008).

(3) When a person is discharged from prison after having served a sentence for a crime, an important cleansing or washing ceremony known as *ucungo* must be performed before the person and their family can begin a new life.

(4) When someone close to a child dies, an adult informs the child about the death by whispering the news while he or she is sleeping. This custom is referred to as *uyubahlebela*.

(5) Marriage usually involves "bridewealth" or "ilobola" (gifts from the kin of the groom to the kin of the bride).

(6) An important bereavement and funeral rite is the practice of bringing the deceased person to the family home for the period before the funeral. During this time, one of the elders speaks to the deceased and explains exactly what is happening and where the person is going. The purpose of this ritual is to keep the deceased informed and at peace, beseech the person to protect the home, and help the family find meaning in their grief and loss. According to Bopape (1995, p. 262) traditional Bapedi mourning and bereavement rituals include "general abstinence from exceptionally joyous activities; 'doctoring' of the grave and funeral preparations; ritual ceremonies for the 'undressing' of mourning clothes and 'spreading' of the clothes of the deceased, and so forth, all of which have a therapeutic function which alleviates the pain of death."

(7) After a highly traumatic or painful event, a cleansing ceremony is held at the place where the event took place. This ritual can allow people from the affected community to collectively acknowledge their pain, to support one another and their need to move forward (Oppong, 1992, as cited in Smith, 2005).

These are all common examples of traditional African religious rituals and practices, which play an important role in the lives of individuals and the community.

Western and South African Worldviews on Healthcare

Spiritual and cultural factors not only influence the meanings attached to different health conditions and beliefs regarding causation, but are also likely to determine which persons are consulted to restore health and well-being. Whether or not one consults a Western health care professional or a traditional healer depends on one's worldview of health.

There are two main worldviews or social constructions of health, illness, disability, and healing: namely, the traditional approach, which is based on Indigenous belief systems, and the so-called modern approach, which is located within a Western medical paradigm.

According to the traditional African worldview, "health is about being 'whole', and refers to the synergies between the individual, the social and the cosmic world" (Kruger, Lifshitz, & Baloyi, 2007, p. 326). Within traditional medicine, diseases and disorders are seen as arising from natural, social, or psychological disturbances that create disequilibrium expressed in the form of physical or mental problems. Traditional healing seeks to restore harmony, balance, and equilibrium, not only through alleviating physical symptoms, but also through re-integrating the person with his or her community, the earth, and the spiritual world. Moreover, the life force can be enhanced through good relations with the family, community, ancestors and God (Kruger et al., 2007, p. 333). Supernatural causes play an important role in explaining health phenomena (Thabede, 2008).

In contrast, Western biomedical or allopathic medicine initially tended to view disease as a form of biological malfunctioning with ill health manifesting in chemical, anatomical, or physiological changes (Ross & Deverell, 2004). Traditionally, the Western medical doctor usually based his or her diagnosis on the patient's medical history, a physical examination, and if necessary, laboratory tests. Healing was viewed as the scientific, rational, and empirical process of correcting disease through appropriate medical, surgical, and chemical interventions (Chalmers, 1996). Prescriptions were given that could only be filled by a licensed dispensing doctor or pharmacist. Moreover, biomedicine had its roots in the Cartesian separation of mind and body (Levers, 2006). However, more recently, there have been attempts by the World Health Organization (WHO, 2002) to integrate the biomedical model with a social model to form a biopsychosocial model, which considers bodily functions and structures, activities performed by an individual, level of participation in societal activities, and the influence of personal and environmental factors on functioning, disability, and health. However, Western thought generally ignores the spiritual dimension and supernatural causes of phenomena.

Western cultures tend to distinguish between physical and mental well-being and approach different types of professionals for help with problems in these two spheres. For example, Westerners or persons of European or American descent tend to seek counselling from professionals such as psychiatrists, psychologists, social workers, and ministers of religion. In contrast, some non-Western cultures do not make any distinction between physical and psychosocial problems. Consequently, they tend to locate psychological feelings in the physical body, in the form of headaches, light-headedness, and other pains. Chalmers (1996, p. 2) elaborates on this theme:

> In contrast with the Western world's separatist approach to health and illness, the African view reflects an integrated, interdependent, totality of all things animate and inanimate, past and present. Underlying this pluralistic but holistic view is a unifying principle and balance between all things.

Western cultures emphasize self-reliance over dependency and the achievement of personal goals over collective ones. In contrast, African cultures embody the philosophy of *ubuntu*, which emphasizes connectedness, relatedness, and interdependence in relation to other people, the earth, and one's ancestors (Wehrly, 1995). The concept of *ubuntu* involves putting people first and reflects the communal values of collective humanity, compassion, solidarity, respect, humility, caring and sharing. In other words, a person is a person through other people (National Heritage Council, 2006). These values are likely to influence whether one consults a health care professional or a traditional healer about problems.

Africans often seek support from elders, family members, friends, and traditional healers before, or instead of, consulting with health professionals (Dlomu, 2000). In some African cultures, the traditional healer is seen as the counsellor and the process of counselling is regarded as a ritual that mobilizes natural or supernatural healing forces on the client's behalf. None of these cultural groups is likely to participate in counselling as part of treatment for an illness or disability. If the disorder is thought to be related to a spiritual cause, it is likely to be treated by confession or other forms of consolation (Battle, 1997, p. 124).

According to the World Health Organization (WHO, 2001), nearly two-thirds of the global population continues to rely upon the health care services of traditional doctors. For example, some Africans who have adopted Christianity may go to church to worship and also go to the graveyard to speak to the deceased family members who have become ancestors. As Thabede (2008, pp. 238-239) explains: "Occasionally one gets the feeling that Africans have a way of dealing in contradictions, incorporating things in their lives that seem to be contradictory, for example, taking a particular problem to church, to the ancestors, to the helping professional and to traditional healers at the same time". Furthermore, in many countries, people from all socio-economic and educational strata utilize Western-based biopsychosocial approaches as well as traditional practices, creating a medical syncretism or pluralism that integrates both models and has implications for the treatment or management of disorders and compliance with therapy, rehabilitation, and medical regimens (Muela, Rubera, Mushi, & Tanner, 2002).

Traditional Healing in the South African Context

Traditional healers play a particularly important role in South Africa where one Western-trained doctor may be responsible for nearly 7,000 people (Couper, 1997). It is estimated that there are between 250,000 and 400,000 traditional healers in South Africa, compared with 23,000 medical doctors, and eight out of every 10 Black South Africans rely on traditional medicine alone, or in combination with Western medicine (Keeton, 2004). For example, Ensink and Robertson (1999) found that 66% of African psychiatric patients in Cape Town, South Africa indicated that they used a combination of medical and Indigenous services for mental health problems. Consequently, South African health care professionals need to be aware of the beliefs and practices of traditional healers in relation to health, illness, and disability, and ways of restoring well-being. The role of traditional healers is an important one throughout the Indigenous South African community and has been recognized by the World Health Organization.

The World Health Organization classifies traditional healers as:

> a group of persons recognized by the community in which they live as being competent to provide health care by using vegetable, animal and mineral substances and other methods based on the social, cultural and religious background as well as the knowledge, attitudes and beliefs that are prevalent in the community regarding physical, mental and social well being and the causation of disease and disability. (WHO, 1978, p.41)

Traditional healers occupy an esteemed position within many Indigenous South African cultures as they are consulted for a wide range of physical, social, and emotional problems and are often expected to assume the multiple roles of medicine healer, physician, priest, psychiatrist, advisor, teacher, diviner, and herbalist (Gregory, 2001).

During the Apartheid era, the 1974 Health Act and its 1982 amendments restricted traditional healers' performance of any act related to medical practices. Nevertheless, despite these laws, traditional healing remained resilient, continued to operate in both urban and rural areas, and served all educational and socio-economic levels (Felhaber & Mayeng, 1997). Soon after the African National Congress (ANC) came to power in 1994, the government formulated the White Paper for the Transformation of the Health System in South Africa (1997), which recognized that traditional healers form part of the broader primary health care team. In September 2004, the South African government promulgated the Traditional Health Practitioners' Bill, which acknowledged the role that traditional healers play in South Africa. The Bill set professional and ethical norms and standards, and required traditional healers to register with a statutory council to ensure strict regulation of their practices (Matomela, 2004).

This legislation supported the stance adopted by the World Health Organization (WHO) on the role of traditional healers in the provision of primary health care in developing regions and has positively impacted the health care in this country.

South African Traditional Healers

African traditional healers are regarded as the guardians of African culture (Hammond-Tooke, 1989). Although they have different names within the different African language groups and regions, one can distinguish between five broad categories of South African traditional healers—namely, diviners, herbalists, prophets or faith healers, traditional surgeons, and birth attendants. While some healers identify themselves primarily as one type of healer, others combine more than one type. (1) *Diviners* form a crucial link between humans and the supernatural. They are chosen by the ancestors and use divination objects and their spiritual mediumistic powers to diagnose the unexplainable and interpret the messages of the ancestors. Their role is mostly that of divination, but they also provide medication for cases that have been diagnosed. They diagnose illness by throwing bones, cards, or stones and consulting the ancestors. The throwing of the bones is sometimes referred to in common parlance as the "floor X-ray" because the ancestors are able to understand the problem from the way in which the bones fall. Some of these diviners are able to go into a trance-like state of altered consciousness, which allows them to commune with the ancestors. (2) *Herbalists,* on the other hand, are ordinary people who have acquired an extensive knowledge of herbal treatments but do not possess occult powers. They are able to diagnose illnesses and prescribe herbs, medication and enemas for a range of ailments, and are expected to be able to provide protection against witchcraft in order to prevent misfortune and bring prosperity and happiness. (3) *The prophet or faith healer* heals and divines within the framework of the African Independent Churches. In their diagnosis and treatment of patients, prophets or faith healers use prayer, candlelight, or water, as well as enemas, and inhalation of the steam of mixed concoctions poured over heated stones (de Andrade & Ross, 2005). (4) *Traditional surgeons* conduct circumcisions of initiates. (5) *Birth attendants* assist with the delivery of babies. For these different healers, there is a strong belief that their power comes from God. Moreover, "religion and magic are not seen as separate, but as aspects of being where all of life is seen as a unitary field and where the spiritual and physical worlds are one" (Moodley & West, 2005, in Kruger et al., 2007, p. 335). Some traditional healers wear modern conventional Western clothing while others use the skins of animals, feathers, and beads as part of their clothing. The colours of the beads have different symbolic meanings. Each healing training school has different adornments, dances, and procedures.

Persons who consult with traditional healers are expected to remove their shoes and hats before entering the consulting rooms, and women are expected not to wear trousers. They do not tell the healer what the problem is; instead, the healer tells the person or family what he or she believes to be the problem. In the past, the term "witchdoctor" was used to portray traditional healers as "the epitome of evil, primeval cunning and the dark forces of barbarism" (Hammond-Tooke, 1989, p. 103) In this way, a negative colonial and Eurocentric bias and cultural hegemony were perpetuated against traditional healers, who were marginalized and treated as "others" (Levers, 2006). However, there has been a move to replace the term "witchdoctor" with "traditional healer" or "traditional medical practitioner," as genuine healers hold paramount the well-being of their patients and eschew all forms of witchcraft. Furthermore, these terms evoke less negative connotations. At the same time, one needs to acknowledge that belief in witchcraft is an important dimension of the African worldview (Thabede, 2008, p. 242).

In general, African traditional healers' skills are acquired by apprenticeship to an older healer, experience of certain techniques or conditions, or by a *calling* by the spirits or the ancestors. Some people are called before they are born, while others are called during childhood or adulthood. The calling can take the form of a dream, a passion, or a feeling. Sometimes the calling makes a person feel sick or brings them ill fortune, leading them to consult with a traditional healer who tells them that they have been "called." The process of initiation as an Indigenous healer is referred to as *ukuthwasa* (derived from the isiXhosa concept of *twasa,* meaning "the emergence of something new") (Hammond-Tooke, 1989). People believe that it is the ancestors who decide who should be chosen to become a healer, and if the calling is not obeyed, the person remains ill or continues to suffer ill fortune until he or she accepts the calling and enters into an apprenticeship with a more experienced traditional healer or *gobela* (Mindset Health, 2006).

After going through a rigorous apprenticeship, which may range from two to 20 years, the graduates attend a ceremony involving a number of tests and rituals over several days, where they each declare their spiritual name and identity. They believe that their power to heal comes though God. Following the graduation ceremony, there is a welcome home ceremony involving a series of rituals that welcome the new traditional healer back to his or her home.

Healing ceremonies often start with cleansing rituals in a consecrated space. The creation of this sacred space is facilitated through rituals such as drumming, dancing, bone throwing, and animal sacrifice. Inhalation of smoke and snuff is also believed to help the healer enter into a heightened physical and psychological trance-like state and commune with the ancestors.

The Value of Traditional Medicine

Traditional medicine, in general, has been shown to have benefits for the South African Indigenous people that include psychological relief from ailments and reduced anxiety through a shared, unquestioned, and unwavering belief in the powers of the healer. The treatment provided by traditional/complementary/alternative healers is viewed by the Indigenous people as holistic as it targets the mind, body, and soul of patients within their family, community, and religious contexts (Levers, 2006). While the efficacy of traditional healing remains contested by conventional medical practitioners, some pharmacological studies have demonstrated the efficacy of herbal substances such as plants used in Borneo for the treatment of malaria and the South African Hoodia plant for the suppression of appetite. Research at the University of California, Los Angeles has shown the effectiveness of Ginkgo biloba for the treatment of memory loss (Aitken, 2003). Hammond-Tooke (1989) acknowledges that it is often difficult to explain why traditional medicine seems to work. He speculates that healing may be promoted by the personal meaning the patient derives from the treatment as well as the connection between the person seeking healing and the healer. A sense of comfort and relief from pain, depression, and despair may also be provided through traditional medicine, even though a cure is not always found. Moreover, traditional healers may be more physically and geographically accessible to populations residing far from centres that dispense Western medicine (Freeman & Motsei, 1992). Their services are also often more affordable, particularly for poor rural families (Aitken, 2003) or for those who live in the poorest parts of developed countries (Levers, 2006). These caregivers are often the first consulted by parents about their children. They enjoy high levels of confidence with local communities, possess significant social capital, and understand the social, cultural, economic, and political context within which they operate (Levers, 2006).

When people have been asked about their reasons for consulting traditional healers, a common response has been dissatisfaction with treatment received from, or negative experiences with, Western, allopathic medical practitioners. Other common themes have been the holistic focus of traditional healing, the healers' close association with cultural, religious, and spiritual beliefs and practices, and the fact that these healers speak their language, spend time with them, and provide explanations for their health conditions.

Ethical Issues in the Application of South African Traditional Healing Approaches within a Western Rights-based Society

According to Mindset Health (2006), African traditional healing is based on the belief that the land's natural resources have nurtured humans and all forms of life since the beginning of time. Consequently, this oldest form of medicine uses natural resources for medicines and treatments. Natural herbs are used as healing agents because of the belief that humans are part of nature and natural products are a gift from the Creator. South African traditional healing is holistic and integrates a combination of approaches such as mental and spiritual guidance, herbal medicine, nutritional therapy, and physical therapy. South African traditional healers have strong ethical principles and believe that it is their duty to develop life in all its forms and to alleviate suffering. They also believe that nature's laws must be obeyed in order to avoid human decline and the destruction of the environment. The natural environment and the people who inhabit the environment are all believed to possess intrinsic worth. South African traditional healers respect the environment and emphasize the need to preserve it and to view it as a sacred entity. Hence, the ethical imperative is not to treat the natural world as a means to an end but as an end in itself.

Moreover, the belief that "in addition to healing methods involving a recovery from bodily ailments, it also involves a social, spiritual and psychological reintegration of the patient into the community of the living and the dead" (Manda, 2008, p. 126), is strongly predicated on the principle of *ubuntu*. The isiZulu concept of *ubuntu* is the foundational doctrine of traditional South African morals and ethics. It emphasizes collective identity as opposed to individual identity, solidarity, caring and sharing, the relatedness between the physical and metaphysical world, the value of interpersonal relationships, and the idea that a person is a person through other persons, *umuntu ngumuntu ngabantu* (National Heritage Council, 2006).

According to Gumede (1990) a Western-trained doctor, both modern healers and traditional healers have the same goal, i.e., to help the sick, to cure illness or relieve pain and suffering, and to comfort the patients and their relatives. Hence, it seems that there should be no conflict between African traditional healing and Western medicine and how human rights are respected among the two practices. However, this issue is discussed in relation to findings from research studies on traditional healing. For example, Dagher and Ross (2004) interviewed a group of traditional healers regarding their views on cleft lip and palate. One belief expressed by several of the traditional healers was that craniofacial conditions signify that the affected individual has been identified by the ancestors to become a traditional healer and that one should therefore not interfere with the ancestor's wishes through surgical intervention. Other healers felt that the affected children should be referred to Western doctors for reconstructive surgery in order to prevent them from being labeled as "witches" as a result of their physical appearance.

These beliefs raise ethical concerns for helping professionals. Health care professionals are expected to respect the cultural beliefs of different groups; however, they also need to consider the rights of affected individuals to receive surgical intervention that could potentially enhance their quality of life and prevent them from being labeled as "witches." Furthermore, what is the responsibility of helping professionals to persons who have already been accused of witchcraft, had their homes burned down, and been chased out of their communities?

A further issue hinges on the finding that has emerged across many studies on traditional healing (Ross, 2008), namely that many disorders and disabilities were perceived as a form of punishment for wrongdoing. Such perceptions are likely to evoke intense feelings of guilt in parents, caregivers, and affected individuals. The question then arises as to whether helping professionals should simply encourage people to work through these feelings in counselling, or whether they have an ethical obligation to provide people with information on the so-called scientific nature and etiology of the condition—information that could run counter to their religious and cultural beliefs. Is it possible to provide such information in a way that still conveys respect for the client's cultural beliefs and values?

Some traditional healers advise persons living with HIV and AIDS or Tuberculosis only to take traditional herbs and not to combine such herbs with antiretroviral (ARV) drugs. In fact, a study conducted by the South African Human Science Research Council in 2008 found that 60% of the 484 patients surveyed in rural KwaZulu-Natal believed that traditional herbs were more effective and safer than ARVs (Mthethwa, 2008). The question then arises as to whether helping professionals employed in health care settings have an ethical obligation to urge patients to continue with their Western medication or to respect their right to choose the health practitioner of their choice and decide what form of treatment they wish to follow.

Implications of Cultural Practices and Rituals for the Helping Professions

These examples highlight the tensions and contradictions between religious and cultural practices and the rights of individuals. According to Holomisa (2007), the basic antagonism between the human rights of mainstream society and an African culture emanates from the fact that while the former believes that the full realization of the human potential lies in the absolute freedom and independence of the individual, the latter espouses the notion of *ubuntu* and the common good, i.e., that no man is an island.

These debates highlight the need for South African helping professionals to re-visit the issue of formulating African models of social work practice that do not rely exclusively on British, European, or American models but which draw on Indigenous best practices, and Indigenous knowledge and culture from the African continent. We need to understand, appreciate, and engage the cosmological, ontological, and epistemological differences that separate Euro-American and African medical and cultural approaches. Mlambo-Ngcuka (in National Heritage Council, 2006: 22) contends that *ubuntu* embodies universal human values that are essentially not in contradiction with values of the diverse communities in South Africa and are found in Christianity, Islam, Judaism, Hinduism, Buddhism, and the Bahai faith (Ross, 2008).

Health practitioners are ethically mandated to exhibit cultural competence in their work with clients. According to Hodge (2006), the development of interventions that are relevant and sensitive to the client's worldview is a foundational principle of cultural competence. In addition, the incorporation of clients' spiritual and cultural beliefs may foster increased client investment in the growth and healing process and increase the likelihood of positive outcomes. As Hodge (2006, p. 163) writes, "If interventions make sense to the client, a greater likelihood exists that the client will be invested in applying the intervention."

In a similar vein, Levers (2006b) emphasizes the need for culturally sensitive, appropriate interventions in Africa and advocates collaboration with traditional healers and the incorporation of African traditional healing within an African approach to counselling. For example, it could be helpful to refer a woman who has been raped to a medical practitioner for antiretroviral therapy while respecting her right to approach a traditional healer who will pray for her and administer various herbs to induce vomiting and diarrhoea, thereby relieving feelings of guilt and pollution.

Levers (2006a) recommends the design of culturally relevant health-related counselling, prevention, and education programmes that take an ecological view of human development into account and are informed by relevant contextual issues such as culture, poverty, gender, migration, domestic violence, civil unrest, and access to health care and social services. Levers (2006a, p. 96) states that pre-service training of African helping professionals:

> ... needs to include an emphasis on contemporary problems in Africa, and problem analysis needs to be linked to Afro-centric models of problem solving. Students need to understand the psychology of Indigenous ways of knowing and encouraged to construct intervention models that address the needs of most Africans in culturally meaningful ways.

Such preparation could lead the way to systemic social service that alters the course of how South African health care services are delivered. These are the types of issues that can be used to encourage students within the helping professions to debate ethical issues in courses on values and ethics. Engagement with these types of ethical dilemmas is not only of relevance to South African health care practitioners but also to other multicultural societies.

The fact that so many people use both health care systems concurrently suggests that African traditional healing and Western allopathic medicine do not necessarily represent incommensurable paradigms but can be combined in the training curricula of health care professionals to form a pluralistic approach to health care. In a similar vein, Moodley (2000, p. 164) posits that including two different health care modalities is possible since "competing and contradictory cures can be held alongside or in tandem with each other without necessarily creating conflict." In the words of Kruger et al., 2007, p. 329), "these fragments of multiple worldviews may merge in unexpected and imaginative ways of relating and living." As Kuokkanen (2006) argues, we need to go beyond Eurocentric conventions of knowledge to include Indigenous ways of knowing and believing.

I concur with Kruger et al., 2007, p. 340) that a pluralistic worldview needs to be informed by the value of *ubuntu*, African notions of connectedness and wider cosmological relatedness, respect for existing beliefs and practices, and the inclusion of Western notions of agency and pro-action (as opposed to reaction and fatalism). Such an approach could potentially allow patients to inform Western doctors that they are consulting with traditional healers without fear of being reprimanded and denigrated; it would allow for reciprocal referrals and for us to be aware of the possible interaction effects of different medications such as antiretroviral and herbal therapy. In this manner, students and graduates may be able to construct intervention models that serve the diverse South African communities in more culturally sensitive and meaningful ways.

References

Aitken, S. (2003). *Biodiversity and health: Conserving our healing resources.* Retrieved from http://www.tc-biodiversity.org.

Battle, D. E. (1997). Multicultural considerations in counseling communicatively disordered persons and their families. In T. A. Crowe (Ed.), *Applications of counseling in speech-language pathology and audiology* (pp. 118-141). Baltimore: Williams & Wilkins.

Chalmers, B. (1996). Western and African conceptualizations of health. *Psychology and Health, 12*, 1-10.

Couper, I. (1997). The future of rural medicine in South Africa. *South African Medical Journal, 87*(3), 290-292.

Dagher, D., & Ross, E. (2004). Approaches of South African traditional healers regarding the treatment of cleft lip and palate. *The Cleft Palate-Craniofacial Journal, 41*(5), 461-469.

De Andrade, V., & Ross, E. (2005). Beliefs and practices of Black South African traditional healers regarding hearing impairment. *International Journal of Audiology, 44*, 489-499.

Dlomu, N. M. (2000). A comparative study of the perceptions and attitudes of psychologists and clients in cross-cultural settings. *MA Psychology Research Report.* Johannesburg: University of the Witwatersrand.

Ensink, K., & Robertson, B. (1999). Patients and family experiences of psychiatric services and African Indigenous healers. *Transcultural Psychiatry, 36*(1), 23-43.

Felhaber, T., & Mayeng, I. (1997). *South African traditional healers' primary health care handbook.* Cape Town: Kagiso Publishers.

Freeman, M., & Motsei, M. (1992). Planning health care in South Africa—Is there a role for traditional healers? *Social Science and Medicine, 34*, 1183-1190.

Gregory, S. (2001). Shamans/traditional healers: Custodians of our people. *Journal of Psychology, 19*(1), 59-64.

Gumede, M. V. (1990). *Traditional healers: A medical doctor's perspective.* Braamfontein: Skotaville.

Hammond-Tooke, W. D. (1974). *The Bantu-speaking peoples of Southern Africa.* London: Routledge and Kegan Paul.

Hammond-Tooke, W. D. (1989). *Ritual and medicines: Indigenous healing in South Africa.* Johannesburg: Donker.

Hodge, D. R. (2006). Spiritually modified cognitive therapy: A review of the literature. *Social Work, 51*(2), 157-165.

Holomisa, P. (2007, April 21). Traditional leaders' perspectives on customary practices, the African renaissance and the new constitution. *Cultural Legislation Indaba.* National Heritage Council. VodaWorld, Midrand.

Keeton, C. (2004, May 9). Sangomas to join medical fraternity. *Sunday Times,* p.4.

Carson, C. (Ed.). (1999). *The autobiography of Martin Luther King, Jr.* London: Little Brown.

Kruger, J., Lifshitz, S., & Baloyi, L. (2007). Healing practices in communities. In N. Duncan, B. Bowman, A. Naidoo. J. Pillay, & V. Roos. (Eds.), *Community psychology: Analysis, context and action* (pp. 323-344). Cape Town: UCT Press.

Kuokkanen, R. (2006). The logic of the gift: Reclaiming Indigenous peoples' philosophies. In T. Bortz-Bornstein & J. Hengelbrock (Eds.), *Re-ethnicising the minds: Cultural revival in contemporary thought* (pp. 101-123). Amsterdam: Rodopi.

Levers, L. L. (2006a). Traditional healing as Indigenous knowledge: Its relevance to HIV/AIDS in Southern Africa and the implications for counselors. *Journal of Psychology in Africa, 1,* 87-100.

Levers, L. L. (2006b). Samples of Indigenous healing: The path of good medicine. *International Journal of Disability, Development and Education, 53*(4), 479-488.

Lubbe, G. J. A. (2004). Health care for people of different faiths. In A. A. Tjale & L. de Villiers (Eds.), *Cultural issues in health and health care: A resource book for Southern Africa.* Cape Town: Juta Academic.

Magubane, P. (1998). *Vanishing cultures of South Africa.* London: Struik Publishers.

Manda, L. D. (2008). Africa's healing wisdom: Spiritual and ethical values of traditional African healthcare practices. In R. Nicolson (Ed.), *Persons in community: African ethics in a global culture* (pp. 125-139). Scottsville: University of KwaZulu–Natal Press.

Matomela, N. (2004). Recognition for traditional healers. *About South Africa>Health.* Retrieved from http://www.southafrica.info/ess_info/sa_glance/health.traditional-healersbill.htm.

Mbiti, J. (1989). *African religions and philosophy.* Pretoria: University of the North.

Midset Health. (2006). Johannesburg, South Africa (A partner of Mindset Network).

Moodley, R. (2000). Representation of subjective distress in black and ethnic minority patients: Constructing a research agenda. *Counselling Psychology Quarterly, 12* (2), 159-174.

Mthethwa, B. (2008, October 12). HIV patients trust in traditional remedies. *Sunday Times*, p.5.

Muela, S. H., Ribera, J. M., Mushi, A. K., & Tanner, M. (2002). Medical syncretism with reference to malaria in a Tanzanian community. *Social Science and Medicine, 55*(3), 403-413.

National Heritage Council. (2006). *Ubuntu Imbizi/Pitso: Reclaiming Ubuntu for a better society Report 2006.* Pretoria: National Heritage Council.

National Heritage Council. (2007, March 16 to 22). Are South Africa's laws on cultural rights and practices in conflict with our democratic Constitution? *Mail & Guardian*, p. 17.

Ross, E. (2008). Traditional healing in South Africa: Ethical implications for social work. *Social Work in Health Care, 46*(2), 15-33.

Ross, E., & Deverell, A. (2004). *Psychosocial issues in health, illness and disability: A reader for health care professionals.* Pretoria: Van Schaik.

Smith, L. (2005). Including cultural and religious rites and practices in emancipatory social work intervention. In R. Lutz (Ed.), *Dialog und diskurs: Zut theorie und praxis der sozialen arbeit.* Oldenburg: Paulo Freire Verlag.

Thabede, D. (2008). The African worldview as the basis of practice in the helping professions. *Social Work, 44*(3), 233-245.

Wehrly, B. (1995). *Pathways to multicultural counseling: A developmental journey.* Boston: Brookes/Cole.

White Paper for the Transformation of the Health System in South Africa. (1997). Pretoria: Government Printers.

World Health Organization (WHO). (1978). The promotion and development of traditional medicine. *Technical reports services, 666.* Geneva: WHO.

World Health Organization (WHO). (2001). *Legal status of traditional medicines and complementary/alternative medicine: A worldwide review.* Retrieved from http://whqlibdoc.who.int/hq/2001/WHO_EDM_TRM_2001.2.pdf

World Health Organization (WHO). (2002). *Towards a common language for functioning, disability and health (ICF).* Retrieved from http://www.who.int/icf/beginners/bg/pdf

Chapter Fourteen

AMANDLA! AWETHU! COMMUNITY HEALTH AND EMPOWERMENT THROUGH HOLISTIC KNOWLEDGE AND HEALTH PRACTICES

By Farah M.C. Shroff and Sundeep S. Dhaliwal

Abstract

This chapter critically explores the increasing popularity of holistic healthcare practices, particularly within Third World societies and with a focus on African societies. We examine the re-integration of traditional and modern health knowledges and how this trend is occurring simultaneously all over the planet. As new diseases and problems arise, holistic healthcare has adapted to meet these challenges. There are many benefits to learning the healing properties of plants, water, naturopathic manipulation, acupuncture, the deep connection between mind, body and spirit, massage therapy techniques, the healing benefits of particular foods, and the salubrious effect of a true healer. As non-Africans, we do not seek to appropriate, nor do we attempt to speak as experts of Africans knowledge forms. Rather, our purpose is to write about congruent trends in holistic medicine around the world, deferring to African scholars, some of whom are publishing other chapters in this book, as the experts in African knowledge forms.

Introduction: Mother Afrika Gave Birth to us All

Afrika is the Mother continent. It is timely to be writing about a revival of Afrikan systems of medicine, for it is time for the Mother continent to regain power on this ailing planet—for the uplifting of peoples everywhere, especially within Afrika and her diaspora. Thousands of years old, Afrikan traditional healing blends mind, body, and spirit. Despite damage created by centuries of European colonialism, Afrikan healers who worked with plants, bone-setters, spiritual healers, birth attendants, and others, were sought out by local people partly because of shared cultural worldviews.

Despite invaders' attempts to destroy traditional medicine, traditional medical practitioners survived and are thriving today, serving 85% of Afrikans throughout the continent (IDRC, 2011; WHO, 2011).

In some cases, people are choosing traditional medicine in conjunction with other systems of medicine and in others, traditional medicine is used on its own; sometimes, traditional medicine is used solo because it is the only affordable option and other times it is because it is the most effective option. Organizations like Pro. Me.Tra (www.prometra.org) and its offshoot, CEMETRA, promote Afrikan traditional systems of medicine through cultural and scientific research as well as medical practice. Through FAPEG, these organizations aim to train healers. They work toward effective holistic treatments for HIV/AIDS and other conditions that have impacted the continent.

The fear-driven and lucrative business of pseudo-traditional healers cannot be ignored when examining the healing industry. It can be easy at times to confuse authentic traditional healers with those who profiteer from the vulnerability and illness of working-class people. However, the rest of this chapter will not focus on these pseudo-healers. Our interest is in finding ways to regain traditional knowledge for the benefit of modern people in Afrika and beyond.

Our interest in holism and holistic health has many purposes. We are interested in documenting the trend toward the resurgence of holistic health around the world, particularly in light of its tremendous healing potential, which has been documented in myriad peer-reviewed articles in medical journals, including systematic reviews (Ernst & Hung, 2011; Ventegodt & Merrick, 2009). We also argue that holism has potential for decolonizing the minds of the peoples of Afrika, Asia, Latin America, the Middle East, and the Original Peoples of the Americas; it is thus part of a larger anti-racism and anti-imperialism project. Finally, when we embrace our cultural ways of knowing the world and our mind/body constitutions, we understand ourselves in a deeper fashion. Knowing ourselves is one of the most important spiritual tasks, and this chapter seeks to explore how holism helps us achieve this.

We have been inspired by the brilliant work of Clem Marshall, Chinweizu, Angela Davis, Thomas Sankara, Maya Angelou, Malcolm X, Bene and Edwin Madanagu, bell hooks, Steve Biko, Marcus Garvey, Tony Morrison, Chinua Achebe, Miriam Makeba, Festus Iyayi, and other Afrikan/diasporic liberation leaders. From them, we have learned about ancient knowledge emanating from traditional Afrikan societies, such as the importance of the ancestors, elders, language, greetings, heart-to-heart communication, and innumerable scientific advancements. These scholars and social actors have taken action to help Afrikans regain self-knowledge, self-love, and power in the world. We are inspired by concepts of Kawaida, Kwanzaa (its seven principles: Umoja, Kujichagulia, Ujima, Ujamaa, Nia, Kuumba, and Imani), Sankofa, and other Afro-centric philosophical conceptualizations. We appreciate the sentiments behind the Swahili word for tradition and reason, *Kawaida*—expounded by Maulana Karenga—because it exemplifies the liberatory use of traditional arts and sciences for healing the modern world. *Kawaida* is much broader than health and healthcare; it embodies the philosophy of Afrika, the Mother Continent, and seeks to heal her children around the planet. Afro-centric explanations of Kwanzaa also resonate within us.

For our title, we chose the Xhosa and Zulu words *Amandla! Awethu!* for their global significance as Afrikan concepts of freedom and power as a result of the anti-apartheid movement. *Amandla! Aweitu!* means power to the people: knowledge is power; healthy people are powerful. There are many reasons that these words resonate with the theme of our work here. Our approach to Afrikan traditional medicine acknowledges the tremendous healing potential of the spirit and the outstanding work done by those who are authentically connected to the spirit. The deepest form of healing is that which is done at the spiritual level; those whose spiritual practices lead them to that profound sense of connection to all life are leaders in the creation of sustainable changes toward community health, human rights, and peace.

Finally, we choose to spell Afrika with a 'k' because we wish to acknowledge and embrace the spelling used by Afrocentric scholars and change makers.

Locating the Authors within the Text

Farah Shroff, PhD: I am a Parsi born in Nairobi, Kenya. Swahili and Kikuyu were two of my first languages, and I also spoke English, Gujarati, and some Hindi as a child. As an adult, I worked as a (volunteer) public health planner and educator in Nigeria where I was also honoured to be a member of Women in Nigeria (WIN); I feel very strongly that South Asians and Afrikans are linked in common struggles for self-determination. Moreover, having seen the destructive divisions between South Asians and Afrikans in both my personal life and in societies around me, I am committed to working toward unity. By and large, South Asians living in Afrika, even those who are oriented toward social justice, have not been in solidarity with our Afrikan sisters and brothers; thankfully this is changing and I look forward to the day when we unbuckle the asphyxiating belt that colonized our bodies and minds! Once we realize that our cultural commonalities are greater than our differences, South Asians will refuse to be the wedge between European imperialists and Afrikans; we will mix more freely with Afrikan peoples, work together, and see that our paths to freedom are similar.

I believe that one of the most powerful roads toward liberation leads to Indigenous knowledge systems; as we get to know ourselves, our worldviews, and our various practices through these ancient knowledge forms, we help to build peace and justice; we also see the commonalities between our worldviews. My work has largely been on South Asian Indigenous knowledge and the linkages that all forms of Indigenous knowledge have with each other. I have a genuine desire to see holistic health practices re-emerge in the modern world, blending old and new in a practical, powerful way to heal this planet. Holistic health systems, in concert with allopathic systems, have the potential to effectively treat many illnesses. Besides working as a researcher and educator, I am also a teacher of yoga, meditation, dance, singing, martial arts, and other creative holistic expressions. In contributing to this important book on Afrikan holistic health practices, I strive to be an ally to Afrikan peoples who are working toward community health, social justice, spirituality, and so forth. In no way do I attempt to be more than an ally. Supporting the work of Afrikan peoples is my role in this struggle.

Sundeep Dhaliwal, MD: I was born in Northern British Columbia and raised among Indigenous North Americans. My early experiences with mind/body interactions stem from my family heritage of Punjab, India. This early exposure helped me understand the traditional South Asian worldviews and the traditional worldviews of other communities. Although a recent graduate of allopathic medical school, I continue to value the role of holistic medicine alongside allopathic understandings of the human body and mind.

Principles of Holism

Holistic worldviews have not been dominant for the past 400 years, but currently a revival of holistic thought forms is taking place in many parts of the world. The purpose of this chapter is to sketch the landscape of holistic philosophical foundations with an emphasis on Afrikan concepts, discuss systems science in this context, and apply these ideas to holistic health in the hope that doing so will increase our understanding of both the conceptual foundations of holism as well as its global applications to health promotion, disease prevention, treatment of ill health, and palliation. We discuss the importance of holism and social justice for developing community health. The article concludes with the recommendation that holistic health care practitioners take social inequities into account so that integrative health care can become a means for individuals to take action for wellness in order to create structural changes toward equitable resource distribution.

The English words 'health' and 'holistic' are semantically related. They both stem from the same root word: the Anglo-Saxon words whole, hale and holy (Pretorius, 2009), and holism is sometimes spelled as wholism to accentuate this semantic connection. Despite the linguistic connection, the word holistic is often used in incongruent ways and has become an umbrella term that is used to encompass anything that is non-reductionist or dualist. In this chapter, the concept of holistic health care will be used interchangeably with alternative or complimentary medicine and will be defined as approaches to well-being and treatment of illness that focus on mind and body. Additionally, the term holistic health care will be used in this chapter to encompass both self-care and practitioner-based care. Holistic self-care encompasses practices such as yoga, meditation, Tai Chi, and Chi Gung. Holistic care provided by professionals encompasses Afrikan bone-setters, spiritual healers, traditional birth attendants, traditional Chinese medicine, Ayurveda, homeopathy, botanical medicine, therapeutic massage, and others.

One principle that holistic schools of thought have in common is that entities and systems in the universe, including humans, are considered part of a unified whole, which cannot be understood by the isolated examination of their separate parts (Dusek, 2006). These parts are actively interrelated. Similarly, matter is interlinked, interconnected, and dynamic; it is constantly changing and it is this transformation that denotes time.

Holistic worldviews do not focus exclusively upon the body or organism but on the larger world—the universe—and are often associated with spiritual or religious thought-forms. At the heart of holism, there is an awareness of the unity and mutual interrelation of all things and events. All things are seen as interdependent and inseparable. This ultimate, indivisible reality is called Ubuntu in southern Afrika, Brahman in Hinduism, Dharmakaya in Buddhism, and Tao in Taoism. Because it transcends all concepts and categories, Buddhists also call it Tathata-Suchness (Deshmukh, 2006), That Which Is, or Is-ness, the sum of all forms.

According to Afrikan holistic worldviews, the cosmos is one, a spiritual totality. Spirit is not separate from matter, as everything is connected (Asante & Mazama, 2009). In Afrikan holistic thought, all things are considered to be related through one divine force (Asante & Mazama, 2009). They are alive, giving and receiving energy, with all life and matter created for a specific purpose. The concept of Ubuntu has been translated as "I am what I am because of who we all are" (Gbowee, 2010), and refers to kindness and other humanitarian values. Ubuntu is found in many Afrikan languages: Shona, Tswana, Rwanada-Rundi, Kitara, Luganda, and others. In the Yoruba tradition, the Creator, Oludumare, is considered to be transcendent, exhibiting the quality of "atérerekáyé (He who spreads all over the world or He who covers the whole world or He makes the whole world feel his presence)" (Omosade, 1996, p.16).

First Nations philosophies are similar to the Ubuntu concept insofar as First Nations peoples see themselves as part of a Sacred Hoop or Circle of Life, not having control over it; they are careful to maintain a balance with life (Hunter et al., 2006). Just as we impact the broad cultural climate in which we live, our physical, emotional, and psychological health is influenced by that very climate. Social harmony thus influences individual well-being in many First Nations cosmo-visions. First Nations healers advise people to see everyone as a family member or friend, thus encouraging social integration (Musqueum Elder Shane Pointe, November 5, 2006, personal communications). The Medicine Wheel, representing harmony and connectivity, takes this concept further. It represents all of creation: all planets, stars, peoples, animals, and plants. It is the basis of community health with the circle symbolizing the cycles of the seasons and of life, and wholeness and perfection. First Nations peoples' healing circles, sweat lodge ceremonies, and other healing rituals are generally performed in a circle. The circle emphasizes togetherness and community unity, without which the individual cannot be well.

The New Physics

Notable physicists such as David Bohm and Fritjof Capra emphasize the similarities between their theories of the indistinguishability of field and force, and the holistic views on mind and matter from spiritual traditions of Buddhism, Confucianism, Hinduism, Taoism, and Afrikan traditional medicine systems. In their work, these scientists emphasize the same foundational notion as holism: that the whole is greater than the sum of its parts. The natural world interacts synergistically. It is thus not possible to fully understand systems by knowing the properties of their individual components (although it is useful to study individual components). Indeed, as stated by Capra (2002), "the basic oneness of the universe is not only the central characteristic of the mystical experience but it is also one of the most important revelations of modern physics. It becomes apparent at the atomic level and manifests itself more and more as one penetrates deeper into matter, down into the realm of subatomic particles" (Gaan, 2005, p. 324).

Holistic Health

The aforementioned concepts of systems science and holism find concrete application in systems of holistic health promotion, disease prevention, treatment of illness and/or palliative care such as bone setting, spiritual healing, yoga, Ayurvedic medicine, herbalism, Chi Gung, Tai Chi, Traditional Chinese Medicine, and Afrikan and Indigenous systems of health care. What connects the diversity of these holistic traditions is that—without exception—they take into account mind, body, the environment, and the interconnection between them. They recognize the interrelationship between human health and the social and physical environments. Holistic health theory is posited on the notion that life force connects all that is alive in the universe, and this energy is responsible for the life of all beings. There is no English word for this concept, but in almost 50 languages around the world it has a name. It is called NTU in Bantu, prana in Sanskrit, chi in Chinese, and mana in Hawaiian. NTU is that which gives us life, or is the vehicle of life, the cosmic breath, the rhythmic oscillation effective on all levels of conditioned existence. Restoring and keeping this life force flowing is one way of keeping people healthy.

Holistic health is typified by the notions that health is a positive state, not merely the absence of disease, and that health is tied closely to familial, social, and cultural environments. Holistic health care is characterized by the belief that successful healing transforms the practitioner as well as the client, and healing includes a spiritual component in the aetiology and treatment of illness. Holistic health care thus understands malfunctions (illness) in the context of the social, cultural, and spiritual environments. Treatment of both body and mind are considered integral (Barnes, Powell-Griner, McFann, & Nahin, 2002).

The body is understood in a unified manner within holistic health perspectives. Injury to one part of the body may thus damage another, seemingly unrelated, part. Kidney malfunction, for example, may result from a damaged heart. If one part of the kidney is injured, another part may take over its functions. Holistic principles maintain that the body has an innate capacity to heal itself, and the role of the physician is firstly to do no harm and secondly, to assist the body in its natural tendency toward balance.

Holistic Health Care: A Growing Trend

While allopathic medicine is useful for the treatment of acute and emergency care needs, holistic health care appears to be more promising for chronic conditions and mental health care, which constitute a majority of health problems; these chronic diseases are leading causes of death and disability around the world (Palmer, 2009). Interest in holistic care in North America is growing among health professionals and the general public. In the United States alone, spending on alternative medicine has increased from $14 billion in the early 1990s to $33.9 billion in 2007. Moreover, 83 million adults in the U.S. are using some form of holistic and alternative medicine (NCCAM, 2011). In Canada, that number is similar, with one study finding that 73% of Canadians have used some form of holistic health care in their lifetime (Esmail, 2007). While studies measure different definitions of holistic health and varying time periods, the overall trend makes it clear that Canadians are increasingly using holistic health care.

The popularity of holistic healthcare is in part due to the increasing dissent with the present system of medical care delivery.

Some people, particularly women, prefer holistic practitioners partly because of practitioner friendliness and interpersonal sensitivity (Barnes et al., 2002; Kelner & Wellman, 1997). Many clients of holistic practitioners value this relatively egalitarian relationship. Other reasons why Canadians are turning to holistic health care practices include fewer side effects, the perceived lack of harm from holistic health care, and the possibility of improved health are (Quan, Lai, Johnson, Verhoef, & Musto, 2008). However, holistic practices are virtually always accessed in conjunction with allopathic practices in North America; very few North Americans, even those who are active proponents of holistic care, use no allopathic medicine.

Holistic Health Care Critically Examined

Most systems of health care, including holistic ones, do not include social health as a major component. This lack of attention to health care is a serious gap in holistic health care practices. Furthermore, within many systems of holistic medicine, patriarchal and classist overtones are apparent. In Chinese medicine, for instance, Yin traditionally means the shady side of a mountain, but is also related to femaleness and inferiority; undcr a patriarchal lens, Yin and women are considered more negatively than Yang. For Taoists, there is no such thing as absolute moral judgments, with neither Yin nor Yan representing good or bad (Brodd, 2009). While this reasoned view (which states that neither Yin nor Yan is good or bad) was probably the original medical understanding, oppressive structures have affected modes of thinking. Most likely, the original writings were not corrupted by hierarchical social structures, but given that medicine and politics are intricately intertwined, have become politicized over time. Upper class, patriarchal, and heterosexist interpretations of holistic health concepts flourish in the literature but are misinterpretations of original teachings (Gyatso & Hakim, 2010; Lad, 2006; Lad & Durve, 2008; Liao, 2006; Lu, 2005).

Furthermore, holism has been embraced by several groups, including those who serve non-holistic ends. Among them are "new age" entrepreneurs who are profiting from the commodification of holistic health, including shamanic healing, hypnosis, trance work, and so forth. Practitioners, who claim to be holistic, profit from the work of others and from the teachings they have gained from South World knowledge forms without crediting the original sources. They may claim to Westernize holistic practices in order to lure customers who know very little about the origins of holism. They may also excuse sexist, heterosexist, classist, and racist behaviour in the social organization of their work, on the grounds that the culture from which it comes is based on oppressive practices. This is a kind of appropriation and misrepresentation of holism, as are the claims made by practitioners masquerading as holistic healers, stating that they can miraculously cure diseases in order to lure vulnerable and ill people into paying large sums of money for unproven therapies.

The critiques of holistic health—that it provides an individualistic solution to problems of health by changing the individual rather than the social causes of illness, and that it carries a victim-blaming ideology (Crawford, 2006)—apply to allopathic medicine as well. Allopathic medicine does not encompass a social and political view of the determinants of health either. In itself, it is not a solid enough argument to dismiss holism. It can, however, be combined with the above arguments of appropriation and class privilege.

Closing Reflections

The concept of holism is international and ancient, stemming from the Mother continent—Afrika. Crossing countries and historical periods, holistic concepts and health practices based on these thought forms flourished for centuries and declined over the past 400 years or so under European colonialism. European domination of the planet brought with it reductionism, dualism, and the Europeans' off-shoot, allopathic medicine. Allopathic medicine has made many useful advances, particularly in acute care. Currently, there is a global re-emergence of holistic thinking and holistic practices, framed within a liberatory lens and embodied by concepts such as Kawaidaa. This chapter analyzed the historical as well as contemporary bases of holism as interconnectedness, unity, and oneness, and their application to holistic health care.

Neither the allopathic nor the holistic model of care attend to social inequities, yet holistic practices generally take into account the many facets of the individual—emotional, social, mental, and spiritual. It is partly for this reason that holistic care is increasingly popular. The peoples of Afrika, Asia, Latin America, and the Middle East, still rely quite heavily on traditional systems of medicine; in many cases this is because of its financial and cultural accessibility. Furthermore, as the health of the individual is clearly linked to her or his income, employment, security, and social status, deepening our understanding of the impact of social inequities on an individual's health will contribute to more efficient and just holistic health care systems. When holistic practices are joined with social justice approaches to working with communities, population health status promises to improve. Moreover, when people's health care reflects their worldview, communities deepen an understanding of who they are—improving self-knowledge and pride.

Major institutions are currently studying alternative medicines, including herbal remedies, bodywork, meditation, dietary changes, and more. Various studies, and some systemic reviews, are available on almost every type of holistic practice, and they typically show good results (Andrade-Cetto et al., 2011; Campbell-Tofte et al., 2011; Hamza et al., 2011; Maude, Woodrow, & White, 2010; Okoli et al., 2008; Schulzke et al., 2011). Working together, there is great potential for holistic health care and allopathic medicine to improve population health. Given that the basis of holistic philosophy is unity and oneness, a health care system that incorporates the most effective aspects of various systems of medicine would have powerful potential to improve population health on many levels—embracing the depth of the concept of Ubuntu. Allopathic medicine has made great advances in population health, particularly in emergency and acute care. If practitioners were to take social inequities into account, this integrative health care could truly become a means for individuals to take action for wellness as well as a means to create structural changes toward equitable resource distribution. We have written elsewhere (Shroff, 1996) about a health care system that incorporates public health approaches and integrates best practices from multi-paradigmatic medical systems.

References

Andrade-Cetto, A., & Wiedenfeld, H. (2011). Anti-hyperglycemic effect of Opuntia streptacantha Lem. *Journal of Ethnopharmacology, 33*(2), 940-943.

Asante, M. K., & Mazama, A. (Eds.) (2009). *Encyclopedia of Afrikan religion* (Vol. 1). Thousand Oaks, CA: Sage Publications, Inc.

Barnes, P., Powell-Griner, E., McFann, K., & Nahin, R. (2004). Complementary and alternative medicine use among adults: United States, 2002. *Seminars in Integrative Medicine, 2*(2), 54-71.

Brodd, J. (2009). *World religions: A voyage of discovery.* Winona, MN: Saint Mary's Press.

Campbell-Tofte, J. I., Molgaard, P., Josefsen, K., Abdallah, Z., Hansen, S., Cornett, C., et al. (2011). Randomized and double-blinded pilot clinical study of the safety and anti-diabetic efficacy of the Rauvolfia-Citrus tea, as used in Nigerian traditional medicine. *Journal of Ethnopharmacology, 133*(2), 402-11.

Capra, F. (2002). *The hidden connections: A science for sustainable living.* New York, NY: Doubleday.

Crawford, R. (2006). Health as meaningful social practice. *Health, 10*(4), 401-420.

Deshmukh, V. D. (2006). Neuroscience of meditation. *The Scientific World Journal, 16*(6), 2239-2253.

Ernst, E., & Hung, S. K. (2011). Great expectations: What do patients using complementary and alternative medicine hope for? *Patient 1:4*(2), 89-101.

Esmail, N. (2007). Complementary and alternative medicine in Canada: Trends in use and public attitudes, 1997-2006. *Public Policy Sources, Number 87.* Vancouver: The Fraser Institute.

Gaan, N. (2005). *Relevance of environment: A critique on international relation theories.* Delhi: Kalpaz Publications.

Gbowee, L. (2010). *It's time to end Afrika's mass rape tragedy.* Retrieved from http://www.thedailybeast.com/articles/2010/04/05/its-time-to-end-Afrikas-mass-rape-tragedy.html

Gyatso, T., & Hakim, C. (2010). *Essentials of Tibetan traditional medicine.* Berkeley, CA: North Atlantic Books.

Hamza, N., Berke, B., Cheze, C., Le Garrec, R., Lassalle, R., Agli, A., et al. (2011). Treatment of high fat diet induced type 2 diabetes in C57BL/6J mice by two medicinal plants used in traditional treatment of diabetes in the east of Algeria. *Journal of Ethnopharmacology, 133*(2), 931-933.

Hunter, L. M., Logan, J., Goulet, J. G., & Barton, S. (2006). Aboriginal healing:

Regaining balance and culture. *Journal of Transcultural Nursing, 17*(1), 13-22.

Kelner, M., & Wellman, B. (1997). Health care and consumer choice: Medical and alternative therapies. *Social Science & Medicine, 45*(2), 203-212.

Lad, V. (2006). *Textbook of Ayurveda: A complete guide to clinical assessment* (Vol.2). Albuquerque, NM: Ayurvedic Press.

Lad, V., & Durve, A. (2008). *Marma points of Ayurveda: The energy pathways for healing body, mind and consciousness with a comparison to traditional Chinese medicine.* Albuquerque, NM: Ayurvedic Press.

Liao, Y. (2006). *Traditional Chinese medicine.* Beijing: China Intercontinental Press.

Lu, H. C. (2005). *Traditional Chinese medicine: How to maintain your health and treat illness.* Laguna Beach, CA: Basic Health Publications.

Maude, R., Woodrow, C., & White, L. (2010). Artemisinin antimalarials: Preserving the "magic bullet." *Drug Development Research, 71*(1), 12-19.

Okoli, C., Akah, P., Onuoha, N., Okoye, T., & Nwoye, A. (2008). Acanthus montanus: An experimental evaluation of the antimicrobial, anti-inflammatory and immunological properties of a traditional remedy for furuncles. *BMC Complementary and Alternative Medicine, 6*(8), 27.

Omosade, A. J. (1996). *Yoruba beliefs and sacrificial rites.* Brooklyn, NY: Athelia Henrietta Press, Inc.

Palmer, S. (2009). Global health in transition. *Center for Communications, Health & the Environment (CECHE).* Retrieved from http://www.ceche.org/programs/globalhealth/globalhealth.html

Pert, C., & Marriott, N. (2007). Everything you need to know to feel go(o)d. Carlsbad, California: Hay House Inc.

Pretorius, S. P. (2009). Is "divine healing" in the "Faith Movement" founded on the principles of healing in the Bible or based on the power of the mind? *HTS Teologiese Studies/Theological Studies, 65*(1),1-7.

Quan, H., Lai, D., Johnson, D., Verhoef, M., & Musto, R. (2008). Complementary and alternative medicine use among Chinese and White Canadians. *Canadian Family Physician, 54*(11), 1563-1569.

Schulzke, J., Andres, S., Amasheh, M., et al. (2011) Anti-diarrheal mechanism of the traditional remedy Uzara via reduction of active chloride secretion. *PLoS ONE,* *6*(3), e18107.

Shroff, F. (2000). Forget reform: We need a revolution! Better health for Canadian women through holistic care. In Diana Gustafson (Ed.), *Care and consequences: The impact of health care reform* (pp. 271-293). Halifax: Fernwood Publishing.

Shroff, F. (1996). *New directions in Canadian health policy: Lessons from holistic medicine.* Unpublished doctoral dissertation, University of Toronto, Toronto, ON.

Ventegodt, S., & Merrick, J. (2009). Meta-analysis of positive effects, side effects and adverse events of holistic mind-body medicine (clinical holistic medicine): Experience from Denmark, Sweden, United Kingdom and Germany. *International Journal of Adolescent Medicine and Health, 21*(4), 441-456.

Weaver, A. J., Vane, A., & Flannelly, K. J. (2008). A review of research on Buddhism

and health: 1980-2003. *Journal of Health Care Chaplaincy, 14*(2), 118-132.

Chapter Fifteen

ETHNO-MEDICINAL PRACTICES AMONG INDIGENOUS ACHOLI[i] COMMUNITY OF UGANDA

By Francis Akena Adyanga, Ph.D Candidate, University of Toronto

Introduction

The main argument in this chapter is that the Acholi people have harnessed from nature medicinal practices that meet their needs within the cultural context of physical healing and spiritual renewal. This is based on their concept of holistic health as including physical and spiritual balance. However, the Indigenous Acholi understanding of good health and a good health care system is undermined by the oppositional forces of modernity and colonization mischaracterizing the Indigenous health care system as backward and illogical. As a unique systematic study of traditional health care practices, the key suggestion in this chapter is that ethno-medical practices make significant contributions to our health and welfare. Thus, we should take seriously the need to remove the stigma associated with colonial labels and integrate ethno-medical practices within the main stream health care system to promote physical and spiritual well-being.

Although traditional medicinal practices are being largely threatened by the forces of modernity in the continent of Africa, the practice coexists informally alongside the modern health care system. African people have a rich history of medicines that are interconnected with spirituality. In most African societies, the practice of medicine is inseparable from divine intervention. This chapter is a reflective analysis of two types of health care systems among the Acholi people: preventative and curative health care practices. The analysis is based on the author's experiences growing up in Northern Uganda as an Acholi native. The reflective analysis is also anchored on informal conversations the author had with two elders in 2013 in Acholi land. Although oral legendii has it that the Luo migrated from the *Bahr el Ghazal* region in Sudan between the 15th and 16th

i [8] The Acholi are an ethnic group occupy most parts of northern Uganda and upper southern Sudan. According to oral historical traditions, they are the descendants of Luo speaking peoples who are believed to have migrated from the Bar el Ghazal region of Sudan before settling in northern Uganda around the fifteenth and sixteenth century.

ii One of the elders named Oola Justino with whom I had informal conversation narrated many legends among the Acholi people. He used the legends to trace the history of the Luo people basing on information passed to him orally.

centuries, they were among the first groups of external migrants to settle in present day Uganda. Upon entry into Uganda, the Luo splintered into several groups, settling in different parts of Uganda and Western Kenya. The groups that settled in northern Uganda are the Acholi, Langi, and Alur. For context specificity, this chapter discusses the traditional health care system among the Acholi people.

The traditional health care system was highly enforced among the Indigenous Ugandan communities for the well-being and continuity of the collective. It is critical to note that traditional medicinal practices involve a complex set of knowledge skills, rootedness in a specific culture, and ability to win trust among the people. Traditional health care practices among the Acholi revolve around specialists such as medicine men/women, diviners/spiritual healers, traditional birth attendants, and bone setters/specialists, among others. Many examples of health care systems enforced include emphasis on personal hygiene, washing hands before eating, sex/marriage education, and maternal education. Some of the health care practices were transferable across clans, cultural and ethnic groups. The health care system focuses on prevention of diseases and also on curative measures. Traditional methods of health care are famous because of their cultural sustainability, admissibility and cost efficacy, coupled with the inaccessibility of the modern health care system in most rural communities. The distinctiveness and sometimes sacredness of knowledge that the health care practitioners command also account for the popularity of traditional health care systems in different communities.

Preventative Health Care Practices

Generally, health care takes different forms among the Acholi people. Everyone, from political leadership to the lay person at the family level, plays a different role. Prevention of ill health is the community's primary objective, with enormous emphasis levied on the good health of children. Historically, to emphasize the importance of children's health, the chief of each community or the clan head ensured that malnutrition was non-existent in the community. The Acholi's understanding has always been that most ill health in children results from poor feeding, which may translate to lack of balanced diet and/or starvation. According to an elder named Oola Justino,[i] from whom I was privileged to learn, the chief in ancient times would visit selected household in his jurisdiction

i Oola Justino is an elderly clan leader and member of the council of chiefs (Ker kal Kwaro) who has accumulated years of experiences related to the Acholi culture. He serves on several cultural committees including but not limited to the cultural justice system to resolve disputes, the community health committee, etc.

at night when the occupants were in a dead sleep. He would travel with his guards, who would be stationed near the courtyard being visited as the chief tip toed to the back of the hut, where he would sit quietly on the veranda listening as the selected family slept. The objective of the chief's clandestine night trip was to undertake his own study of whether or not the suspected family was getting enough food. When the chief did not hear a significant level of farting (passing gas) coming from the sleeping family, he would invite the family to his palace during the day and inquire as to whether they had enough food in the house or not. Also, a release of food from the central granaries (storage device) would immediately be ordered for the family. Then, it if was rainy season, the family would be required to plant peas, millet and sorghum for their future sustenance. The chief was not just a political and religious figure for the area under his command; he also catered for the good health of the community. According to Oola, the significance of the night trips to suspected households was to ensure that preventative disease measures were in place. This is because, kwashiorkor—a common occurrence in children—was linked to starvation and poor diet.

Curative Health Care System

The curative community health care system among the Acholi centers on the expertise of two types of healing systems. The first is medicinal (herbal) practices. Acholi ethno-medical practices are local-centered approaches to physical healing and spiritual renewal. They have been the cornerstone of preserving community health and welfare for time immemorial. Their significance has been weakened, but not destroyed, by several forces of modernity. A traditional doctor's knowledge of ailments is derived intuitively, from physically examining the patient's body for symptoms or by the patient telling the doctor the invisible symptoms for internal ill health. When the ill health is identified, treatment plans usually follow. However, the existence of unequal power relations is deeply embedded in treatment plans (Akena, 2011), whereby doctors make autonomous decisions as they treat patients.

Patients usually take submissive roles and try as much as possible to avoid questioning doctors' authority. Belief in the medicinal practitioner takes center stage where the patient is concerned; this is reinforced by the deep rooted trust, respect, and confidence that the community has built in the doctor over a long period of time. Questioning doctors' authority may be interpreted as doubting or challenging their knowledge. A renowned anticolonial theorist, Fanon (1959) presented a similar picture within the context of Algeria when he stated that:

> In a non-colonial society, the attitude of a sick man in the presence of a medical practitioner is one of confidence. The patient trusts the doctor; he puts himself in his hands. He yields his body to him. He accepts the fact that the pain may be awakened or exacerbated by the physician, for the patient realizes that the intensifying of suffering in the course of examination may pave the way for peace in his body. (p.123)

In extending the same line of argument as Fanon, Oola states that confidence in traditional medical practitioners is based on the community's long term observation of the practitioners' training and experiences. Practitioners usually receive their training over an extended period of time before they qualify to practice medicine. Sometimes their mentors start training them from childhood, and they remain assistants until the death of their mentors. When the mentor dies, the trainee inherits the office but still remains under the close scrutiny of the community and other practitioners until the people confide in him/her. This complex training process is very vital in ensuring that those who practice medicine act professionally in maintaining community health and well-being. The sense of accountability for lives lost due to professional misconduct is highly enforced. It's against this background that herbal practitioners make referrals when patients' health conditions are complex and beyond his/her medicinal knowledge. In present times, the referral process takes a different form: from one traditional healer to another or from traditional healers to hospitals specializing in Western modes of treatment.

Another female elder with whom I interacted (named Ladur) gave an example of herbs used for curing different sicknesses among the Acholi people. Below, I have captured some of the herbs that she uses on regular basis to treat her patients.

1. Measles, locally known as *anyongo* in the Acholi language, is a common disease in children. In the past, there were medicine men and women who specialized in treating measles. Laduri is one such herbal specialist. She said that when a patient brought to her; she examines all physical and non-physical symptoms to rule out other diseases. Once measles is confirmed, she gives the patient herbs to boost his/her appetite before the patient is put on measles' herbs. The measles herb is called *pedu wii akuru*. It's taken from soft grass roots, crushed and mixed with cold water.

i Ladur is a female elder who is also a traditional doctor. She specializes in treating measles and snake bites. She has been serving her community for over twenty years. At 70 year old, she is mentoring her son with the hope that the medicinal practice will carry on even after her death.

The patient takes the mixture for four days, and usually, full recovery is attained.

2. The elderly medicine woman also identified camel foot tree roots that she uses for treating wounds. Its botanical name is *piliostigma thonningii*. The local name for this herb is *te ogali matar*. Piliostigma thonningii tree roots are dug out, crushed, and allowed to dry. Later, they are crushed further into powder form and administered directly onto the wounds. This powder dries the wounds within two days and complete healing is normally attained after five days. During the five days of administering the powered herbs, Ladur also makes bandages from the fibre of the camel foot roots. The soft bandages are used to cover the wounds every day after cleaning and applying the powdered herbs. The bandages must be changed twice daily (in the morning and evening).

3. Lastly, Ladur identified *centosema puberbcens*, a plant from which an herb for treating snake bite is extracted. The local name for this herb is "agaba." It is a mixture of extracts from centosema puberbcens' stems and roots. The outer layer of the stem is extracted, washed, and assorted with fresh roots. Then it is crushed, mixed with lukewarm water, and given to the patient to drink at a volume of at least 100ml (based on the size of the tiny bottle she showed me) once a day. The patient will drink this herb for about five days and recover. She claimed that there are immediate indications of whether or not the herb will work. When a patient drinks the first dosage of the herb and vomits, this is a positive sign because vomiting brings out the excessive venoms that have spread into other body organs, like the intestines. In a related work (Akena, 2011); I have witnessed this treatment first-hand when my mother was bitten by a snake. We took her to a male herbalist. After she was given the herb to drink, she vomited a yellowish substance and the herbalist was happy with this outcome. In the same way, Ladur confirmed that everyone she has treated of snake bites in the last 15 years responded by vomiting after taking the first dose. The medicine woman also said that in the event that her medicine failed to cure someone, she would see it as exacerbation of visible and invisible symptoms and make referrals either to other healers or to a government hospital (referring to modern medical facilities).

According to Ladur, herbal treatments are given to patients at no cost. However, in most cases when full recovery is registered, patients usually return to express their gratitude; in the process, they bring gifts such as chickens, grains, soap, salt, etc. During my visit to this healer, I was fortunate enough to meet some of the patients who came for treatment as well as a few former patients who claimed to have been healed. It was reassuring hearing their stories and high opinions of this traditional herbal practitioner.

Spiritual Health Care System

The second type of traditional healer is the spiritual healer/doctor. These doctors interweave spiritual powers with medicinal practices to dispel evil spirits (depending on diagnosis) and derive holistic healing for patients. The Acholi and other African societies have unique worldviews in which the spiritual and universal worlds exist in harmony. Most Ugandan communities have a profound belief in the existence of a Supreme Being called God and other supernatural powers called spirits (both good and evil). Evil spirits radiate ill health that comes with varying degrees of suffering. Among the Acholi people, for example, *twoo Rubanga* (hunchback) is believed to be caused by an evil spirit called *jok Rubanga*. It therefore takes the specialty of the spiritual healers/doctors to dispel hunchback. To effectively carry out their role in maintaining community health, the spiritual healers/doctors have shrines from where they evoke the spirits of the ancestors or departed family members to disclose the concealed source of ill health and guide them to the appropriate therapeutic mechanism. According to Oola, the Acholi worldview is that no sickness comes from nowhere. All ill health must be associated with a cause and consequence. Therefore the root causes of every illness must be established and addressed accordingly. The objective is to avoid the spread of the sickness or its reoccurrence. In most cases, when a family member falls sick, the spirits of the ancestors are consulted to find out if there are hidden causes.

Families may carry out the work of a spiritual healer/doctor on a smaller scale. For instance, many families have small private shrines from where living family members offer foods and drinks to departed family members to maintain their presence among the living as well as to protect the living members from tribulation. In the event of natural calamities such as measles, poor harvests or total crop failure, impotency/infertility etc. in the family, the affected family would first consult the ancestors in their small shrines for the source of the disaster and how to address it. If it turned out that the spirit of an ancestor or any dead family member was angry with living family members, and hence caused the disaster to show his/her frustration, any grievances would be addressed through the offering of sacrifices. Sometimes, a local brew called *kwete* would be offered to the spirit by pouring it on the floor of the shrine (libation) to appease the angry spirit.

Over the years, Acholi community health care systems have made significant contributions to the well-being of the people. There was once no stigma associated with the traditional health care system because the community understood and valued the ethos and principles of health care, as pointed out by Wane (2011). She argued that one must understand and appreciate the beliefs, values, symbols, myths, and socio-cultural components that are associated with African traditional healing practices. This is because, in many cases, aspects of Indigenous practices are appropriated without acknowledgement through written text or media, and in the process, their authenticity is lost.

Among some clans, it is believed that spiritual healers have the power to disclose the source of the ill health and then transfer such ailments to their own bodies before casting them out. Elsewhere in Uganda, the Baganda of Southern and central Uganda have spiritual healers whose healing power puts the healers at the centre of cure for patients. In agreement, Kyewalyanga (1976) illustrated that:

> The ritual of transferring illness to an animal was performed by medicine man (omusawo). The medicine man would rub some grass on the sick man, and then tie this grass to the animal. He drove the animal to the wasteland where he killed it, and the meat was his own payment. If the sick person was so poor that he would not afford a goat, a fowl was taken as scapegoat. In this case, the grass was rubbed on the body of the sick man, and the medicine man personally took it to the wasteland. After this ritual, the sick person was supposed to recover. (p.126)

There are many accounts/testimonies by people who gained healing from hunchback or tuberculosis of the spine after being treated by these doctors. A belief in the existence of God and holy spirits has a corresponding belief in the existence of evil spirits and their ability to disorganize mankind. The interlacing of spirituality and herbal practices is thus required to dispel evil from possessed patients. Castle (1966) explicitly testified this from observation during his time teaching at Makerere University in Uganda. He observed that:

> It is difficult for the Western observer to realize how deeply this influence penetrates into the daily life of the family. The spirits

> of a deceased grandparent or aunt may possess any member of the family who disturbed their rest. I have known a Makerere undergraduate student deeply perturbed by the conviction that he was possessed by the spirit of his grandfather. Taylor cites the case of an educated girl suffering from what the European doctors diagnosed as acute hysteria for which lengthy treatment was advised. But her father thought otherwise, took her home under the conviction that 'the sickness is from her aunt', and returned her to school cured in two weeks by the local practitioner in magic. (p. 31)

In Africa, the existence of certain phobic conditions that are related to mystical causation of ailments—which are beyond the scope of modern science and thus require the intervention of African native doctors for remedy—cannot be underestimated. The practice of spiritual healing has been widely misunderstood and castigated by early European explorers and missionaries referring to it as witchcraft and sorcery, but to the African people, it is the interlacing of spirituality and herbal practices for community health. The labelling and consequent dismissal of the works of spiritual healers/doctors by the Western education system renders their efforts futile and accounts for the contemporary low perceptions of these doctors among educated and pious Africans. Despite this, Sertima (1983) respectfully reminds us that

> Western-trained doctors who have studied the traditional medicine-man concede that the African doctor has a profound knowledge of human body and anatomy. He usually gives careful diagnosis, beginning with a history of the disease, followed by a thorough physical examination. (p. 23)

Among the *Acholi* people of northern Uganda, several medicinal practices exist to cater to the well-being of the community. For example, people consume specific wild fruits with the conviction that doing so reinforces the body's immunity against multiple diseases. The most common of the fruits are Lantana trifolia and Ampelocissus Africana. These fruit, with the Acholi names of *bel-winyo* and *olok*, respectively, are known to have antioxidants which are a perfect deterrent to most liver diseases and cancer, and also help with weight loss. A study conducted by Badakhshan et al. (2011) on the toxicity of Lantana camara methanol extract on male and female mice at the University of Malaysia provides substantive evidence of the effectiveness of these plant species. After administration of a single dose of leaf extract in an acute toxicity test, the female mice lost body weighs while the male mice lost organ mass, particularly for kidney and heart. Although the study was conducted to determine the toxicity of the leaf, its effects on the male mice provide clues to its toxicity. In addition to losing organ (kidney and heart) weight, the mice were found to have developed minor liver damage. This suggests that the Lantana camara/ trifolia have antioxidants which the *Acholi* people have long known to use for the enhancement of the body's immunity against cancer and other heart diseases. Perhaps this explains why cases of cancer occurrences among the *Acholi* people and other African groups are minimal.

Elsewhere, Sertima (1983) introduced us to Nigerian root bark Annona senegalensis, which has been found to possess strong anti-cancer properties. He argued that the Nigerian root-bark could provide a breakthrough in cancer treatment. In many Ugandan as well as other African societies, the use of different herbs grew organically due to outbreaks of sickness. When there was an outbreak, certain individuals gained the insight into the remedy through dreams or were intuitively guided to it. It was not apparent that every herb prescribed to patients for specific ill health derived cure since others would still be at trial stages. In the period when the existence of modern laboratories for testing medicinal effectiveness was unheard of, such experimentations were done directly on the patients. Trial and error was therefore an effective way to establish the validity of the herbs.

In Africa, like in other continents during the early centuries, there existed a substantial number of doctors who were committed to finding curative measures for different diseases of their times. However, the lack of modern technology as we have in the 21st century centered their efforts to trial and error, which would either succeed or fail, with failure signifying the extensive loss of lives. For example, the sleeping sickness pandemic was rampant in Africa during the 18th and 19th centuries, and native African doctors were already involved in the struggle to bring it to an end before the European counterparts joined this struggle. Sleeping sickness is caused by two germs, trypanosoma brucei rhodesiense and trypanosomoa brucei gambiense.i Tsetse flies are known to be the major carriers of these infectious germs. When an infected fly bites the victims, the infection spreads through victims' blood and develops into full blown sickness. Hattersley (1968) traced the entry of European doctors in the fight against sleeping sickness to 1906 after two Europeans succumbed to the disease in Uganda. One of these was the head of the Botanical Department of the Uganda Administration, Mr. Mahon, whose work in

---

i Centre for Disease Control. Parasites - African Trypanosomiasis (also known as Sleeping Sickness). http://www.cdc.gov/parasites/sleepingsickness/health_professionals/

the Botanical Gardens at Entebbe lay in one of the most thickly infested districts. The other was Lieutenant Tullock, a member of the sleeping-sickness commission. Following the death of these two Europeans, Professor Koch and two assistants were sent to Uganda in 1906 on a special mission financed by the German government at an estimated cost of £ 6,000 plus an offered reward of £ 8,000 from the King of Belgium for anyone who could discover sleeping sickness' remedy (p. 134).

Although African native doctors were, by that time, already heavily involved in searching curative measures for the pandemic, no mention was made of their efforts. Even the Sleeping Sickness Commission that was sent to Uganda paid no attention to the local initiatives that were already in place to combat the plague. Hattersley's descriptions of the treatment method used by Professor Koch depict a trial and error mode. He argued that, thought Professor Koch's method was able to provide short term relief to patients, it largely failed to attain total healing for the victims of sleeping sickness. He asserted:

> His method of treatment was to inject hypodermically a preparation of atoxyl.... Professor Koch made an admixture of aniline with the preparation of arsenic, which enabled the latter to be increased to several amounts of ordinary dose. He found that this preparation freed the blood temporarily from all trypanosomata. As he himself stated before the German Emperor, when he injected 0.5 grams of atoxyl he found trypanosomes in the blood after five days; if he injected double doses..., he could not encounter any of the parasites in the blood for a long time. They then endeavoured to obtain still better results and increase the dose to 1 gram, injecting that quantity about every seventh day..... After a while the doctors had a great surprise. More than twenty of their patients became blind, and this was apparently not temporary but permanent.... Professor Koch himself appears to agree that his treatment is open to grave doubts; but he believes that if it can be adopted in the first stage, atoxyl can certainly cure. (p. 135)

It is clear that Professor Koch and his team were investigating sleeping sickness cures not due to compassion for the African victims suffering from the disease, but due to their natural desire for the cause of scientific discovery then driven by the hefty financial reward from Koch's home government of Germany and from the Belgian king. The trial and error strategy used was normal and logical; hence, the respective community had no problem with it. What is problematic, however, is the deliberate predisposition to exaggerate the failure/futility of African native doctors' efforts at that time, mythicizing them as sorceries, satanic worship, and primitive. For fairness to reign in society and in the education system, the examination of African efforts in science and medicine must be weighted and valued on the same analytical scale as the evolution of European scientific and medicinal practices.

In the domain of surgery, the Baghisu of eastern Uganda have long practiced, and continue to practice, the lighter surgical procedure of *imbalu* (circumcision) of every male youth. Although this is a cultural initiation practiced into adulthood, the scientific skills used in the procedure are quite astonishing. Without any painkiller given to the candidate, the surgeon is able to carefully place the edge of his surgical blade at the right spot to cut off the male foreskin without causing damage to the soft tissue. After the surgery, the surgeon then invites the herbal man or woman to apply medicines usually extracted from plants fibres on the wound. Imbalu thus signifies a well-organized principle of specialization that draws on expertise in different segments of science. Usually the patients' healing time frame for this procedure is more or less equivalent to that of patients circumcised by Western trained medical doctors. Sertima (1983) reminds us that surgery also seems to be an area in which African doctors attained a level of skill comparable with, and in some respect superior to, that of Western surgeons up until the 20th century.

It was not until recently that the Ugandan government formally recognized the significance of this generational practice and adopted it into its health care system. Studies (some conducted in Rakai District—Western Uganda) indicate that circumcised men have a 60% reduced risk of contracting HIV/AIDS. In 2008, the US government, under President Bush's program for AIDS treatment and prevention, made circumcision free for every male in Uganda. Also, according to the *New York Times* (2011), male circumcision appears to help protect a man's sexual partners against cervical cancer. In an offshoot of a landmark study of 1,200 heterosexual couples in Uganda involving circumcision and AIDS, researchers reported to *The Lancet* that having a circumcised partner reduced a woman's risk of catching human papillomaviruses by about 25 percent. Such viruses lead to genital warts and cervical cancer. The different studies in the present times have validated some of the traditional science practices by African communities. As a result, massive campaigns have been launched by Uganda's government for every male child, youth, and adult to be circumcised as a strategy to reduce HIV/AIDS. The recognition and integration of some elements of Acholi health care practices in the main stream health care system would therefore play a significant role in promoting public health.

Conclusion

The evolution of the health care system among the Acholi and other African societies has experienced enormous challenges right from the time of the colonial encounter. The colonization of African societies was followed by the subjugation of their health care system, which was subsequently labeled as satanic practices. However, suppression of this generatinal health care knowledge did not completely purge it from African societies. Instead, this health care system went undercover. The practices continued alongside the Western health care system that became the only formally acceptable form of health care. In the book *A Dying Colonialism*, Fanon (1959) articulates how traditional medicine persisted despite its being banned from Algerian society during French colonial rule. Therefore, as more people continue to use traditional health care system regardless of stereotypical inferences attached to it, there is an urgent need to establish appropriate systems of quality control and open space for its inclusion beside the dominant health care system. Implementing quality control measures and opening space for traditional health care system would promote community health. It would also ensure that the best practices and the most sustainable health care systems are made available in the most affordable manner. It is therefore incumbent upon every country in Africa to adopt an inclusive and sustainable method of preserving the culture-friendly practices of traditional health care along with the dominant health care practices. The scarcity of the modern health care facilities across Africa thus calls for the institutionalization of appropriate traditional health care practices that offer a more culturally relevant health care system.

References

Akena, F. A. (2011). The dialectics of Western Christianity and African spirituality. In Wane N., Manyimo E., & Eric R. (Eds.), *Spirituality, education and society: An Integrated Approach* (pp. 111-127). Sense Publishers.

Badakhshan, M. P., Lachimanan Y. L., & Sreenivasan, S. (2011). Cytotoxicity and oral acute toxicity studies of Lantana camara leaf extract. Molecules, 16, 366-374.

Castle, E. B. (1966). Growing up in East Africa. London: Oxford University Press.

Centre for Disease Control. Parasites—African Trypanosomiasis (also known as Sleeping Sickness). Retrieved from http://www.cdc.gov/parasites/sleepingsickness/health_professionals/

Fanon, F. (1959). *A Dying Colonialism*. New York: Groves Press.

Hattersley, C. W. (1968). *The Baganda at Home*. The Religious Tract Society.

Kyewalyanga, F. (1976). Traditional religion, custom, and Christianity in Uganda as illustrated by the Ganda with some references to other African cultures and Islam. Freiburg im Breisgau.

New York Times (2011). Uganda: Male Circumcision May Help Protect Sexual Partners Against Cervical Cancer.

Sertima, I. V. (1983). Blacks in science. Ancient and modern. *Journal of African Civilizations, 5*(1&2).

Wane, N. (2011). The Kenyan herbalist ruptures the status quo in health and healing. In G. J. S. Dei (Ed)., *Indigenous philosophies and critical education: A reader* (pp. 280-298). New York: Peter Lang.

Contributors

Francis Akena Adyanga got his PhD from the Department of Humanities, Social Sciences and Social Justice Education (HSSSJE) at the Ontario Institute for Studies in Education (OISE), University of Toronto in 2014. His research interests include Indigenous knowledge, anticolonial education, spirituality and schooling, education in emergencies, and post emergencies contexts. He is also a certified teacher with the Ontario College of Teachers (OCT), currently teaching with the York Region District School Board. He is also a course instructor in the Initial Teacher Education Porgram (ITE) at OISE.

Dr Akwasi Asabere-Ameyaw is a Professor and Vice Chancellor of the University of Education, Winneba, with a Doctor of Philosophy degree in Zoology from the University of Cape Coast, Ghana, with a specialization in fish biology, fish stock assessment, and aquatic biology. Over the past few years, he has developed a keen interest in environmental education and the contextualization of the teaching of science and technology.

Mary Ashiedu, PhD Candidate, in the Department of Humanities, Social Science, Social Justice Education, Ontario Institute for Studies in Education, University of Toronto. She is also a full time teacher.

Edna Aryee**,** M.A., MPhil is completing her Ph.D. in Clinical/Counselling and Forensic Psychology in the Department of Applied Psychology and Human Development at the University of Toronto/OISE. She is also admitted into the **Collaborative Graduate Program in Women's Health also at the University of Toronto.** Ms. Aryee recently completed her clinical and forensic internship/residency with Correctional Service of Canada and the Forensic Behaviour Clinic in Kingston, Ontario. Edna currently works with the Forensic Consultation Services at the Centre for Addiction and Mental Health. Edna has extensive skills in clinical assessments, including personality assessments, cognitive assessments, risk assessments, psycho-legal and psycho-immigration assessments. In addition, she is a competent clinician providing therapy to both clinical and forensic populations including individuals, couples, families and groups. Her **research and clinical interest includes women's health, HIV risk prevention, forensic rehabilitation, and culture and psychopathy among** people of African descent. Her recent publications include, "The psycho-spirituality among African-Canadian women living with HIV/ AIDS in Ontario" and "I was raped: A study on the psychological effect of rape on Liberian and Ghanaian women residing in Ghana."

Natasha Burford, M.A. is a student in the Department of Humanities, Social Science, Social Justice Education, Ontario Institute for Studies in Education, University of Toronto. She is also a full time teacher.

Dr. George J. Sefa Dei is Professor in the Department of Humanities Social Science, Social Justice Education, Ontario Institute for Studies in Education, University of Toronto (OISE/UT). His teaching and research interests are in the areas of anti-racism, minority schooling, international development, Indigenous philosophies, and anti-colonial thought. He has researched and written extensively in these areas. His most recent books include *Indigenous Philosophies and Critical Education: A Reader* (Peter Lang Publishing, 2011); *Teaching Africa: Towards Transgressive Pedagogy* (Springer Publishers, 2010); *Fanon and Education: Pedagogical Challenges*, co-edited with Marlon Simmons (Peter Lang Publishing, 2010); *Fanon and the Counterinsurgency of Education* (Sense Publishers, Rotterdam, 2010); and *Learning to Succeed: Improving Educational Achievement for All* (Teneo Press, 2010). In July 2007, he succeeded the occupant of the stool [Odikro] of Asokorekuma and was installed as a traditional chief in Ghana. His stool name is Nana Sefa Atweneboah I the Adomakwaahene of the town of Asokore, near Koforidua in the New Juaben Traditional Area of Ghana.

Dr. Edmund J. Kayombo, PhD, is a research fellow at the Muhimbili University of Health and Allied Sciences in the Institute of Traditional Medicine. His research interests include public health with a focus on population issues, Indigenous knowledge (IK) with special in traditional socio-cultural practices related to reproductive health, traditional medicine with its practitioners, Indigenous food, policy issues, and the legal framework of IK.

Dr. Regine Uwibereyeho King is an Assistant Professor at the University of Manitoba. She graduated from the Factor-Inwentash Faculty of Social Work, University of Toronto, in November 2011, with a one-year CIHR post-doctoral fellowship in social aetiology of mental illness based at the Centre for Addiction and Mental Health. She obtained her masters of education in counseling psychology and community development from the Ontario Institute for Studies in Education, University of Toronto.

King was born and raised in Rwanda, where she witnessed and survived the 1994 genocide. She then worked as a co-ordinator and facilitator of a trauma healing program through World Vision Rwanda, bringing together the Hutu and Tutsi for mutual healing. She moved to Canada in 2000, where she worked as a mental-health counselor and a community activist through public speaking. Her research interests include mental health, survivors of organized violence, cross-cultural mental-health interventions, forgiveness and reconciliation processes. Her doctoral research involved mental-health and trauma healing interventions in post-genocide Rwanda and her post-doctoral research has focused on refugee mental health in Toronto.

Sumaya Laher is a psychologist specializing in the field of psychological assessment. Her doctoral and subsequent research into personality, psychometrics, and assessment is instrumental in pioneering the usage and interpretation of key instruments in South Africa. It also has real implications for equity and redress, given the complexities of the South African context. In addition, Sumaya contributes actively to research on Indigenous knowledge systems with her work on traditional healing systems, particularly those proposed by Islam, Hinduism, and African approaches. Sumaya also supports emerging scholarship and plays an active role in getting students to undertake and publish research.

Joash Abere Migosi is a career educationist for a period of not less than 15 years. He is a graduate of the Catholic University of Eastern Africa, Nairobi, and Moi University in Eldoret. His research areas of interest centre on the management of higher education in developing countries. His PhD thesis focused on the research productivity of a university faculty in Kenya. Dr. Migosi now teaches on a part-time basis at Moi and Egerton Universities in Kenya. He has served as an Assistant Director of Research in the Directorate of Research Management and Development in the Ministry of Higher Education Science and Technology. He is currently the Head of the Department of Educational Management and Policy Studies at South Eastern College, University of Nairobi, Kenya.

Dr Roy Moodley, Ph.D; is Associate Professor in Clinical/Counselling Psychology at the Ontario Institute for Studies in Education at the University of Toronto. His research and publication interests include traditional and cultural healing; multicultural and diversity counselling; race, culture and ethnicity in psychotherapy; and masculinities. Roy co-edited *Transforming Managers: Gendering Change in the Public Sector*

(1999); *Carl Rogers Counsels a Black Client: Race and Culture in Person-Centred Counselling* (2004); *Integrating Traditional Healing Practices into Counselling and Psychotherapy* (2005); and *Race, Culture and Psychotherapy: Critical Perspectives in Multicultural Practice* (2006).

Simon Murangiri is a traditional healer and medical herbalist in Kenya. He has been practicing Indigenous Healing using herbs for more than twenty years. He grows his own herbs and he is widely consulted.

Dr. Erica Neeganagwedgin, PhD, is currently an Assistant Professor at the Centre for World Indigenous Knowledge and Research at the Athabasca University.

Dr. Tom Mongare Ndege is a visiting scholar at the Center for Integrative Anti-Racism Studies (CIARS), University of Toronto. He is a Senior Lecturer, Moi University. He is a widely published scholar with an immense commitment to issues related to often ignore human phenomena. He has more than 20 publications in the form of books, journal articles, conference presentations, and monographs. In all these he has drawn extensively from his African ancestry, which has given him the humility, determination, and generosity to share ideas, concepts, and knowledge that promote human well-being. His commitment to preserving these values has thus supplied him significant motivation to contribute to the understanding of different African institutions. In this respect, Dr. Ndege has engaged education, health, land, and governance as key pillars of African progress. Through his extensive teaching experience, he has come to identify the poisoning of these pillars as the genesis of all ills that afflict Indigenous people. The healing of these pillars thus anchors the vision of his scholarship. Holistic rather than piecemeal presentation of this vision is the hallmark of his writing, which continues to emphasize the greatness of social values over private interests.

Professor Meki Nzewi lectures in African Music at the University of Pretoria. As a cultural scientist, he has undertaken an interactive study of the creative theory and performance practice underlying African traditional musical arts for over 36 years. He has written copiously on all musico-philosophical aspects of African music, and has published four books and 34 articles and philosophical essays on African music, dance, and drama. He has written, composed, and produced five music-theatre works, seven musicals, three operas, and three poetic-dance theatre works. His other compositions include works for orchestra, choir, solo voice, drums, and other ensembles. In 2001, the English Chamber Orchestra gave the world premiere of his newest orchestral work during a tour of South Africa. Prof. Nzewi has also published literary works including three plays, a novel, and poems, and has written and produced works for TV and radio. As a master drummer, he has performed and given workshops throughout Europe and Africa. He is also the founder and co-director of the Ama Dialog Foundation for African traditional arts in Nigeria. His creative philosophy and practice aim at continuing the traditional multi-disciplinary approach to creativity, performance, and presentation.

Dr. Emilio Ovuga is a Professor of Psychiatry and Mental Health, Faculty of Medicine, Gulu University, Uganda. Dr. Ovuga is the Dean at the Faculty of Medicine, Gulu University, Uganda, and Project Coordinator of the ENRECA Gulu Project. He is currently the Principal Investigator at Gulu University in a study of neurocysticercosis and epilepsy in Sub-Saharan Africa involving Uganda and Zambia in Africa. Dr. Ovuga is also currently Team Leader for a Ugandan team of researchers on a school-based pilot study for the World Psychiatric Association (WPA) as part of a multi-national collaborative study on creating awareness of child and adolescent mental health problems in Kampala District schools. Dr. Ovuga has published widely. His research interests include community level mental health conditions, awareness, coping mechanisms, and service provision. Dr. Ovuga has a PhD in Public and Mental Health, Stockholm, 2005; MA in Medicine (Psychiatry), Makerere University, 1981; and MBChB, Makerere University, 1976.

Kai ner Maa Pitanta, M.A.; is a Naturalpath & Health practictioner. He is an African Indigenous Scholar who specializes in African Indigenous Education. He is among the few Africans who own and operate an Afrocentric school in Toronto.

Professor Kolawole T. Raheem worked as a Senior Researcher in the University of Jyväskylä, Finland, for more than a decade before becoming the Deputy Director of the Center for School and Community Science and Technology Studies (SACOST) in the University of Education, Winneba, Ghana. His lectures deal with environmental management and education—mainly waste management. He also researches and lectures on Indigenous science activities, seeking new approaches to environmental management for sustainable development in Africa. He is a founding member of the Board of the Centre for Environmental Science Education (CESE), Lagos State University, Nigeria. Professor Raheem's special areas of research are environmental education, waste management, Indigenous science knowledge, and production of contextualised materials for teaching and learning science in West African schools. He is also a consultant to some Non-Governmental Organisations involved with environmental issues in Africa and Europe.

Dr. Eleanor Ross has a BA in Social Work, MA in Social Work (cum laude) and PhD from the University of the Witwatersrand (Wits) in South Africa. She has worked in the areas of crime prevention, substance abuse, and with the deaf community. She has also been employed as a lecturer in the Departments of Speech Pathology and Audiology as well as Social Work, and is currently Professor of Social Work and Head of the Department of Social Work at Wits. Eleanor Ross has been involved in various research projects and has approximately 80 local and internationally accredited publications. Her research interests include ethics and culture, with particular reference to traditional healing.

Dr. Izumi Sakamoto is Associate Professor of Social Work at the University of Toronto. A former Fulbright Scholar, she received and MSW, MSc (Social Psychology) and PhD. (Social Work & Psychology) from University of Michigan and a BA and MA from Sophia University (Jochi Daigaku), Japan. Dr. Sakamoto's teaching focuses on empowerment, anti-oppression, globalization, community organizing, qualitative research, and community-based and arts-informed research. With four grants from the Social Sciences and Humanities Research Council of Canada (SSHRC) as Principal Investigator, Dr. Sakamoto's research has focused on the experiences of skilled immigrants, exploring the negotiation of multiple identities, equity and access to social services, and the reconceptualization of "acculturation" and "integration."

Dr. Immaculate Wamimbi Tumwine, PhD, is a Canadian, born in Uganda, where she worked for 15 years as a lecturer and consultant. Prior to immigrating to Canada in 1996, she was a Communications Officer at the Association of African Universities, whose Secretariat is based in Ghana. She has carried out numerous consulting assignments including health-related research for non-governmental organizations and international agencies. An advocate for low-income communities, Immaculate currently works as Projects Coordinator at the Ontario Council of Agencies Serving Immigrants. Her publications include The Training Needs of Non-Academic Staff and The Current Providers of

Middle Management Training in African Universities. In A. Schofield (Ed.), *The United Nations Educational* (1996); Strengthening the Skills of Middle Management in Universities: The Training and Development of Middle Managers in Higher Education. In *New Papers on Higher Education* (1996); Rural Ugandan Women and the Technological Race to the 21st Century.

Dr. Njoki Nathani Wane, PhD, is a Professor at the University of Toronto, Department of Humanities, Social Science, Social Justice Education at the Ontario Institute for Studies in Education. She is the current Special Adviser on the Status of Women at University of Toronto as well as the current Director of the Office of Teaching Support at OISE (OTSO) and Co-Director of the Centre for Integrative Anti-Racist Research Studies (CIARS). For the last twenty years she has been researching, writing and teaching in the areas of Black feminisms in Canada, African feminisms, African Indigenous knowledges, anti-racist education in teacher education, African women and spirituality, anti-colonial thought, and ethno-medicine. Her co-edited books include *Spirituality, Education & Society: An Integrated Approach* (with Energy Manyimo & Eric Ritskes) and *The Politics of Cultural Knowledge* (with Arlo Kempf and Marlon Simmons), with both published by Sense Publications in 2011. Her co-authored articles include Wane and Sutherland (2010). African and Caribbean Indigenous Healing Practices and their Relevance to Counselling and Psychotherapy: Research Findings from Kenya & Grenada, in Moodley & A. George (Eds.), *Alternative Counseling & Healing.* Other recent publications include: Reading Fanon Differently: Black Canadian Perspectives (2010), in G. Dei (Ed.), *Fanon and the Counterinsurgency of Education*; Traditional Healing Practices: Conversations with Herbalists in Kenya (2010), in D. Kapoor & E. Shizha (Eds.), *Contemporary Asian and African Indigenous Knowledge and Learning: Essentialisms, Continuities and Change*; Spirituality: Pedagogical Tool for Feminism & Activism (2012), in *Canadian Journal of Women Studies*; Grandmothers: Othermothering Responsibilities in Kenya Rural Communities (2011), in the *Journal of Revista De Investigacion Social*; Black Canadian Feminism Thought: Perspectives on equity and Diversity in the Academy (2009), in *Indigenous Education*; Cultural Resistance: a Decolonizing Project (2009), in *Curriculum Inquiry*; *Journal of Race, Ethnicity and Education*; Mapping the Field of Indigenous Knowledge in Anti-Colonial discourse: A Transformative Journey in Education (2008), in the *Journal of Race, Ethnicity and Education.*